Diabetes Care

Published and forthcoming Oxford Care Manuals

Stroke Care: A Practical Manual (2nd Edition)
Rowan Harwood, Farhad Huwez, and Dawn Good

Multiple Sclerosis Care: A Practical Manual
John Zajicek, Jennifer Freeman, and Bernadette Porter (eds)

Dementia Care: A Practical Manual
Jonathan Waite, Rowan H Harwood, Ian R Morton, and David J Connelly

Headache: A Practical Manual
David Kernick and Peter J Goadsby (eds)

Diabetes Care: A Practical Manual (2nd Edition)
Rowan Hillson

Preventive Cardiology: A Practical Manual
Catriona Jennings, Alison Mead, Jennifer Jones, Annie Holden,
Susan Connolly, Kornelia Kotseva, and David Wood

Neuromuscular Disorders in the Adult: A Practical Manual
David Hilton-Jones, Jane Freebody, and Jane Stein

Cardiovascular Disease in the Elderly: A Practical Manual
Rosaire Gray and Louise Pack

Motor Neuron Disease: A Practical Manual
Kevin Talbot, Martin R. Turner, Rachael Marsden, and Rachel Botell

Breast Disease Management: A Multidisciplinary Manual
John Winstanley, Hugh Bishop, James Harvey, Sue Down, and
Rachel Bright-Thomas

Diabetes Care: A practical manual

Second Edition

Dr Rowan Hillson MBE, MD, FRCP

National Clinical Director for Diabetes,
England 2008–2013

OXFORD
UNIVERSITY PRESS

OXFORD
UNIVERSITY PRESS

Great Clarendon Street, Oxford, OX2 6DP,
United Kingdom

Oxford University Press is a department of the University of Oxford.
It furthers the University's objective of excellence in research, scholarship,
and education by publishing worldwide. Oxford is a registered trade mark of
Oxford University Press in the UK and in certain other countries

First Edition published 2008
Second Edition published 2015

Impression: 1

Published in the United States of America by Oxford University Press
198 Madison Avenue, New York, NY 10016, United States of America

British Library Cataloguing in Publication Data
Data available

Library of Congress Control Number: 2014943832

ISBN 978–0–19–870563–5

Printed in Great Britain by
Ashford Colour Press Ltd, Gosport, Hampshire

For Kay and Rodney Hillson

Acknowledgements

I wish to thank the following for their help.

This book would not have been possible without the support of my family, my patients, my colleagues in Diabeticare, and my colleagues around The Hillingdon Hospital, and nationally who have taught me so much.

I particularly wish to thank my family for their patience and encouragement, and, alphabetically:

for the first edition Pat Bacon, Carol Candlish, Ruth Chalmers, Anne Currie, Deb Datta, Mark Edwards, David Evans, Mary Jurd, Sandra Ross, Gill Ruane, Pat Smith, Dai Thomas, and the anonymous but most helpful GP reviewer, and the pharmacology reviewer engaged by OUP.

for the second edition Lisa Bradbury, Damian Fogarty, Donal O'Donoghue, Debbie Hicks, June James, Christine Jones, Gerry Rayman, Benjamin Wiles and the anonymous but very helpful and constructive reviewers engaged by OUP.

I thank Helen Liepman, Eloise Moir-Ford, James Oates, Kate Wilson, Janet Walker, Fiona Chippendale, and colleagues from Oxford University Press.

I am grateful to the Diabetic Medicine, Wiley, the DVLA, eMIMS (electronic Monthly Index of Medical Specialties), NICE, and Springer-Verlag for permission to use material.

Contents

Introduction

Who is this book for?

- All health care staff in any discipline, e.g. doctors, nurses, dietitians, podiatrists, physiotherapists, occupational therapists, speech and language therapists, psychologists, pharmacists, health care assistants, medical secretaries, managers and care planners, and others
- Primary, community, secondary, NHS, or private care services
- Are you a person with diabetes who wants to learn more, or a family member of a person with diabetes? This book is written for health staff but many patients will find it of interest

For example:

- Do you see people with diabetes?
- Are you a GP or practice nurse working in primary care running your own diabetic clinic?
- Do people with diabetes ask for your advice?
- Are you a diabetologist or a GP with a special interest in diabetes who teaches other staff about diabetes?
- Are you a nurse working in A&E?
- Are you working on a hospital ward or clinic caring for diabetic patients—often or sometimes?
- Are you a doctor admitting emergency patients?
- Have you just started work with a diabetes team in a hospital?
- Are you a student of medicine, nursing, dietetics, podiatry, physiotherapy, occupational therapy, biochemistry?

Diabetes

Diabetes is a common long-term condition. Some numbers for 2012/2013:

- The International Diabetes Federation (IDF) estimated that there were 382 million people with diabetes worldwide
- Half were undiagnosed
- 56 million live in Europe, 20 million undiagnosed
- 3.2 million live in the UK
- 15 % of UK hospital beds occupied by people with diabetes
- Primary care prescriptions for glucose-lowering drugs in England cost £764 million
- Nationally total UK expenditure on people with diabetes has been estimated at ~ 10 % of national health expenditure
- Diabetes prevalence rises every year in every country
- Where 2013–14 information is available, numbers have already increased

Why write this book?

- Everyone with diabetes deserves the highest standards of personalized diabetes care, no matter where, when or by whom they are cared for.
- Everyone caring for people with diabetes must be trained in diabetes and know the limits of their knowledge. They must have opportunities to extend those boundaries and to keep up to date.
- Everyone, people with diabetes and healthcare professionals, must have prompt access to expert advice.

There are many diabetes textbooks. This is a pocket book, an aide memoire, a quick guide. The aim is to help those caring for diabetes to manage most patients themselves, and to recognize and refer those who need specialist care. References will lead you to more detailed descriptions of specialist care.

Diabetes is compatible with many years of healthy living but can also be more lethal than cancer. It is a multi-system disorder of which one manifestation is raised blood glucose. Because the complications of diabetes are so varied, and often hidden, the underlying influence of the diabetes may be ignored. Each complication may be managed as a 'one-off'. It is crucial that people with diabetes have integrated continuity of care from a team who know them well, and whom they can trust to monitor them to reduce risk factors for complications, and to detect and manage complications and emergencies.

No book or guideline can provide perfect advice suitable for every patient. This manual is a general guide but you must tailor the care of each diabetic patient to that person's individual condition and situation. A particular patient's condition may mean that advice in this manual is not applicable or that the situation is not covered. Ask the specialist diabetes team for advice. Agree local protocols for your practice, hospital, or district. Diabetes is a very rapidly moving field so it is important to keep up to date. All drug information and dosages should be confirmed for your particular patient using a current BNF. Be alert for changes in clinical management algorithms.

Patients' stories are imaginary, based on general experience.

References are brief. No responsibility can be taken for the content of websites or for sequelae of using them (or not using them).

This book represents the author's personal views only.

Symbols and abbreviations

➔	cross reference
ﾉﾞ	website
⚠	warning
~	about/circa
<	less than
>	more than
≥	equal to or greater than
≤	equal to or less than
=	equals or equal to
x	times (e.g. 2x = two times)
999	call emergency ambulance
A&E	Accident and Emergency Department
ABCD	Association of British Clinical Diabetologists
ABPI	ankle:brachial pressure index
ABPM	ambulatory blood pressure monitoring
ACE	angiotensin-converting enzyme
ACR	albumin:creatinine ratio, microalbumin:creatinine ratio
ACS	acute coronary syndrome(s)
ADA	American Diabetes Association
ADAG	HbA$_{1c}$-derived average glucose—see EAG
AF	atrial fibrillation
AGE	advanced glycosylation end-products
ALT	alanine aminotransferase
AMBG	assisted monitoring of blood glucose
AMI	acute myocardial infarction
antiGAD-Ab	glutamic acid decarboxylase autoantibodies
APHO	Association of Public Health Observatories
ARB	angiotensin receptor blocker
ARDS	adult respiratory distress syndrome
AST	aspartate aminotransferase
BDA	British Diabetic Association (now Diabetes UK)
BHS	British Hypertension Society
BMI	body mass index; weight/height^2 (kg/m^2)
BNF	British National Formulary (most recent edition)
BNFC	British National Formulary for Children (most recent edition)
BNP	serum B-type natriuretic peptide
BP	blood pressure

BSPED	British Society for Paediatric Endocrinology and Diabetes
CABG	coronary artery bypass graft(ing)
cal	calorie; in this book = kilocalorie
CAPD	continuous ambulatory peritoneal dialysis
CCG	clinical commissioning group
CEMACH	Confidential Enquiry into Maternal and Child Health (became CMACE—Centre for Maternal and Child Enquiries)
CF	cystic fibrosis
CG	clinical guideline
CGM/CGMS	continuous glucose monitoring system
CHO	carbohydrate
CK	creatine kinase
CKD	chronic kidney disease
CO_2	carbon dioxide
COPD	chronic obstructive pulmonary disease
CRP	C-reactive protein
CSII	continuous subcutaneous insulin infusion
CT scan	computed tomography scan
CVD	cardiovascular disease
CVP	central venous pressure
DAFNE	Dose Adjustment for Normal Eating
DAN	diabetic autonomic neuropathy
DCCT	Diabetes Control and Complications Trial
DDA	Disability Discrimination Act
DESMOND	Diabetes Education and Self-Management for On-going and Newly Diagnosed
DIDMOAD	diabetes insipidus, diabetes mellitus, optic atrophy and deafness
DISN	diabetes inpatient specialist nurse
DKA	diabetic ketoacidosis
DPP-4	dipeptidylpeptidase-4
DSFT	multidisciplinary diabetes specialist footcare team
DSME	diabetes self-management education
DSN	diabetes specialist nurse
DST	multidisciplinary diabetes specialist team
DVLA	Driver and Vehicle Licensing Agency
EAG	estimated average glucose
EASD	European Association for the Study of Diabetes
ECG	electrocardiogram
ED	erectile dysfunction
eGFR	estimated glomerular filtration rate in mls/min/1.73 m^2

EHIC	European Health Insurance Card
EMA	European Medicines Agency
EPP	Expert Patients Programme
EQA	external quality assurance
ESC	European Society of Cardiology
FBC	full blood count
FDA	Food and Drug Administration (USA)
FEV	forced expiratory volume
FPT	foot protection team
FR	fixed rate
FRIII	fixed rate intravenous insulin infusion
FVC	forced vital capacity
FEV1	forced expiratory volume in 1 sec
G6PD	glucose-6-phosphate dehydrogenase
GAD-Ab	glutamic acid decarboxylase autoantibodies
GDM	gestational diabetes mellitus
GI	gastrointestinal
GIT	gastrointestinal tract
GLP	glucagon-like peptide
GMC	General Medical Council
GPwSI	GP with a special interest
HAPO	hyperglycaemic and adverse pregnancy outcomes
HbA_{1c}	Haemoglobin A_{1c}
HBPM	home blood pressure monitoring
HCP	healthcare professional
HCSIC	Health and Social Care Information Centre
HDL	high-density lipoprotein (cholesterol)
HDU	high dependency unit
HHS	hyperglycaemic hyperosmolar state
HIV	human immunodeficiency virus
HONK	hyperosmolar non-ketotic hyperglycaemic state (see HHS)
HPS	Heart Protection Study
HR	hazard ratio
hr	hour
HRG	Healthcare Resource Group
HRT	hormone replacement therapy
HSE	Health Survey for England
IADPSG	International Association of Diabetes and Pregnancy Study Groups
ICU	intensive care unit (see ITU)
IDF	International Diabetes Federation

IFCC	International Federation of Clinical Chemists
IFG	impaired fasting glucose
IGT	impaired glucose tolerance
IHD	ischaemic heart disease
IM	intramuscular
INR	International Normalized Ratio
IRMA	intra-retinal microvascular anomalies
IT	Information Technology
ITU	intensive therapy unit (see ICU)
IUCD	intra-uterine contraceptive device
IUS	intra-uterine system
IV	intravenous or intravenously
JBDS	Joint British Diabetes Societies Inpatient Care group
JBS3	Joint British Societies' Guidelines on the Prevention of CVD in Clinical Practice: Risk Assessment
LADA	latent autoimmune diabetes of adulthood
LDL	low-density lipoprotein (cholesterol)
LFT	liver-function test/liver enzymes
LGV	large-goods vehicle
LH	luteinizing hormone
LoS	length of stay
MAOI	monoamine oxidase inhibitor
mcg	microgram
mg	milligram
MHRA	Medicines and Healthcare Products Regulatory Agency
MIDD	maternally inherited diabetes and deafness
MIMS	Monthly Index of Medical Specialties
min(s)	minute(s)
mm Hg	millimetres of mercury (measurement of blood pressure)
mmol/l	millimoles/litre
mmol/mol	millimoles/mole
MODY	maturity-onset diabetes of the young
MRI	magnetic resonance imaging
MRSA	meticillin-resistant Staphyloccocus aureus
MSU	midstream urine
mth(s)	month(s)
NaCl	sodium chloride
NaDIA	National Diabetes Inpatient Audit
NAFLD	non-alcoholic fatty liver disease
NASH	non-alcoholic steatohepatitis
NDA	National Diabetes Audit

NDIS	National Diabetes Information Service
NG	nasogastric or nasogastrically
NGSP	National Glycohemoglobin Standardization Program
NHS	National Health Service
NICE	National Institute of Care Excellence
NPDA	National Paediatric Diabetes Audit
NPID	National Pregnancy in Diabetes Audit
NPSA	National Patient Safety Agency
NSAID	non-steroidal anti-inflammatory drug
NSF	National Service Framework
NSTEMI	non-ST elevation myocardial infarct
OA	osteoarthritis
OCP	oral contraceptive pill
OCT	optical coherence tomography
OGTT	oral glucose tolerance test
OR	odds ratio
OSA	obstructive sleep apnoea
PAD	peripheral arterial disease
PCI	percutaneous coronary intervention
pCO_2	arterial carbon dioxide level
PCOS	polycystic ovarian syndrome
PCR	protein:creatinine ratio
PCV	passenger-carrying vehicle
PDE5i	phosphodiesterase type-5 inhibitors
PDR	proliferative diabetic retinopathy
PEF	peak expiratory flow
PGV	passenger-carrying vehicle
PIL	patient information leaflet
PO	oral or orally
pO_2	arterial oxygen level
POCT	point-of-case testing (near patient)
POD1	post-operative day one
PPAR-γ	peroxisome-proliferator-activated receptor-gamma
PSA	prostate-specific antigen
QOF	Quality and Outcomes Framework
RCOG	Royal College of Obstetricians and Gynaecologists
RCOphth	Royal College of Ophthalmologists
RCPCH	Royal College of Paediatrics and Child Health
RCT	randomized controlled trial
SC	subcutaneous
SCI-DC	Scottish Care Information—Diabetes Collaboration

SD	standard deviation
SDB	sleep-disordered breathing
SGLT2	sodium-glucose co-transporter 2
SHBG	sex hormone-binding globulin
SMBG	self-monitoring of blood glucose
SPC	summary of product characteristics
SPK	simultaneous pancreatic and kidney transplant
SRCh	state-registered chiropodist
SSRI	selective serotonin-reuptake inhibitors
STEMI	ST elevation myocardial infarction
TDD	total daily dose
TFT	thyroid function test
TIA	transient ischaemic attack
U&E	urea and electrolytes (in UK practice, plasma urea, sodium, potassium, and creatinine)
UKTIS	UK Teratology Information Service
ULN	upper limit of normal
UTI	urinary tract infection
VC	vital capacity
VEGF	vascular endothelial growth factor
VIA	variation in inpatient activity
VR	variable rate
VRIII	variable rate intravenous insulin infusion
vs	versus
WBCC	white blood cell count
WHO	World Health Organization
wk(s)	week(s)
YDC	young diabetic clinic
YHPHO	York and Humber Public Health Observatory
yr(s)	year(s)

Chapter 1

Is it diabetes?

The path to diagnosis

Diabetes presents in many forms to different people in different fields. The person to whom it presents or the place in which it is diagnosed affects initial assessment and management. Once you suspect the diagnosis of diabetes, confirm it, tell the patient the diagnosis, and explain what happens next.

Presentations

The way in which the diagnosis comes to light influences the patient's attitude to his/her condition. Those with thirst and polyuria want relief from their symptoms and may be more likely to comply with treatment than those patients who feel well (Box 1.1).

> **Box 1.1 Presentations of diabetes**
> - Patient-initiated
>   - Symptoms of hyperglycaemia (e.g. thirst, polyuria)
>   - Symptoms of diabetic tissue damage
>   - Symptoms of conditions causing diabetes (e.g. steroid excess)
> - Unrelated symptoms leading to general biochemical screen
> - Screening
>   - Well-person health check (state decreed or patient request)
>   - Insurance medical
>   - During training in glucose testing (e.g. nurse)
>   - Employment medical

Symptoms of diabetes

Toilet, thirsty, tired, thinner (Diabetes UK)

Thirst, polydipsia, and polyuria
- Severe thirst, including at night. A few patients, often elderly, ignore their thirst for fear of increasing urination. This causes dehydration and may precipitate hospital admission. Sugary drinks worsen hyperglycaemia.
- Polyuria (frequent passage of large volumes of urine, usually dilute).
- Nocturia with sleep disturbance.
- Urinary incontinence, bed-wetting, or sodden nappies (children).
- Stress incontinence.
- Urinary retention in men with prostatism.
- The severity of the polyuria, or the thirst and polydipsia, may not match the degree of hyperglycaemia.
- Polyuria without glycosuria is not due to diabetes mellitus. Seek other causes.

Weight loss
- Some weight loss is due to dehydration. The rest is due to reduction of adipose tissue by fat and muscle breakdown to fuel gluconeogenesis.
- Obese patients may be pleased, not realizing that weight loss is because of diabetes. On treatment, lost weight may be regained.
- Classically, the weight loss of diabetes mellitus is associated with normal or even increased appetite. A few patients crave sweet foods.
- Cachexia may develop rapidly in patients with type 1 diabetes who were slim to start with or in whom the diagnosis has been delayed.
- Some patients with type 2 diabetes do not lose weight.
- In patients with steroid-induced diabetes the weight gain of steroid excess may balance the weight loss of untreated diabetes.

Tiredness and malaise
- Tiredness is an insidious but frequent symptom.
- Treated patients may now recognize previous non-specific malaise.
- People may complain that the patient is irritable and hard to live with.

Bowel symptoms
- Dehydration may cause constipation, perhaps severe in the elderly.
- Lack of pancreatic enzyme may cause steatorrhoea.

Recurrent or refractory infections
- Boils, cellulitis, abscesses. Consider nasal carriage of *Staphylococcus aureus.*
- Candida may recur despite antifungals—thrush or balanitis.
- Recurrent urinary tract or chest infections.

Visual disturbance
- Changes in blood glucose concentrations may alter the refractive index of the lens, aqueous humour, and cornea, and cause blurred vision.
- New spectacles may be useless once the hyperglycaemia resolves.
- Additional symptoms relating to tissue damage are discussed later in the chapter and in Chapters 14 and 15.

Paraesthesiae
- Pins and needles in hands and feet; may resolve on treatment of the diabetes.
- Peripheral nerve damage may persist or worsen.

Pruritus
Pruritus vulvae is a common presenting feature caused by candidal infection. Generalized pruritus is not a feature of diabetes alone. There are other causes including, rarely, pancreatic malignancy.

Cramp
Patients with uncontrolled diabetes often complain of cramp, especially in the legs. If persistent it can be relieved by quinine sulfate.

Symptoms of diabetic tissue damage

These will be discussed in the relevant sections. Diabetes can remain undetected for many years and its first manifestation may be a myocardial infarction or a foot ulcer. The higher the fasting glucose at presentation of type 2 diabetes, the more likely the patient is to have tissue damage later (*Diabetes Care* 2002; **25**:1410–17; doi:10.2337/diacare.25.8.1410)

Box 1.2 Symptoms of diabetes
- General
  - Thirst and polydipsia
  - Polyuria
  - Weight loss
  - Tiredness, malaise, irritability
  - Constipation
  - Visual disturbance, e.g. blurring
  - Paraesthesiae
  - Pruritus
  - Cramp
- Tissue damage. Any form of diabetic tissue damage may present. The more common ones are
  - Ischaemic heart disease
  - Peripheral arterial disease
  - Cerebrovascular disease
  - Neuropathy
  - Cataract or retinal disease
- Conditions causing diabetes
  - Steroid excess (iatrogenic) is the most common

No symptoms

It is estimated that 800 000 people in the UK have undiagnosed diabetes. In 2011 the Health Survey for England among people > 16 yrs of age found that 2.3 % of men and 2.2 % of women had undiagnosed diabetes while 7.0 % men and 4.9 % of women had diagnosed diabetes ℘ <http://www.hscic.gov.uk/catalogue/PUB09300/HSE2011-Ch4-Diabetes.pdf>. This may not mean that the patient is unaware of the diagnosis—some may be ignoring symptoms (Boxes 1.1 and 1.2). About 10 % of type 2 patients are asymptomatic.

Diabetic tissue damage begins long before diabetes is actually diagnosed: 30–50 % of patients with newly recognized type 2 diabetes (➲ p. 17) have tissue damage already. Diabetes UK used linear regression analysis of an audit of 155 000 type 2 patients to calculate the number of years before diagnosis that complications (and hence diabetes) began to occur. The audit suggested a 10-yr delay in diagnosing diabetes (Diabetes UK, 2000). It also indicated that large-vessel complications started 20 yrs before diagnosis. People with diabetes progress from impaired fasting glucose (IFG) and/or impaired glucose tolerance (IGT) to frank diabetes over a period of years. Symptoms occur only with frank diabetes. It is essential to identify patients with all degrees of glucose intolerance as early as possible to allow risk-reduction care.

Screening and risk assessment

There is no single screening method for diabetes that fulfils requirements for a universal screening test. Focus on people likely to have diabetes or to be at high risk of this. Some populations may be at high risk.

Finger-prick capillary glucose tests are quick and simple but may be inconclusive. Warn patients that a negative test does not always exclude diabetes. Only laboratory venous blood glucose or HbA$_{1c}$ measurements should be used formally to diagnose diabetes (➔ p. 8).

Tests for diabetes must be performed with care.

Urine screening is not recommended. Some people with diabetes do not have glycosuria. A post-prandial urine sample is more likely to detect diabetes. A low renal threshold for glucose can cause glycosuria in those without diabetes (renal glycosuria).

> A 10-year-old boy was brought to a diabetes information stand at a show. A voluntary screening group had just diagnosed diabetes on the basis of a finger-prick glucose level over 11 mmol/l. His distraught mother begged for help. She was clutching a large sticky lolly, confiscated because 'diabetics can't eat sweets'. After a thorough handwash his finger-prick glucose was 4 mmol/l.

Identifying people at high risk of diabetes or with diabetes

Use the lists in Box 1.3 to identify people to be tested for diabetes or to undergo a risk assessment. NICE PH38 Preventing Type 2 diabetes: risk identification and interventions for individuals at high risk, which can be found at ℘ <http://www.nice.org.uk/PH38> includes a useful flow diagram.

NHS Health Checks (previously 'vascular checks') are offered to adults in England aged between 40 and 74 yrs not on a GP register for cardiovascular or renal disease, or diabetes. About 15 million people will be checked. The checks, commissioned by local authorities, will be offered every 5 yrs. The aim is to identify people at high risk of diabetes in order to offer them preventive lifestyle advice. About 20 000 people with previously undiagnosed diabetes are likely to be found. ℘ <http://www.healthcheck.nhs.uk/>

Use validated diabetes risk assessments or validated questionnaires

Examples:
- Diabetes UK/Leicester Risk Score, ℘ <https://www.diabetes.org.uk/Riskscore/>
- Qrisk®2 and QDiabetes® scores, ℘ <http://qintervention.org/>
- Cambridge score. *Diabetes Care* 2004; **27**:116–22; doi:10.2337/diacare.27.1.116

Test then act

Offer everyone you test healthy lifestyle advice. Those at high risk of diabetes should have intensive help with diet, exercise, and smoking cessation, and should be re-checked annually. Re-check those at lower risk at least every 5 yrs.

Box 1.3 People who should be tested for diabetes

- Anyone presenting with symptoms of diabetes
- Those with hypertension
- Those with ischaemic heart disease/cerebrovascular disease/peripheral arterial disease
- People with tissue damage known to be associated with diabetes
- Everyone attending A&E or an Emergency Admissions Unit
- Patients attending medical/surgical, renal, vascular, or eye services
- Individuals from South Asian or Chinese ethnic groups ≥ 25 yrs and BMI > 23 kg/m²
- People found to be at high risk of diabetes on risk assessment or questionnaire (see later in chapter)
- Those with impaired fasting glucose or impaired glucose tolerance
- Those with conditions known to cause or to be associated with diabetes (e.g. endocrinopathies, polycystic ovarian syndrome)
- On medication known to be associated with diabetes (e.g. steroids, thiazides, antiretrovirals)
- Patients who have had past gestational diabetes
- Pregnant patients (➔ p. 345)
- Those with severe mental health disorders
- Hypertriglyceridaemia
- First-degree relatives of patients with type 2 diabetes
- Those with a learning disability

People who should have a risk assessment for diabetes

- All adults aged 40 and above, except pregnant women
- People aged 25–39 yrs of South Asian, Chinese, African–Caribbean, Black African, and other high-risk Black and minority ethnic groups, except pregnant women.
- Those with waist circumference:
  - ≥ 94 cm men, other than Asian men
  - ≥ 90 cm Asian men
  - ≥ 80 cm women
- BMI > 25 kg/m²

The Diabetes UK risk score can be used for anyone > 18 yrs except pregnant women.

Expanded from recommendations of Diabetes UK Position Statement for Early Identification of Type 2 Diabetes, July 2006, and NICE PH38.

Making the diagnosis

The diagnosis of diabetes has major implications for the individual, not only with regard to changes in lifestyle and the introduction of self-monitoring and medication, but also with regard to employment, insurance, driving, sports, and hobbies. Therefore it is essential to prove the diagnosis at the outset.

There is no perfect 100 % reproducible test to diagnose diabetes. Blood sugariness (glycaemia) is a continuum, as is height. WHO defines the cut-off points for the blood sugariness that diagnose diabetes. The cut-offs are the levels of glycaemia at which prevalence of diabetic retinopathy rises rapidly. ℘ <www.who.int/diabetes/publications/en/>

Tests used are laboratory venous glycosylated haemoglobin—haemoglobin A_{1c} (HbA$_{1c}$), fasting (FBG) or random glucose, or oral glucose tolerance test (OGTT) (Table 1.1). Fasting means no caloric intake for at least 8 hrs. Plain water may be drunk. Point of care (finger-prick tests) can be used for an initial check only if the methodology conforms to national external quality assurance (EQA) standards and the diagnosis must be confirmed by a laboratory test. Oral glucose tolerance test (Table 1.4) is rarely necessary nowadays except in pregnancy.

Table 1.1 Glucose vs HbA$_{1c}$

	Glucose (mmol/l)	HbA$_{1c}$ (mmol/mol)
The patient	Requires fasting—concordance varies Needs 2nd visit, may default OGTT takes 2+hrs, sample timing precision varies, glucose dose unpalatable	Can have test straightaway Simple No fasting
Biological variations within the person	FBG varies day-to-day (an FBG of 7 can vary from 6.2 to 7.8 in one person) 2-hr OGTT readings better predict mortality and morbidity but: OGTT results vary 16.7 % within a person in addition to variation in glucose levels	Very little day to day variation
Biological variations between different people	Higher in elderly, South Asian, and African–Caribbean groups Not affected by red cell turnover	Affected by red cell turnover, e.g. severe anaemia (iron deficient, haemolysis), homozygous haemoglobinopathies Higher in elderly, South Asian, and African–Caribbean groups (+4 mmol/mol)

(Continued)

Table 1.1 (Cont.)

	Glucose (mmol/l)	HbA_{1c} (mmol/mol)
Preanalytical variation	Reflects glycaemia today Varies with food (today and recent, especially OGTT), exercise, stress, medications, acute illness, etc. FBG higher in am than pm Affected by posture, sampling site (capillary 20–25 % higher than venous), venous stasis Unstable in tube: plasma glucose falls by 5–7 % / hr, e.g. value of 7 falls to 6.1 in 2 hrs at room temperature even in fluoride Whole blood values (e.g. finger prick) 11 % lower than plasma	Reflects glycaemia for past 2–3 months Does NOT reflect rapidly rising glucose Does not vary with food, stress, exercise, time of day Not unstable
Analytical variation	High precision Within EQA limits in UK	Lower precision but within EQA limits in UK
Cost	Cheap OGTT has high staff costs	More expensive

Table 1.2 Possible diagnoses

Diagnosis	Clinical evidence and/or risk score	Laboratory venous blood test HbA_{1c} in mmol/mol Glucose in mmol/l
Lower risk of diabetes*	No	HbA1c < 42 (< 6 %) Fasting glucose < 5.6 Random or 2-hr OGTT glucose < 7.8
High risk of diabetes	Yes	As above
High risk of diabetes	Yes or no	HbA_{1c} 42–47 (6.0–6.4 %) Impaired fasting glucose (5.6 – 6.9) Impaired glucose tolerance OGTT: fasting glucose < 7.0 AND 2 hr glucose 7.8–11.0
Diabetes	Yes or no	HbA_{1c} ≥ 48 (≥ 6.5 %) Fasting glucose ≥ 7.0 (×2 if no symptoms) Random glucose (×2 if no symptoms) ≥ 11.1 OGTT glucose 2 hr ≥11.1

*Everyone is at some risk of diabetes and should follow healthy lifestyle advice.

Glucose has been the standard for centuries, first by tasting urine, and later by blood analyses. In 2011, WHO stated that HbA_{1c} could 'be used as a diagnostic test for diabetes providing that stringent QA tests are in place and assays are standardized to criteria aligned to the international reference values, and there are no conditions present that preclude its accurate measurement.'

Which test?

As with any patient and condition, consider severity of symptoms, clinical condition, and need for same-hour or same-day action. Untreated and undiagnosed type 1 diabetes can kill rapidly, especially in children (Table 1.3). Consider this possibility first. As with all situations in which the blood glucose level is likely to have risen rapidly, test blood glucose. (HbA_{1c} may be raised but a normal HbA_{1c} does not exclude diabetes.) The UK guidance is discussed in Figures 1.1 and 1.2.

Situations in which testing HbA_{1c} is not appropriate for diagnosing diabetes (do it as a baseline for treatment monitoring if the blood glucose is in the diabetic range; after treating anaemia if relevant) are:

- Patients < 18 yrs old (likely to have type 1 diabetes)
- Suspected type 1 diabetes all ages
- Pregnant now or < 2 mths earlier
- Diabetes symptoms for < 2 mths
- Acutely ill patients at high risk of diabetes
- Medications started or increased < 2 mths earlier that can cause raised glucose, e.g. corticosteroids, antipsychotics, antiretrovirals. Check HbA_{1c} annually in those on stable dosage for > 2 mths
- Pancreatic injury or surgery < 2 mths earlier
- Severe anaemia, e.g. iron deficient or haemolytic
- Homozygous haemoglobinopathy, e.g. sickle cell or thalassemia
- <2 mths after blood transfusion
- Renal failure associated with anaemia, especially if on erythropoietin
- Human immunodeficiency virus infection
- Splenectomy

If unsure, check with your local laboratory.

Table 1.3 Diagnosing type 1 Diabetes

Person presents with one or more symptoms suggestive of diabetes:
- Thirst, polydipsia
- Polyuria, new-onset bedwetting
- Weight loss
- Recurrent infections
- Patient, carer, or family member suspects diabetes

Assess the patient and perform finger-prick blood glucose

Patient ill* and finger prick glucose ≥ 11.1 mmol/l

(*e.g. vomiting, dehydration, confusion, hypotension, collapse)

⚠ Diabetes likely. Possible diabetic ketoacidosis

ADMIT VIA 999 AMBULANCE IMMEDIATELY

Patient not ill but finger prick glucose ≥ 11.1 mmol/L

Diabetes likely

⚠ Seek diabetes specialist advice same day especially if ketones present in blood or urine

Send venous sample to laboratory for glucose and HbA_{1c} analysis but do not wait for result. Call paediatric or medical on call team if specialist unavailable

Patient not ill and glucose 7.0–11.0 mmol/L

Diabetes possible.

Send venous sample to laboratory for glucose and HbA_{1c} analysis. (HbA_{1c} confirms diabetes if ≥48 mmol/mol—but result < 48 mmol/mol does not exclude diabetes.) Tell patient or carer to contact GP straightaway if symptoms worsen:

Review within three days

Patient not ill and glucose below 7.0 mmol/L

Diabetes unlikely:

Review if symptoms persist

People who are increased risk of developing type 1 diabetes

Autoimmune Family History e.g. type 1 diabetes, thyroid disease, coeliac disease, pernicious anaemia, Addison's disease.

Reproduced from with permission of Wiley from W G John, Use of HbA1c in the diagnosis of diabetes mellitus in the UK. The implementation of WHO guidance 2011. (*Diabet. Med.* 2012; **29**, 1350–7 doi: 10.1111/j.1464-5491.2012.03762.x) ©

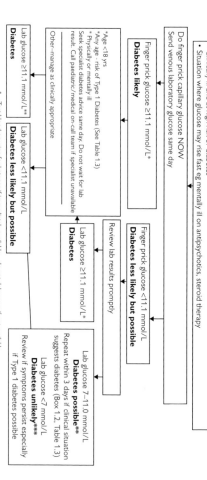

Fig. 1.1 Patients who may need urgent treatment

Reproduced with permission of Wiley from W G John, Use of HbA1c in the diagnosis of diabetes mellitus in the UK. The implementation of WHO guidance 2011. (*Diabet Med* 2012; 29: 1350–7; doi 10.1111/j.1464-5491.2012.03762.x).©

The content of the figure:

- All aged under 18 years
- Symptoms of diabetes for under 2 months
- Clinically ill and at high risk of diabetes
- Situation where glucose may rise fast eg mentally ill on antipsychotics, steroid therapy

Do finger prick capillary glucose NOW
Send venous laboratory glucose same day

Finger prick glucose ≥11.1 mmol/L*
Diabetes likely

Finger prick glucose <11.1 mmol/L*
Diabetes less likely but possible

*Age <18 yrs
*Any age - risk of Type 1 Diabetes (See Table 1.3)
*Physically or mentally ill

Seek specialist diabetes advice same day. Do not wait for lab result. Call paediatric/medical on-call team if specialist unavailable

Other - manage as clinically appropriate

Review lab results promptly

Lab glucose ≥11.1 mmol/L**
Diabetes

Lab glucose <11.1 mmol/L
Diabetes less likely but possible

Lab glucose ≥11.1 mmol/L*
Diabetes

Lab glucose 7–11.0 mmol/L
Diabetes possible**
Repeat within 3 days if clinical situation suggests diabetes (Box 1.2, Table 1.3)

Lab glucose <7 mmol/L
Diabetes unlikely***
Review if symptoms persist especially if Type 1 diabetes possible

*   Test blood or urine for ketones if immediately available – do not delay care if not available
**   Repeat lab tests if no symptoms but do not delay care of ill patients
***   HbA1c confirms diabetes if >48 mmol/mol – but result <48 mmol/mol does not exclude diabetes here

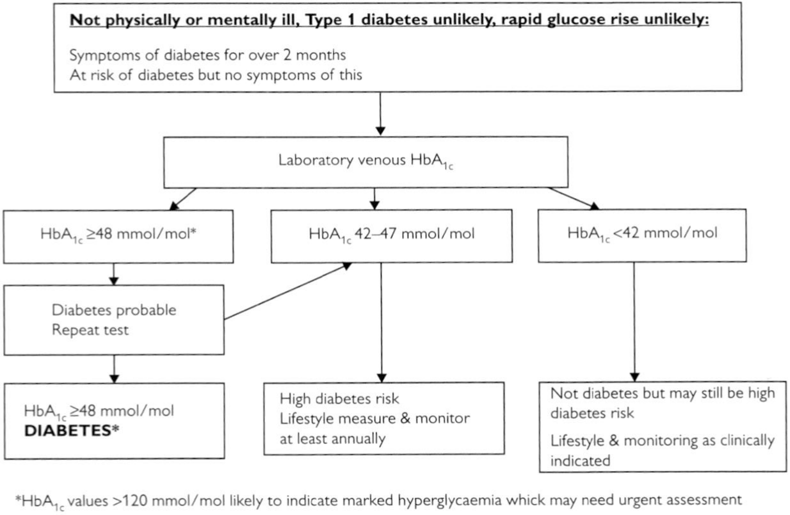

Not physically or mentally ill, Type 1 diabetes unlikely, rapid glucose rise unlikely:

Symptoms of diabetes for over 2 months

At risk of diabetes but no symptoms of this

↓

Laboratory venous HbA$_{1c}$

| HbA$_{1c}$ ≥48 mmol/mol* | HbA$_{1c}$ 42–47 mmol/mol | HbA$_{1c}$ <42 mmol/mol |

HbA$_{1c}$ ≥48 mmol/mol*
↓
Diabetes probable
Repeat test
↓
HbA$_{1c}$ ≥48 mmol/mol*
DIABETES*

HbA$_{1c}$ 42–47 mmol/mol
↓
High diabetes risk
Lifestyle measure & monitor
at least annually

HbA$_{1c}$ <42 mmol/mol
↓
Not diabetes but may still be high
diabetes risk
Lifestyle & monitoring as clinically
indicated

*HbA$_{1c}$ values >120 mmol/mol likely to indicate marked hyperglycaemia which may need urgent assessment

Fig. 1.2 Non-urgent situations in adults > 18 yrs old.

Reproduced with permission of Wiley from W G John, Use of HbA1c in the diagnosis of diabetes mellitus in the UK. The implementation of WHO guidance 2011. (Diabet Med 2012; 29: 1350–7; doi: 10.1111/j.1464-5491.2012.03762.x.) ©

Table 1.4 The oral glucose tolerance test (OGTT) (75 g)

Ask the patient to eat his/her normal diet. If the dietary carbohydrate is less than 125 g daily, the patient should eat 150 g daily for the three days before the test.

Fast the patient overnight for 10–14 hours. He/she should eat nothing, drink only water, and should not smoke during this time nor during the test.

The patient should be sitting at rest during the test.

Take a venous blood sample for plasma glucose estimation. Test the urine for glucose.

Give the patient 75 g glucose dissolved in 250–350 ml water to be swallowed over 5–15 min. (420 ml Original Lucozade® can be used.)

Two hours after the start of the test take another venous blood sample for plasma glucose estimation. Test the urine for glucose.

Ensure all samples are labeled with the patient's name, the time, and the date. Ensure that the request card(s) mirrors this labelling.

Interpreting the results of the oral glucose tolerance test

	Venous plasma glucose concentration (mmol/l)		
	Fasting		2 hrs after glucose load
Diabetes	≥ 7.0	or	≥ 11.1
Impaired glucose tolerance (IGT)	< 7.0	and	7.8–11.0
Impaired fasting glucose (IFG)	6–6.9	and	< 11.1

Table 1.5 Impaired glucose tolerance (IGT) High risk of future diabetes

OGTT:	Fasting venous plasma glucose < 7 mmol/l
	Two-hour venous plasma glucose 7.8–11.0 mmol/l

Not a benign condition

This condition is associated with a substantial risk of future diabetes (about 10% per annum). In overweight people appropriate diet and exercise greatly reduce the risk of developing diabetes. IGT is also associated with increased risk of cardiovascular disease.

Check for cardiovascular disease—heart, brain, peripheries

Check and treat risk factors

Smoking

Blood pressure

Weight

Lack of exercise

Fasting cholesterol (total, HDL, LDL)

Triglyceride

(Continued)

Table 1.5 IGT (Cont.)

Tell the patient:

'Your body is not using glucose properly. You do not have diabetes although this condition may lead to diabetes. Healthy eating, so your weight is normal for your height, with regular exercise will reduce your risk of developing diabetes.'

Give them a copy of the results. Explain the risk of diabetes and heart and circulatory disease (and what both of these are). Warn the patient to seek a blood glucose test if he/she experiences thirst, increased urination, weight loss, thrush/ perineal irritation, undue tiredness; or if he/she is ill, injured, or pregnant. Provide intensive healthy lifestyle advice.

Recheck HbA$_{1c}$ or fasting glucose annually

Fasting venous plasma glucose at OGTT < 6 mmol/l—recheck annually; repeat OGTT if 6–7 mmol/l.

Fasting plasma glucose at OGTT 6–7 mmol/l—follow impaired fasting glucose pathway.

This guideline was adapted by the author from the Diabetes UK Guidelines, June 2000, with the help of Dr Dai Thomas, The Hillingdon Hospital.

Table 1.6 Impaired fasting glucose (IFG) High risk of future diabetes

OGTT:	Fasting venous plasma glucose 6–7 mmol/l
	Two-hour venous plasma glucose below 11.1 mmol/l

This category identifies people likely to develop diabetes. Patients can have both IFG and IGT and such patients have a high risk of diabetes and should be followed closely.

Check for cardiovascular disease—heart, brain, peripheries

Check and treat risk factors

Smoking

Blood pressure

Weight

Lack of exercise

Fasting cholesterol (total, HDL, LDL)

Triglyceride

Tell the patient:

'Your blood sugar is higher than normal but not in the diabetic range. You may develop diabetes although this process can be slowed by early treatment.'

Explain what diabetes is. Give the patient a copy of their results. Warn the patient to seek a blood glucose test if he/she experiences thirst, increased urination, weight loss, thrush/perineal irritation, undue tiredness; or if he/she is ill, injured, or pregnant. Provide intensive healthy lifestyle advice.

(Continued)

Table 1.6 IFG (Cont.)

Recheck fasting glucose

Recheck fasting venous plasma glucose in three months, then every 6 months. If IFG *and* IGT, check every three months, long term. If IFG persists do an OGTT annually or HbA_{1c}.

Consensus awaited

The patient cannot be officially diagnosed as diabetic until he/she has a fasting glucose > 7.0 mmol/l or a 2 hr glucose > 11.0 mmol/l or HbA_{1c} ≥48 mmol/mol.

This guideline was adapted by the author from the Diabetes UK Guidelines, June 2000, with the help of Dr Dai Thomas, The Hillingdon Hospital.

Metabolic stress

In patients whose blood glucose levels suggest diabetes but who are under a metabolic stress, such as an infection, myocardial infarction, surgery, or a course of steroid treatment, check HbA_{1c} now (≥ 48 mmol/mol strongly suggests diabetes, < 48 mmol/mol does not refute it). Repeat diabetes tests at least six weeks after the patient has recovered to confirm the persistence of diabetes. You may need to treat the high glucose – get specialist advice.

Ill patients

Do not delay treatment of severely hyperglycaemic and clinically ill patients because laboratory confirmation is unobtainable or slow. In unwell patients, if the finger-prick glucose concentration is ≥11.1 mmol/l, wash another of the patient's fingers with plain water, dry well, and repeat the finger-prick glucose. If hyperglycaemia is confirmed, treat the patient accordingly (as previously discussed), but send a pre-treatment blood sample to the laboratory for blood glucose estimation

Pregnancy

Many authorities consider that these diagnostic criteria for blood glucose also apply to pregnant women. However, different criteria are sometimes used in pregnancy (➔ p. 346).

Retrospective diagnosis of diabetes

Occasionally, a doctor is presented with a patient in whom oral hypoglycaemic treatment for diabetes has already been started without proper confirmation of the diagnosis. This should not occur if the guidelines are followed. If the patient is seen within six weeks of starting medication, the finding of a raised HbA_{1c} (➔ p. 12, Figure 1.2) provides support for the diagnosis of diabetes. Sometimes oral hypoglycaemic treatment has to be stopped to allow clarification of the diagnosis.

Types of diabetes

There are 3.2 million people with diabetes in the UK (Table 1.7). About 10 % of all diabetic patients have type 1 diabetes. Among adults with apparent type 2 diabetes, 10–25 % are likely to have latent autoimmune diabetes of adulthood (LADA) or type 1 diabetes. Just under half of all cases (47 %) of type 2 diabetes can be attributed to obesity. York and Humber Public Health Observatory (YHPHO) have produced local and national prevalence estimates for total diabetes in NHS districts: <http://www.yhpho.org.uk/resource/view.aspx?RID=154049>

The same glycaemia criteria apply to the diagnosis of all types of diabetes. The two main types are type 1 (previously called insulin-dependent diabetes or juvenile-onset diabetes) and type 2 (previously called non-insulin-dependent or maturity-onset diabetes). It can be very difficult to decide what type of diabetes a patient has; treat the patient and the glucose and seek specialist advice. The need for insulin treatment does NOT define diabetes type. Time sometimes provides the answer. Beware LADA; such patients may suddenly develop diabetic ketoacidosis (DKA).

People with type 1 diabetes are usually (but not always):
- under 40 yrs
- slim
- ketosis-prone
- islet-cell antibody, and/or glutamic acid decarboxylase autoantibodies (antiGAD-Ab) positive
- have rapid onset of symptoms (often severe)
- unable to survive without insulin treatment

People with type 2 diabetes are usually:
- over 40 yrs (but it is increasing in younger people)
- overweight
- not ketosis-prone
- islet cell or antiGAD-Ab negative
- have variable onset of symptoms (often slow and less severe)
- able to survive without insulin treatment, but often require it over time
- have a family history of type 2 diabetes

Type 1 diabetes

Type 1 diabetes appears to have three general forms of onset:
- Type 1*a* Usually occurs in young people. There are symptoms over weeks or months, with high glucose, high HbA_{1c}, ketones and islet cell or antiGAD-Ab antibodies present. Type 1a may also present as late onset autoimmune diabetes (LADA) in apparent type 2 diabetic patients. Patients with LADA may manage on tablets for years but have positive anti-GAD antibodies and ultimately need insulin. Parental diabetes is uncommon.
- Type 1b Some patients have features of type 1a but are antibody negative.
- Type 1c A few patients may have very rapid onset with normal or only slightly raised HbA_{1c} but high ketones. This is rare and dangerous.

Surgical removal of the pancreas, inflammatory damage, or pancreatic trauma produces insulin-deficient diabetes—like type 1 but without the autoimmune connotations, and usually with deficient pancreatic enzymes.

Type 2 diabetes

Most diabetic patients in the UK have type 2 diabetes. Type 2 diabetes is a multi-factorial condition. Multiple genes have been implicated in various combinations with significant interaction with environmental factors. TCF7L2 shows the strongest association (*Diabetologia* 2007; **50**:1–4; doi: 10.1007/s00125-006-0507-x). Type 2 diabetes is largely a diagnosis made when other forms have been excluded and it includes multiple variants, most with unclear cause.

Most patients have metabolic syndrome. While many can be managed by diet, exercise, and oral hypoglycaemics, many come to need insulin. Type 2 diabetes is usually a combination of relative insulin lack and insulin resistance.

Early-onset type 2 diabetes is an unusual variant which starts between 25 and 40 yrs. Glucose intolerance is found in 90 % of parents and 68 % of siblings. It is associated with obesity. Insulin is often needed and microvascular complications are common.

Monogenic diabetes/maturity onset diabetes of the young (MODY)

A subset of people with type 2 diabetes have monogenic diabetes, the preferred name for maturity-onset diabetes of the young (MODY). This affects 30 000–60 000 people in the UK. MODY is used here as the familiar term. This usually starts in those under 25 yrs old. Glucose intolerance is found in 50 % of parents and 50 % of siblings. MODY is slowly progressive and seldom needs insulin. Six gene defects have been identified (87 % of all MODY patients):

- HNF1-α (70 % all MODY patients; sulfonylureas very effective)
- Glucokinase: uncommon, mild glucose rise, rarely needs medication
- HNF1-β (including renal cysts and diabetes)
- HNF4-α (variable age of onset, 30 % will need insulin)
- IPF1
- NeuroD1

For more information and contacts for advice, see ✆ <http://www.diabetesgenes.org>. Seek advice before arranging tests or family screening for suspected MODY.

Maternally inherited diabetes and deafness (MIDD)

This mitochondrial disorder in men and women, inherited via the female line, affects up to 300000 people in the UK. It is usually diagnosed in middle age, although it can affect any age. Most patients are short and not overweight. MIDD can usually be treated with tablets at first (avoid metformin) although many people need insulin within two years. About 75% of patients develop deafness. Patients may also have heart rhythm problems, myopathy, kidney and eye disease, and constipation. Seek expert advice about testing and family screening. For further information and contact details for advice, see: ✆ <http://www.diabetesgenes.org>

✆ <http://www.diabetesgenes.org/sites/default/files/midd_or_maternally_inherited_diabetes_15.05.12.doc>

Table 1.7 Types of diabetes
N.B. Anyone with any type of diabetes may need insulin treatment. The use of insulin does NOT define the type of diabetes.

Type	Comment
Type 1	Islet cell damage—autoimmune or rarely idiopathic
	Severe or absolute insulin lack
Type 2	Insulin resistance and/or relative insulin lack to varying degrees
	Multifactorial
Gestational	
Other	Monogenic diabetes
	Mitochondrial diabetes and deafness
	*Abnormal insulin action, e.g. severe insulin resistance or lipoatrophy
	Pancreatic damage, e.g. pancreatitis/injury/tumour/surgery Cystic fibrosis Haemochromatosis Fibrocalculous damage
	Endocrine: Pituitary—acromegaly, Cushing's Adrenal—Cushing's/Conn's syndrome, phaeochromocytoma, Glucagonoma/somatostatinoma Thyroid overactivity Polyglandular autoimmune syndrome
	Drugs, e.g. Corticosteroids, thiazides, antipsychotics, antiretrovirals
	Infections, e.g. congenital rubella, cytomegalovirus
	Rare auto-immune variants

*Syndromes, e.g. Down's, Wolfram, Alström, Turner, porphyria.

We await the WHO classification. A comprehensive report is available from the American Diabetes Association Diabetes Care, 2012, 35, Supplement 1.

Note that in the UK there are nationally commissioned specialist services for some of these conditions ℛ <http://www.specialisedservices.nhs.uk/services>.

Other forms of diabetes

Some patients are difficult to classify but can still be treated on clinical and biochemical assessment. African–Caribbean patients presenting in DKA may have ketosis-prone type 2 diabetes or type 1b diabetes. There is a sub-Saharan variant. Tropical diabetes is rarely seen in the UK. It is associated with pancreatic calculi (fibrocalculous) and, sometimes, with malnutrition. People with insulin-resistance syndromes may have acanthosis nigricans and unusual body-fat distribution. Those in whom diabetes is part of a complex syndrome may have deafness, early visual problems, and other physical abnormalities.

Inheritance of diabetes

Much more is known about this complex topic than in the past. Diabetes—a high blood glucose—is the endpoint of thousands of different genetic and environmental interactions. Genetic studies have identified multiple genes linked in various ways to type 1 and type 2 diabetes. Diabetes-related genetic testing should not be undertaken without specialist advice because 'over-the-counter' online testing can be misleading and can easily cause anxiety. For background information, see the following, but note that this is a rapidly moving field: ✍ <http://www.who.int/genomics/about/Diabetis-fin.pdf>.

Type 1 diabetes

An identical twin has a ~ 30 % chance of developing type 1 diabetes if his/her twin has it. The sibling of someone with type 1 diabetes has ~ 8 % chance of developing diabetes (this can be better predicted if HLA typing is done). A child with an affected mother has a ~ 1–4 % chance of developing diabetes, with an affected father a ~ 6 % chance. If both parents have type 1 diabetes, the risk is ~ 6–12 %. The risk increases if the parent's diabetes was diagnosed aged < 11 yrs. These figures should be compared with the frequency of type 1 diabetes in the population as a whole, which is about 1 %.

Type 2 diabetes

The chance of inheriting type 2 diabetes is harder to assess as some individuals do not develop the disease until they are in their eighties. We now know that many genetic and environmental factors interact to produce type 2 diabetes. There is virtually 100 % concordance of type 2 diabetes in identical twins. It is estimated that ~ 25 % of the relatives of someone with type 2 diabetes have had, have, or will eventually develop diabetes. If one parent has type 2 diabetes, ~ 15 % of the children will eventually develop it; if both parents have type 2 diabetes the risk may be as high as 75 %. The frequency in the population as a whole is ~ 4 % and rising.

MODY is dominantly inherited; i.e. 50 % of children will have it.

Miscoding, misclassification, and misdiagnosis of diabetes

Classification of diabetes is much more complex than previously believed. If in doubt about the type of diabetes, explain to the patient that he or she has diabetes but it may take a little time to clarify exactly which type. Glucose-lowering treatment and management of any risk factors or complications can continue. Typing is important for optimal management, especially glucose-lowering. If in doubt seek specialist advice. Misunderstandings may lead to wrong diagnoses being recorded. In particular, insulin treatment in people with type 2 diabetes may be recorded as type 1. Investigation of routinely collected primary care data showed that 2.2% of people had been misdiagnosed, 2.1% of people misclassified, and 0.9% miscoded. (*Diabet Med* 2012; **29**:181–9. doi: 10.1111/j.1464-5491.2011.03419.x.).

C-peptide

Pancreatic islet cells produce insulin attached to C-peptide. On release into the circulation the insulin and C-peptide separate. The presence of C-peptide is a sign that the patient is making his or her own insulin. At diagnosis people with all types of diabetes may be making some insulin—usually much less in type 1 than type 2. As diabetes progresses insulin production falls. There is increasing evidence that C-peptide measurement may help inform difficult diagnoses or treatment decisions. Absent or very low C-peptide indicates the need for insulin treatment. For example, post-meal urinary C-peptide:creatinine ratio < 0.2 nmol/mol indicates absolute insulin deficiency and mandatory insulin treatment (likely type 1, especially in long-standing diabetes); < 0.6 nmol/mol suggests type 1 diabetes/ unlikely to respond to non-insulin treatments. In children or young people, > 1.1 nmol/mol at diagnosis suggests monogenic·or type 2 diabetes. (*Diabet. Med.* 2013; **30**:803–17; doi: 10.1111/dme.12159).

Diabetes in remission

After pancreatic transplant or bariatric surgery, patients may be normogly-caemic on no glucose-lowering treatment. They may be told that their diabetes is cured and be taken off the diabetes register at the GP surgery. But diabetes is not just sugar trouble. High glucose levels in the years before the procedure may still be driving diabetic tissue damage (➲ pp. 180, 245–9). For example, although in future years retinopathy may stabilize or improve, it can still worsen in the year or so post-operatively. Furthermore, if the graft fails or weight is regained, the hyperglycaemia will return.

Patients should be coded as 'diabetes remitted' or 'diabetes in remission', and they must still attend annual diabetes review, and must remain on the retinal screening list.

Summary

- There are many paths to the diagnosis of diabetes and many patients are asymptomatic
- Check finger-prick glucose immediately in symptomatic patients.
- Use targeted screening, although most of the population will fulfil one or more criteria
- Remember that a one-off screening glucose test is not foolproof
- Confirm the diagnosis formally with laboratory venous glucose or HbA$_{1c}$ tests
- Differentiate between diabetes and high risk of diabetes
- Remember that those at high risk (including IFG and IGT) can progress to diabetes, and carry excess cardiovascular risk. Warn patients and advise on lifestyle measures
- Classify diabetes if possible—usually type 1 or type 2
- Remember unusual versions of diabetes. Seek specialist advice if suspected
- Do not delay treatment whilst trying to type the diabetes. Treat the patient and the glucose

Useful reading

Handbook for vascular risk assessment, risk reduction and risk management 2012 ℳ <http://www.screening.nhs.uk/publications>
IDF 2013 Diabetes Atlas 6th edn ℳ <http://www.idf.org>

Chapter 2

Assessing a person with diabetes

Emergencies

Box 2.1 Emergencies

Danger signs

Start urgent treatment. Consider urgent hospital admission. Seek specialist/ hospital advice immediately.

- Any impairment of conscious level
- Clinically ill
- Vomiting
- Hyperventilation
- Severe dehydration
- Low blood pressure
- Fever
- Foot or leg infection or gangrene
- Patients with any concomitant severe illness, especially infection
- Child under 18 yrs
- Pregnant woman
- Blood glucose > 20 mmol/l (some patients tolerate high glucose levels well but it can be difficult to decide who needs urgent help)

Urgent management

These patients need urgent assessment and management but in the absence of danger signs can usually be managed out of hospital.

- Severe symptoms
- Profuse urinary ketones
- Marked weight loss
- Under 30 yrs of age

For both groups consider giving *adults* 4–8 units fast-acting insulin subcutaneously (intramuscularly or intravenously if shocked) immediately if the diagnosis of diabetes is secure and the blood glucose level is > 20 mmol/l. If hypotensive or shocked, iv fluids are required first. (see Chapters 12 and 24, (➲ pp. 213–31, 417–43)).

Information needed by the diabetes care team

Much of this may seem basic information, but items are frequently omitted, to the detriment of patient care. This causes extra work and delays. Diabetes is a lifelong condition and it has a major impact on social and family life. Robust and regularly updated information is essential. Much of this information is already available in practice or hospital records. GPs may feel that this information is much too detailed, but because about half of all patients with newly diagnosed type 2 diabetes have complications at diagnosis, it is important to make a thorough initial assessment.

Demographic
- Name
- Address
- Telephone (day and night) and mobile numbers
- Name and contact details of carer, if relevant
- E-mail address if patient wishes (N.B. remember, information transmitted this way is not be secure)
- Date of birth
- NHS number
- Practice/hospital record number
- Does patient want copies of letters? If so, delivery address

Practical
- Current occupation
- Language spoken (if not English, note name and address of interpreter)
- Hearing, visual, speech, or other communication problems
- Comprehension problems (e.g. Down's syndrome)
- Mobility problems or other physical disabilities
- Religious or other beliefs which may influence treatment (e.g. vegetarian, non-beef/pork eating, no blood products, prefers to see female staff, etc.)
- Names and contact details of health or social care professionals, e.g. social worker

Clinical history
- Patient's main concerns
- Presentation of diabetes, symptoms, and duration (➲ p. 2)
- Previous medical history:
  - large-vessel disease, e.g. myocardial infarct, stroke
  - small-vessel disease, e.g. renal disease
  - endocrine disorders, e.g. thyroid
  - autoimmune disorders, e.g. pernicious anaemia
  - conditions likely to need steroid treatment or diuretics
  - obstetric history, e.g. gestational diabetes, big babies
  - pancreatitis
  - carcinoma pancreas
  - pancreatic or major abdominal surgery, trauma
  - other rarer linked conditions (➲ p. 27)

- Family history
  - diabetes
  - heart/arterial disease
  - endocrine
  - autoimmune disease
  - other inherited disease (⊃ p. 27)
- Family circle/support from friends.
- Women of child-bearing potential—are they planning pregnancy, risking it, using contraception or sterilized?
- Social history. Accommodation: stairs, council/state, residential/nursing home, detention centre/prison
- Education: to help tailor explanations and introduction of self-care
- Occupation. What does it involve? The diagnosis may have important financial implications.
  - sedentary
  - physically strenuous
  - risky, e.g. water or heights
  - shift work
  - feet at risk, e.g. building sites
  - armed forces
  - handles gun, e.g. police
  - driving—car, large-goods vehicle, passenger vehicle
  - flying
- Leisure activities:
  - energetic, e.g. football, dancing
  - potentially hazardous, e.g. martial arts, sub-aqua diving, rock climbing, horse riding
- Diet (in general—the dietitian will check in detail)
- Exercise
- Smoking (ask about bindi or hookah in relevant groups)
- Alcohol:
  - consider pancreatitis and malabsorption
  - check liver function and triglyceride
  - warn about hypoglycaemia with glucose-lowering medication
- Prescribed drugs:
  - steroids
  - oral contraceptives
  - thiazides
  - tricyclics
  - atypical antipsychotics
  - antiretrovirals
  - β-blockers (impair hypoglycaemia warning)
- Street drugs: used by one in four young people. Injecting drugs increases risk of hepatitis B/C and HIV.
- Allergy/adverse drug reactions. Sulfonamide allergy precludes sulfonylurea use. Most diabetic patients will need antibiotics sometimes.
- System review—do not skimp. Consider evidence of diabetic tissue damage.
- Does the patient have regular dental care?

Clinical examination

General observations

- Conscious level. Impaired? Consider hypoglycaemia (if on glucose-lowering medication), diabetic ketoacidosis, hyperosmolar hyperglycaemic state, stroke.
- Personality, psychological and educational factors. These will influence impact of diabetes and ability to self-care.
- Fever? (Infection common, not excluded by normal temperature).
- Weight and height, body mass index.
- Abdominal circumference—central vs general obesity? Central obesity—seek other metabolic syndrome features.
- Dehydration.
- Clues to causes of secondary diabetes, or associated syndromes:
  - alcoholic pancreatic disease (common)
  - polycystic ovarian syndrome (common)
  - steroid excess, including iatrogenic (common), or lack (rarer)
  - thyroid disease (common)
  - acromegaly
  - haemochromatosis
  - Down's syndrome
  - cystic fibrosis
  - Wolfram's syndrome
  - hypogonadal syndromes, e.g. Kleinfelter's, Turner's, Prader–Willi, Laurence–Moon–Biedl
  - ataxia telangiectasia
  - dystrophia myotonica
  - congenital rubella
  - lipoatrophic conditions
  - Freidreich's ataxia
  - Huntington's chorea

Skin (⮕ pp. 294–5)

- Skin infections, e.g. boils, cellulitis, ulcers, fungi (common)
- Diabetic dermopathy (quite common)
- Necrobiosis lipoidica diabeticorum (rare)
- Vitiligo
- Jaundice
- Stigmata of hyperlipidaemia (e.g. xanthomata, corneal arcus in under 50s)

Thyroid

Always examine the thyroid: enlargement?
General thyroid status

Breast (⮕ p. 295)

Diabetic mastopathy
Breast carcinoma (*Int J Cancer* 2007; **121**:856–62; doi: 10.1002/ijc.22717)

Cardiovascular system

Usual assessment, particularly:
- pulse rhythm—atrial fibrillation (common)
- hypertension (common)
- postural hypotension (overtreated hypertension, autonomic neuropathy, dehydration)
- left ventricular hypertrophy (hypertension)
- systolic murmur (aortic sclerosis, mitral regurgitation—previous myocardial infarct is common)
- peripheral pulses weak or missing (peripheral arterial disease common)
- ankle or sacral oedema—cardiac failure (common), nephrotic syndrome

Respiratory system

- Breathlessness—chest infection, cardiac failure (common)
- Asthma or chronic obstructive airways disease: on steroids?
- Hyperventilation—diabetic ketoacidosis (uncommon)

Abdomen

- Obese (is obesity general or central?)
- Scaphoid (severe weight loss if hyperglycaemic, or pancreatic cancer)
- Hepatomegaly: alcohol, non-alcoholic fatty liver, haemochromatosis
- Kidneys: tender—pyelonephritis; bruits—renal arterial stenosis
- Bladder tenderness—urinary tract infection
- Epigastric tenderness—severe ketosis
- Genitalia—vulvovaginitis (common) or balanitis from candidiasis

Nervous system including eyes (➲ pp. 268–3, 274 and 280–4)

- Eyes
  - cataract
  - retinopathy
  - reduced acuity is a late sign of diabetic eye disease
- Hearing
  - deafness hinders education unless recognized
  - deafness common—can be due to mononeuropathy, infection; rarely congenital rubella, Wolfram's syndrome, etc.
- Cranial nerves
  - stroke
  - mononeuropathy
- Limbs
  - peripheral sensory neuropathy
  - mononeuropathy
  - paresis or other evidence of new or old stroke
- Autonomic neuropathy
  - postural hypotension

Joints and ligaments (➲ pp. 296–7)

- Dupuytren's contracture
- Cheiroarthropathy
- Charcot joints
- Arthritis: may make injections difficult or limit dexterity/mobility
- Arthritis: may be on steroid treatment

Feet and legs (⟳ pp. 301–5)

- Gait: mobility
- Shoes (distorting or distorted)
- Foot hygiene
- Previous surgery or amputation
- Deformities
- Skin: dry, cracked, blisters, blemishes, colour (red, white, purple, blue, black)
- Pressure areas
- Old or current ulcers
- Circulation and pulses, feet hot or cold
- Sensation: monofilament, light touch, pin-prick (Neurotip), position, vibration

When finished

- Record your findings. Negative findings are important—record them
- Feed back to the patient

Information from others

Partners/relatives

Amplification of history if necessary

Information from other health care professionals

- Diagnostic glucose concentrations—if you did not make the diagnosis confirm it before starting lifelong treatment
- Amplification of clinical history

Share findings

- With patient:
  - discuss diagnostic and clinical findings
  - encourage patient to keep copies of this information
- With relevant health care professionals

Patient folder (paper or electronic)

Many different versions. The simplest is an envelope folder containing:

- information about help and rescue
- information about diabetes care (GP, clinic, etc.)
- appointment card
- glucose diary if required
- personalized health targets
- copies of laboratory and other test results, including X-ray report
- photocopy of ECG (important)
- relevant information leaflets

There are a number of investigations to diagnose diabetes as shown in Box 2.2.

Box 2.2 Investigations
- Finger-prick capillary blood:
  - glucose
  - HbA_{1c} (if device with full QA available)
  - ketones if emergency attender and/or ill/vomiting and glucose >11 mmol/l; or if appears well and glucose >15 mmol/l
- Urine:
  - dipstick glucose, ketones, protein, blood, leucocytes, nitrite
  - laboratory microalbumin:creatinine ratio (ACR)
- *Fasting laboratory venous blood (non-fasting if emergency attender or already on insulin):
  - fasting glucose (if diagnosis unproven but could use HbA_{1c})
  - fasting cholesterol, HDL, LDL, triglyceride*
  - urea and electrolytes
  - creatinine
  - liver function
  - calcium and albumin
  - thyroid function
  - haemoglobin A_{1c}
  - full blood count
  - consider adding C-reactive protein (infection?), urate (gout?)
  - add tissue transglutaminase once if < 18 yrs
- Chest X-ray if chest signs or symptoms, recent immigrant, Asian
- Foot X-ray if ulcer, possible infection, or injury
- ECG if chest pain, or if age > 40 yrs (ECG changes are common at diagnosis; future cardiac events are common)

*Fasting (nothing to eat/drink except plain water for 12 hours pre-test) not essential (➲ pp. 251–2)

This chapter assumes that the person has untreated diabetes. This system can also be used to reassess someone with known diabetes. Full assessment takes at least 30 min. Full dietetic assessment takes another 30 min.

Summary
- Is the patient ill? Always assess for danger signs and treat promptly.
- Is the patient high risk—child or pregnant woman?
- Obtain a full history on first encounter. Get to know your patient.
- Detailed examination is important.
- It takes up to an hour to assess a new diabetic patient fully.
- Every patient needs investigations.
- Start the record which will follow the patient for the rest of his/her life.
- Share your findings with the patient and with relevant health care professionals.

The aims of diabetes care

Introduction

To enjoy life to the full and stay well

The aim should be for a person with diabetes to enjoy life to the full without diabetes or its care causing problems now or in the future. This means avoidance of acute glucose emergencies and long-term diabetic tissue damage. It also means as little interference as possible with the patient and his or her life from the process of diabetes care and clinical supervision.

Many people with diabetes simply want to 'get back to normal'. Normality is hard to define; each person will have his or her own personal definition. It is devastating to discover that one has a permanent illness which may disable or kill, which requires inconvenient, uncomfortable, and sometimes complex treatment, and which may impact on one's job, driving, insurance, and family life. It is misleading and unfair to paint too rosy a picture of life with diabetes, but neither should carers depict too gloomy a future. Help people with diabetes to get back towards their version of normal life as soon as possible. If this is not feasible, then provide them with sympathetic and practical support through their disappointment and frustration. Help them to build a new 'normality'.

Diabetes education (➲ Chapter 4, pp. 55–66)

People with diabetes need to understand what diabetes is, what it means for them personally, and what may happen in the future. They need to learn what they themselves can do to reduce the likelihood of glucose problems and tissue complications, and what their diabetes team can do to help them. They should understand how best to use their medication and related technology, how to cope with common difficulties and emergencies, how to seek help, and how to make the most of health resources. Relatives and friends also want to learn and help.

Education is a continuous process, and so there must be opportunities for learning during every interaction with health care staff—and in between. People need revision sessions and opportunities to extend and update their knowledge.

Appropriate accessible care

Appropriate accessible high-standard evidence-based health care

Each person with diabetes should be able to access diabetes care when and where they need it. Distant surgeries or clinics, too few diabetes-trained staff, poor public transport, tired and stressed staff, lack of continuity of staff, and lack of expert advice out of hours are some examples of barriers to care. Some can be resolved by increasing resources, and some by additional training

Daisy has lived alone since her husband died. She is 81, walks with a stick, and is blind in one eye. She has peripheral arterial disease and arthritis, and has had several falls. She takes gliclazide for her type 2 diabetes. Her BMI is 24 kg/m² BP 165/95, and HbA$_{1c}$ 70 mmol/mol (8.6 %).
    Malcolm is a successful 32-yr-old businessman. He has had diabetes for 5 yrs which is treated with gliclazide. He works long hours and regards his job as stressful. He enjoys playing football at weekends. His BMI is 24 kg/m², BP 165/95, and HbA$_{1c}$ 70 mmol/mol (8.6 %).

Staff delivering diabetes care should know about diabetes, in depth. Obvious? Apparently not. Many patients are looked after by healthcare staff who have had no special training in diabetes care. Nowadays this is not acceptable. There is a clear evidence-based blueprint for diabetes care (➲ pp. 36, 45–9). Everyone caring for diabetic patients should follow this blueprint to the best of his or her ability and keep up to date. As numbers of patients rise resources must be used efficiently, primary and secondary care must communicate well and avoid duplication or omission. Staff should be supported with good training, updating, and good working conditions.

Each patient is unique

Clearly Malcolm and Daisy are very different. One is elderly and frail, the other young and energetic. One has plenty of time for herself, the other is in a stressful time-consuming job. One finds finger-prick glucose measurements difficult, the other easy. One does not drive and cannot use a bus, the other has a car. Both have elevated BPs and poor glucose balance. So what factors influence the targets set for Daisy and Malcolm? Think about it.

If it doesn't work for me, it doesn't work

The care plan clinicians produce must be acceptable to the patient and he or she must feel that it will work for him or her. As with all patients, consider their previous knowledge of their condition and its care, their attitudes, their expectations, their emotional state, their educational level, and factors which may impede understanding.

Physical factors

Factors affecting understanding (e.g. dementia, metabolic disarray), movement and mobility (arthritis, stroke, amputation), sensation (neuropathy), balance (stroke, postural hypotension), concentration (malaise from persistent hyperglycaemia, pain), vision (cataract, retinopathy), and hearing (diabetic deafness) can all impede care, as can comorbidities. For example, do not aim for a BP of < 130/80 in someone with postural hypotension.

Practicalities

Modern diabetes care means that the patient must be reviewed more often than was deemed necessary in the past. He or she needs to be able to get to the surgery or clinic easily. If not, the care should go to the patient. Consider using telephone (landline or mobile), texting, e-mail (with appropriate confidentiality warning), and services like Skype®. Many areas have specialist helplines. However, it is often those patients who have most difficulties in seeing or hearing or using the phone who cannot get to the surgery, and who have the most co-morbidities.

Patients who are well off find it easier to look after their diabetes than those who are not so fortunate, but diabetes is more common among socially deprived groups. Glucose monitoring meters are not yet available on the NHS and so may have to be bought, although some meters can be provided free by healthcare professionals (see BNF). It is easier to enjoy an appetizing diabetic diet if one can afford interesting food. Advise low-income patients to check if they are eligible for any benefits. Diabetes team members may be able to advise on economical and healthy food. With more frequent check-ups, patients may worry that they may lose their jobs, those with young families may find it hard to find babysitters, and students may miss school or college. Late evening or weekend surgeries are valued by patients but have to be staffed.

NHS care arrangements are complicated, especially with disabilities such as amputation. Links between different health services, and between health and social care are essential. Diabetic patients are often under the care of multiple medical teams. Daisy, for example, sees her GP, the diabetic clinic, the eye clinic, the vascular clinic, the rheumatologist, and the orthopaedic clinic. She has an appointment for care of the elderly about her falls. She sees a chiropodist separately, has a social worker, and her son recently arranged a visit to an osteopath. One healthcare professional should act as a keyworker for such patients and coordinate care.

Evidence-based diabetes care for adults

There can be few chronic disorders which offer as much scope for preventive healthcare as diabetes (Box 3.1). This section summarizes some evidence from the many studies, but it is worth noting that '[e]vidence-based advice depends on the existence of primary source evidence. This emerges only from clinical trial results in highly selected patients, using limited strategies. It does not address the range of choices available, or the order of use of additional therapies. Even if such evidence were available, the data would show median responses and not address the vital question of who responded to which therapy and why. Patient-centred care is defined as an approach to "providing care that is respectful of and responsive to individual patient preferences, need, and values and ensuring that patient values guide all clinical decisions".' (*Diab Care* 2012;35:1364–79; DOI: 10.2337/dc12-0413)

There is clear evidence that good diabetes care reduces diabetic tissue damage, and some evidence that it reduces mortality. Do not endanger patients in the search for the 'perfect' glucose or 'perfect' BP. However, with care, patients can achieve considerable improvements in both without major physical or emotional side effects. The world of research is very different from the busy clinic with too many patients and too few staff. The resourcing of modern diabetes care is a national issue. Focus on the key care issues for each patient and try to deliver them as efficiently and kindly as possible.

Personalized goals

The aim of diabetes care is to return the patient to as close a non-diabetic state as is safe and practical for that particular person. Suggested goals must be tailored to individual patients' clinical and personal needs. It is the combination of risk factors that cause diabetes complications, so treat them all.

This book is about adults. Children also need careful diabetes care, aiming for safe, near normalization of parameters, but this has particular risks. Children should be cared for by specialist paediatric diabetes teams.

The goals cited here are supported by the literature and by the relevant specialist societies. They will not be achievable in some patients and care is needed in their application. There is increasing evidence that there is no threshold effect for BP or glucose provided that they remain within physiological levels (i.e. providing sufficient blood and glucose supply to the brain and body—no fainting and no hypoglycaemia respectively), and avoid adverse effects of drugs. There appears to be no threshold effect for cholesterol either, although research continues. Risk reduction will also be discussed in later chapters on complications of diabetes.

The UKPDS risk engine is based on people with diabetes ✒ <http://www.dtu.ox.ac.uk/riskengine/>. Do not use risk engines that are not diabetes-specific in people with diabetes. Diabetes itself is such a risk that it renders these inappropriate.

Box 3.1 General goals for preventive care in diabetes

Tailor to the patient

- No smoking
- *BMI 18.5–24.9 kg/m^2
- 150 min/wk moderate intensity aerobic exercise
- BP (without postural hypotension)
  - 130/80 in most patients
  - 120–129/75–80 in kidney, eye or cerebrovascular disease
- Assessment of the need for statin therapy (Box 3.2)
- **Fasting lipids
  - Total cholesterol < 4 mmol/l or a 25 % reduction, whichever is lower (use LDL goal if HDL > 1.4 mmol/l)
  - LDL cholesterol < 2 mmol/l or a 25% reduction, whichever is lower
  - Fasting triglyceride < 2.3 mmol/l
- Fasting and premeal plasma glucose 4–7 mmol/l without hypoglycaemia; i.e. if safe
- HbA$_{1c}$ 48–58 mmol/mol (6.5–7.5 %) without hypoglycaemia i.e. if safe (➔ p. 109)
- No high glucose emergencies
- Urine albumin-to-creatinine ratio normal (➔ p. 92)

* BMI unhelpful in very muscular people. BMI upper limit in Asian/African–Caribbean or Chinese people = 23 kg/m^2.

**Fasting may cause hypoglycaemia in insulin or sulfonylurea-treated patients and is not essential unless triglycerides are raised. These lipid values are not necessary to guide treatment as current evidence advocates statin treatment for most people with diabetes regardless of cholesterol levels (see Box 3.2).

Guidance adapted from NICE CG 87, NICE PH 46, NICE Quality Standard, JBS3, and ADA/EASD position statement (➔ pp. 51–3).

Stop smoking!

- People with diabetes who smoke have at least the same risk of morbidity and mortality as non-diabetics who smoke, probably greater.
- People with diabetes who smoke have about four times the risk of dying from cardiovascular disease (CVD) as those who do not.
- Give smokers support in stopping—stop smoking groups/courses
- Vigorously discourage young people with diabetes from starting smoking
- Nicotine may alter the rate of insulin absorption, so monitor glucose after stopping. The insulin dose may need to be adjusted, as it may for those changing to e-cigarettes (safety evidence in diabetes awaited).
- Nicotine replacement products, or bupropion or varenicline can be used in people with diabetes. Check for diabetes complications first.
- Medications to assist cessation require care or avoidance in patients with CVD. Reduce doses of bupropion or varenicline in renal impairment. Glucose should be monitored in all. There is a risk of suicidal behaviour with varenicline. Note that depression is common in people with diabetes.

Blood pressure (BP) control (see also Chapter 14)

For clinical management, (➲ pp. 257–8)

CVD is the most common cause of death in diabetic patients. Reducing BP greatly reduces the risk of diabetic and cardiovascular events, both fatal and non-fatal. Be constantly aware of the risk of postural hypotension. There is considerable evidence of the benefits of lowering BP.

Start antihypertensive treatment in people with diabetes aged < 80 yrs if clinic blood pressure is 140/90 mmHg or higher and subsequent ambulatory blood pressure monitoring (ABPM) daytime average or home blood pressure monitoring (HBPM) average blood pressure is 135/85 mmHg or higher.

First, vigorously encourage lifestyle measures with weight reduction as needed; a low sodium, high potassium diet; moderate alcohol only; and regular exercise.

In UKPDS 38, tight BP control with medication produced a mean BP 144/82 mmHg vs 154/87 in the less tight control group. The tight control group showed a 24 % reduction in diabetes-related endpoints, 32 % reduction in deaths due to diabetes, 44 % reduction in strokes, and 37 % reduction in microvascular endpoints.

In 2012, a meta-analysis found that intensive BP treatment reduced stroke but not non-fatal myocardial infarction or mortality. Microvascular disease (e.g. nephropathy) was not included in the meta-analysis. UKPDS 38 showed substantial reduction in urinary albumin excretion and retinopathy.

NICE Clinical Guideline 87 (2009) advocates a target of < 130/80 if kidney, eye, or cerebrovascular damage, and BP 140/80 for others. The Joint British Societies 2014 guidance (JBS3) advises maintaining BP at 130/80 for patients with type 1 diabetes (with consideration of 120/75–80 if aged < 40 yrs with microalbuminuria). JBS3 states: '[l]owering systolic blood pressure (BP) in the majority of type 2 diabetes patients to around 130 mmHg appears beneficial. Pursuing lower targets does not reduce coronary event rates, although stroke incidence may be modified.' (JBS3 *Heart* 2014; **100**:ii1–ii67. doi:10.1136/heartjnl-2014-305693). Most patients with diabetes need treatment.

Angiotensin-converting enzyme (ACE) inhibitors (captopril (UKPDS), enalapril (ABCD), fosinopril (FACET, HOT), ramipril (HOPE/MICRO-HOPE)), perindopril + indapamide (ADVANCE), β-blockers (atenolol (UKPDS)), and diuretic agents (bendroflumethiazide (UKPDS), hydrochlorothiazide (not available on its own in UK) (Syst-EUR)) are effective and do not produce adverse metabolic effects in diabetic patients. ACE inhibitors possibly have benefits in addition to BP lowering. ACE inhibitors and diuretics are often combined.

Angiotensin receptor blockers (ARBs) reduce CVD endpoints. Losartan reduced cardiovascular events and total mortality vs atenolol (LIFE), and also reduced end-stage renal failure vs placebo (RENAAL). Irbesartan reduced end-stage renal failure vs amlodipine and placebo (IDNT).

Calcium-channel blockers showed variable results. Felodipine (HOT) and nitrendipine (unavailable in UK) (Syst-EUR) were safe and effective. Amlodipine ± perindopril reduced cardiovascular endpoints more than atenolol ± thiazide, and was less diabetogenic in non-diabetics. (ASCOT).

ALLHAT showed no difference in cardiovascular endpoints between chlortalidone, amlodipine, lisinopril, and doxazosin, but there was less heart failure on chlortalidone.

Most patients need several drugs to control the blood pressure.

Microalbuminuria

Measure laboratory urinary microalbumin:creatinine ratio (ACR) in every patient every year. Microalbuminuria warns that diabetes has damaged the kidneys and renal failure will follow. The rate of progression to renal failure can be slowed by prompt and vigorous treatment. Risk factors for progression are:

- male sex
- family history
- South Asian or African–Caribbean
- smoker
- BP > 125/75
- HbA_{1c} > 53 mmol/mol (7 %)
- dyslipidaemia
- retinopathy
- type 1 diabetes onset aged < 20 yrs

Trandolapril given to reduce BP to 120/80 reduced development of microalbuminuria vs verapamil (BENEDICT). Enalapril showed a reduction in development of microalbuminuria in normotensive diabetic patients (*Ann Int Med* 1998; **12**:982–8). Ramipril (HOPE and MICRO-HOPE) and losartan (LIFE 2004) are licensed for use in microalbuminuria with or without hypertension. MICRO-HOPE and HOPE demonstrated the benefit of ramipril in reducing deterioration of renal function in diabetic patients with early nephropathy/microalbuminuria, although it was thought that much of this effect was due to BP lowering. Captopril (type 1 diabetes), lisinopril, and ramipril are licensed for use in diabetic nephropathy.

The decrease in albuminuria was significantly greater with losartan vs atenolol in the LIFE study. Losartan is licensed in treatment of diabetic nephropathy in type 2 diabetes, as is telmisartan. Irbesartan is licensed for use in hypertensive diabetic patients, including those with renal disease, following IRMA-2 in which irbesartan appeared to have an effect upon albumin excretion apart from BP lowering. Valsartan had a similar additional benefit when compared with amlodipine ± other agents as needed to achieve the same BP lowering effect (MARVAL).

Prescribe an ACE inhibitor or an ARB in nephropathic patients even if the patient is normotensive, and in hypertensive patients keep BP <130/80 without postural hypotension. Do not combine ACE inhibitors and ARBs as this increases side effects (ONTARGET).

Lipid lowering (see also Chapter 14)

For clinical management see (➲ pp. 261–3).

A rigorous low-fat, high-fibre, weight-normalizing diet reduces lipids. Good glucose control also reduces lipids (DCCT 1995; UKPDS 39). However, lifestyle measures are not enough. The evidence of the benefit of statins is overwhelming, even in patients with 'normal' cholesterol levels (Box 3.2).

Box 3.2 Cholesterol lowering

Type 1 diabetes mellitus

Statins* should be offered in type 1 diabetes for the following categories:

- All patients with type 1 diabetes aged ≥ 50 yrs.
- The majority aged 40–50 yrs, unless short duration of diabetes (< 5 yrs) and absence of other CVD risk factors.
- Those aged 30–40 yrs with any of the following features: long duration of diabetes (20 yrs) and poor control (HbA$_{1c}$ > 9 % (75 mmol/mol)), persistent albuminuria (> 30 mg/day) or eGFR < 60 ml/min, proliferative retinopathy, treated hypertension, current smoking, autonomic neuropathy, total cholesterol (> 5 mmol/L) with reduced HDL-cholesterol (< 1 mmol/L for males and < 1.2 mmol/L for females), or central obesity, or with a family history of premature CVD (< 50 yrs).
- Those aged 18–30 yrs should receive statins if persistent albuminuria is detected, with caution exercised in women of child bearing potential.

Type 2 diabetes mellitus

Statin* therapy is recommended for all patients with type 2 diabetes above age 40 irrespective of cholesterol level.

- Intensive statin is recommended for diabetes patients with existing CVD, and those with persistent proteinuria or CKD with eGFR 30–60 mL/min. Intensive statin treatment is also recommended for patients who do not achieve non-HDL-cholesterol targets.
- Statins should also considered for patients with type 2 diabetes under 40 yrs of age if there is evidence of persistent albuminuria, eGFR < 60 ml/min, proliferative retinopathy, treated HBP, or autonomic neuropathy.
- Fibrates, used as monotherapy or in combination therapy, have not been shown to provide overall cardiovascular benefit in type 2 diabetes, and should not be prescribed routinely for CVD risk reduction.
- Fibrates show promise in prevention or treatment of retinopathy in type 2 diabetes in a manner independent of lipid-lowering action.

*Note extensive list of drug interactions with statins including hypotensive or CVD drugs and antibiotics—see BNF.

JBS3 Heart 2014;100:ii1–ii67. doi:10.1136/heartjnl-2014-305693

The five-year Heart Protection Study (HPS) included 5963 people with diabetes who did not satisfy existing criteria for cholesterol-lowering therapy in 1994. The study compared simvastatin 40 mg with placebo. There was a 22 % reduction vs placebo in cardiovascular events in those on simvastatin, with a 33 % reduction in those without overt vascular disease at outset, and a 27 % reduction if low-density lipoprotein-cholesterol < 3 mmol/l at the outset. HPS also showed that there was no significant difference in elevation of liver enzyme or of muscle enzyme between the two groups.

CARDS showed a reduction in ACS, coronary revascularization, and stroke, regardless of initial lipids, with atorvastatin vs placebo. In DAIS, micronized fenofibrate reduced coronary arterial narrowing in diabetic patients with coronary artery disease vs placebo.

A meta-analysis (CTT 2010) of 170,000 participants (with and without diabetes) in 26 trials showed that statins reduced myocardial infarction and stroke. All-cause mortality fell by 10 % per 1 mmol/l reduction in LDL cholesterol and the risk of CVD fell by 21 %. People with type 2 diabetes showed similar benefits to non-diabetics. The effect was less marked in type 1 diabetes, perhaps because of smaller numbers.

There are fewer studies of lowering triglyceride or raising HDL, although both are risk factors for CVD. Gemfibrozil increased HDL and reduced triglyceride and reduced CVD mortality (N Engl J Med 1999; **341**:410–18; doi: 10.1056/NEJM199908053410604). In FIELD fenofibrate significantly reduced CVD events in people with type 2 diabetes with low high-density lipoprotein (HDL) cholesterol or hypertension. Those with marked dyslipidemia (elevated triglycerides > 2.3 mmol/l and low HDL cholesterol) were at the highest risk of CVD. Fasting triglycerides should be < 1.7 mmol/l.

Blood glucose control (see Chapters 7–13)

Glucose control is a particularly challenging part of diabetes management. Intensive blood glucose control reduces the development and progression of diabetes complications (DCCT, UKPDS) but increases hypoglycamia. Hyperglycaemia may worsen pancreatic damage—glucose toxicity.

In DCCT (1993), intensively treated type 1 diabetic patients had a mean blood glucose of 8.6 mmol/l compared with 12.8 mmol/l in the conventionally treated group. Intensive therapy reduced the risk of developing new retinopathy by 76 %, and slowed progression by 54 % in those with pre-existing retinopathy. Overall, intensive therapy reduced occurrence of microalbuminuria by 39 %, overt proteinuria by 54 %, and clinical neuropathy by 54 %. The benefit persisted post-trial even though glucose levels rose (DCCT 2000). There was a trend towards reduction of CVD during the original study, and long-term follow-up (DCCT 1995, 2005) showed a significant reduction of 42 % in CVD in the intensive therapy group.

In UKPDS (34), intensive treatment with metformin in overweight type 2 patients produced a median HbA_{1c} of 57 mmol/mol (7.4 %) compared with 64 mmol/mol (8.0 %) in those treated conventionally. Intensive treatment with metformin reduced any diabetes-related endpoint by 32 %. In UKPDS (33), intensive treatment of type 2 patients with sulfonylurea or insulin reduced HbA_{1c} to 53 mmol/mol (7.0 %) compared with 63 mmol/mol (7.9 %) with conventional treatment. This reduced any diabetes endpoint by 12 %. Post-trial, at 20 yrs, despite the HbA_{1c} returning to that of the control group once the study ended, mortality was lower in the intensive glucose control groups than the control group (13 % less on sulfonylurea/insulin, and 27 % less on metformin).

ACCORD studied the effect of very intensive glucose control in type 2 diabetes. That group (HbA$_{1c}$ < 42 mmol/mol (6.0%)) had more hypoglycaemia and more deaths (14/1000/yr vs 11/1000/yr) than the standard group (HbA$_{1c}$ 53–63 mmol/mol (7–7.9 %)) (*BMJ* 2008; **336**: 407; doi: http://dx.doi.org/10.1136/bmj.39496.527384.DB).

The larger ADVANCE study (11,140 patients with type 2 diabetes) used gliclazide and other drugs to reduce HbA$_{1c}$ to 48 mmol/mol (6.5 %) vs 56 mmol/mol (7.3 %) in a standard control group. this intensive glucose control reduced combined major macrovascular and microvascular events by 10 %, primarily due to 21 % relative reduction in nephropathy. There was no significant difference in mortality (intensive control 8.9 % vs standard control 9.6 %). A later analysis (2012) showed threshold effects—risks of macro- or microvascular disease or death were the same in the intensive vs control groups below HbA$_{1c}$ 53 mmol/mol (7.0 %) for macrovascular events and death, and 48 mmol/mol (6.5 %) for microvascular events. Above this for every ~ 11 mmol/l (1 %) higher HbA$_{1c}$ level the risk of events rose by 38 % for death, 38 % for macrovascular disease, and 40 % for microvascular disease.

Intensive blood glucose control increased the frequency of hypoglycaemia in ADVANCE and DCCT, but careful blood glucose monitoring, good access to knowledgeable advice, and appropriate treatment adjustment can reduce this. Quality of life was no different between intensively and conventionally treated patients. Intensive glucose lowering did not appear to have an adverse effect upon cognitive function in DCCT.

Thus reducing the HbA$_{1c}$ reduces the risk of diabetic tissue damage but potentially increases the risk of adverse effects. Aim to return the blood glucose towards that observed in non-diabetics but not under 4 mmol/l in patients on glucose-lowering medication. Consider aiming for a fasting blood glucose between 4 mmol/l and 7 mmol/l and a level up to 10 mmol/l after food, if safe for that individual patient. The NICE Quality Standard (➲ pp. 47–8) suggests that HbA$_{1c}$ should be between 48 mmol/l and 58 mmol/mol (6.5–7.5 %) tailored to the patient's needs. For a detailed discussion of glucose-lowering agents, see Chapters 8 and 9.

The main risk is of hypoglycaemia (➲ pp. 181–90)). A post-hoc analysis of ACCORD showed that hypoglycaemia occurred at all HbA$_{1c}$ levels and was most frequent with poor glycaemic control (*BMJ* 2010; **340**:b5444; doi: 10.1136/bmj.b5444).

Teach all patients on glucose-lowering treatment how to recognize and treat hypoglycaemia. Teach them how to adjust their treatment to reduce the risk of further hypoglycaemia. Patients with varied timetables, meals, exercise, emotions, and varied compliance are particularly at risk of hypoglycaemia, as are children and the elderly. Educational background and ease of understanding medical advice may also be relevant. Any patient who has had one hypoglycaemic attack is likely to have more. Some patients will be unable to achieve a normal glucose without hypoglycaemia. If this is the case, work together towards the best compromise between safety now and good health long term.

Normalize weight

See (➲ pp. 78–80)

Obesity increases insulin resistance, BP, and cardiovascular risk. Weight reduction reduces symptoms of diabetes and reduces the treatment needed to normalize blood glucose, BP, and lipids. Encourage weight loss in people with diabetes (Canadian Task Force, 1999).

The aim is a BMI between 18.5 kg/m^2 and 25 kg/m^2 (23 kg/m^2 for Asian/African–Caribbean or Chinese people). Waist circumference provides a better estimate of adiposity and should be < 102 cm in men (< 92 cm in Asian men); and < 88 cm in women (78 cm in Asian women).

In general, the most effective weight-reduction strategy combines dietary advice (see Chapter 5), regular exercise (see Chapter 13), and long-term help in changing everyday weight-gaining habits. Very-low-calorie diets are successful but these require expert supervision for safety (*Diabetologia* 2011; **54**:2506–14; doi 10.1007/s00125-011-2204-7).

Most drugs to aid weight loss have been withdrawn because of side effects. Orlistat is available over the counter. It inhibits pancreatic lipase and therefore induces fat malabsorption (with frequent embarrassing gastrointestinal side effects if patients do not adhere to a low- fat diet).

Bariatric surgery is effective in weight reduction and improving glucose control in obese diabetic patients.

UK bariatric surgeons audited their data for 2009/10; 6537 operations were analysed. In-hospital mortality was 0.1 %, and surgical complication rate for primary surgery was 3.6 %. At one year patients lost 57 % of their excess weight. Two years post-operatively 85.5 % of the diabetic patients no longer needed glucose-lowering medication.

Identification and treatment of tissue damage

The main thrust of diabetes care must be prevention of problems, but in reality much effort is needed to detect and slow progression of diabetic tissue damage. Up to half of all patients with type 2 diabetes have obvious tissue damage at the time of diagnosis. Diabetes UK's audit data and regression calculations showed that the onset of coronary heart disease culminating in myocardial infarction is 20 yrs pre-diagnosis, stroke 12 yrs, nephropathy 18 yrs, amputation 7 yrs, and retinopathy 7 yrs (➲ p. 4). ⚠ At least half of the patients with diabetes on any practice list will have overt tissue damage. Every person with diabetes must be assumed to have hidden tissue damage.

Many diabetic complications have specific treatments and their progress can be slowed by redoubled preventive care (see Chapters 14 and 15). It is essential to test for any hint of tissue damage early. This means rigorous checks by the patient (reporting visual change, foot problems, etc.) and by healthcare professionals. Standards for monitoring are described in the relevant chapters of this book. Record negative information (e.g. normal foot pulses, no retinopathy) as well as positive findings. Check tissue damage annually at present (note that there is no evidence to support a 12-month interval as being any better than a shorter or longer one). Checks should probably be carried out more often. The main difficulty lies in the silence of much severe tissue damage until it is too late to prevent disability.

Delivery of good diabetes care

Annual review

Everyone with diabetes should have a full review by someone trained in the assessment of people with diabetes at least once a year (Box 3.3).

Box 3.3 Annual review

- Who is the patient? Age? Child/teenage/adolescent/adult?
- Woman of child-bearing potential?
- How is the person feeling? Any symptoms?
- Life events? Births, deaths, marriages, separations? Moves? Job? Hobbies?
- Emotions. Check for depression or anxiety and manage appropriately if present.
- Driver? If yes, check knowledge of safe driving with diabetes. Told insurance company and drivers' licensing agency?
- Diet. If unhealthy or overweight, provide appropriate advice and dietetic referral as required. Ideally, everyone with diabetes should see a dietitian annually.
- Exercise? Advise if insufficient.
- Smoker? If yes, help them stop.
- Alcohol? If excessive, help them reduce/stop.
- Hospital attendances or admissions? For diabetes, e.g. hypoglycaemia, high glucose/diabetic ketoacidosis. For non-diabetes, reason.
- Symptoms of cardiovascular disease, eye problems, neuropathy, foot problems, sexual dysfunction, other complications.
- Woman. Periods? Planning pregnancy? Contraception?
- Glucose control: SMGB (self-monitoring of blood glucose), hypoglycaemia.
- BP (including home monitoring, if done).
- Full foot assessment: shape, skin, pulses, sensation. Refer any problems to podiatrist.
- Cardiovascular examination if any hint of cardiac disease.
- Examine other systems if any relevant symptoms.
- Finger-prick or laboratory glucose ($\pm$ ketone).
- Laboratory HbA$_{1c}$, cholesterol, HDL, LDL, triglycerides, urea, electrolytes, creatinine, eGFR if relevant, LFT, thyroid function. Full blood count + vitamin B12 (if on metformin or otherwise relevant).
- Urine laboratory microalbumin-to-creatinine ratio (ACR).
- Ensure patient has had visual acuity check and digital photographic retinal screening by a recognized service, and obtain the results.
- Check patient knows what and how to monitor.
- Diabetes education and revision.
- Check patient knows where and how to seek help.
- Any questions?
- Date of next appointment.
  Give the patient a copy of the annual review.

Diabetes register: audit and recall system

See (➲ pp. 460–2).

In order to deliver good diabetes care, each unit or practice needs to know who has diabetes within their area of responsibility and what care they have had. This means a keeping a register with audit facilities. Establish a recall system for annual review and, optimally, reminders for interim check-ups. Non-attenders have a high rate of complications and should be pursued in a constructive way.

There is an English and Welsh national diabetes audit (NDA) programme: ✍ <http://www.hscic.gov.uk/nda>.

Scotland has SCI-DC: ✍ <http://www.sci-diabetes.scot.nhs.uk/>

Local support

There should be a local forum for supporting district-wide diabetes care. In the past this was the Local Diabetes Services Advisory Group. There should be representation from all those involved in receiving, providing, and purchasing diabetes care throughout the district. Such a group can be a major force in communication, education, and improving resources.

Cost-effectiveness

Many health service financial cycles are annual. Diabetic complications take years to become apparent, and so the immediate benefits of intensive management can rarely be demonstrated to a financial manager planning the following year's budget. Both DCCT and UKPDS demonstrated the long-term cost-effectiveness of intensive diabetes care.

DCCT (1996) concluded that intensive rather than conventional therapy for 120 000 people with type 1 diabetes in the USA would gain 920 000 yrs of sight, 691 000 yrs free from end-stage renal disease, 678 000 yrs free from lower-extremity amputation, and 611 000 yrs of life.

In UKPDS 41, intensive management of type 2 diabetic patients 'significantly increased treatment costs but substantially reduced the cost of complications and increased the time free from complications'. They calculated that, with intensive care, the patient would gain 1.14 yrs (confidence interval 0.69–1.61) of event-free time (an event being a diabetic complication, including death). This did not include the non-medical and social benefits such as fitness to work.

National Service Framework for diabetes: summary of standards (England 2003–13)

Prevention of type 2 diabetes

Standard 1

The NHS will develop, implement, and monitor strategies to reduce the risk of developing type 2 diabetes in the population as a whole, and to reduce the inequalities in the risk of developing type 2 diabetes.

Identification of people with diabetes

Standard 2

The NHS will develop, implement, and monitor strategies to identify people who do not know they have diabetes.

Empowering people with diabetes

Standard 3

All children, young people, and adults with diabetes will receive a service which encourages partnership in decision-making, supports them in managing their diabetes, and helps them to adopt and maintain a healthy lifestyle. This will be reflected in an agreed and shared care plan in an appropriate format and language. Where appropriate, parents and carers should be fully engaged in this process.

Clinical care of adults with diabetes

Standard 4

All adults with diabetes will receive high-quality care throughout their lifetime, including support to optimize the control of their blood glucose, blood pressure, and other risk factors for developing the complications of diabetes.

Clinical care of children and young people with diabetes

Standard 5

All children and young people with diabetes will receive consistently high-quality care and they, with their families and others involved in their day-to-day care, will be supported to optimize the control of their blood glucose and their physical, psychological, intellectual, educational, and social development.

Standard 6

All young people with diabetes will experience a smooth transition of care from paediatric diabetes services to adult diabetes services, whether hospital- or community-based, either directly or via a young people's clinic. The transition will be organised in partnership with each individual and at an age appropriate to and agreed with them.

Management of diabetic emergencies

Standard 7

The NHS will develop, implement, and monitor agreed protocols for rapid and effective treatment of diabetic emergencies by appropriately trained health care professionals. Protocols will include the management of acute complications and procedures to minimize the risk of recurrence.

Care of people with diabetes during admission to hospital

Standard 8

All children, young people, and adults with diabetes admitted to hospital, for whatever reason, will receive effective care of their diabetes. Wherever possible, they will continue to be involved in decisions concerning the management of their diabetes.

Diabetes and pregnancy

Standard 9

The NHS will develop, implement, and monitor policies that seek to empower and support women with pre-existing diabetes, and those who develop diabetes during pregnancy to optimize the outcomes of their pregnancy.

Detection and management of long-term complications

Standard 10

All young people and adults with diabetes will receive regular surveillance for the long-term complications of diabetes.

Standard 11

The NHS will develop, implement, and monitor agreed protocols and systems of care to ensure that all people who develop long-term complications of diabetes receive timely, appropriate, and effective investigation and treatment to reduce their risk of disability and premature death.

Standard 12

All people with diabetes requiring multi-agency support will receive integrated health and social care. See:
 <http://www.gov.uk/government/publications/national-service-framework-diabetes>

NICE Quality Standard for diabetes in adults (NICE QS6)

Statement 1. People with diabetes and/or their carers receive a structured educational programme that fulfils the nationally agreed criteria from the time of diagnosis, with annual review and access to ongoing education.

Statement 2. People with diabetes receive personalised advice on nutrition and physical activity from an appropriately trained healthcare professional or as part of a structured educational programme.

Statement 3. People with diabetes participate in annual care planning which leads to documented agreed goals and an action plan.

Statement 4. People with diabetes agree with their healthcare professional a documented personalised HbA_{1c} target, usually between 48 mmol/mol and 58 mol/mol (6.5 % and 7.5 %), and receive an ongoing review of treatment to minimize hypoglycaemia.

Statement 5. People with diabetes agree with their healthcare professional to start, review, and stop medications to lower blood glucose, blood pressure, and blood lipids in accordance with NICE guidance.

Statement 6. Trained healthcare professionals initiate and manage therapy with insulin within a structured programme that includes dose titration by the person with diabetes.

Statement 7. Women of childbearing age with diabetes are regularly informed of the benefits of preconception glycaemic control and of any risks, including medication that may harm an unborn child. Women with diabetes planning a pregnancy are offered preconception care and those not planning a pregnancy are offered advice on contraception.

Statement 8. People with diabetes receive an annual assessment for the risk and presence of the complications of diabetes, and these are managed appropriately.

Statement 9. People with diabetes are assessed for psychological problems, which are then managed appropriately.

Statement 10. People with diabetes at risk of foot ulceration receive regular review by a foot protection team in accordance with NICE guidance.

Statement 11. People with diabetes with a foot problem requiring urgent medical attention are referred to and treated by a multidisciplinary foot care team within 24 hours.

Statement 12. People with diabetes admitted to hospital are cared for by appropriately trained staff, provided with access to a specialist diabetes team, and given the choice of self-monitoring and managing their own insulin.

Statement 13. People admitted to hospital with diabetic ketoacidosis receive educational and psychological support prior to discharge and are followed up by a specialist diabetes team.

Statement 14. People with diabetes who have experienced hypoglycaemia requiring medical attention are referred to a specialist diabetes team.

Reproduced with permission from NICE.

✑ <http://publications.nice.org.uk/diabetes-in-adults-quality-standard-qs6/list-of-statements>

Care essentials/processes

The NDA reports local and national results for nine basic care processes performed annually to detect risk factors for complications or the early signs complications. These are:

- BP
- BMI
- Foot check
- Smoker?
- Retinal screening (up to and including 2011–12)
- Laboratory blood HbA_{1c}, creatinine, and cholesterol
- Laboratory urine microalbumin:creatinine ratio

Diabetes UK lists 15 care essentials: (🔗 <http://www.diabetes.org.uk/15-essentials>) which include the nine mentioned:

1. HbA_{1c}
2. BP
3. Cholesterol
4. Retinal screening
5. Foot check
6. Kidney check (blood creatinine and urinary microalbumin:creatinine ratio)
7. Weight and waist circumference
8. Stop smoking support if required
9. Care planning
10. Diabetes education
11. Specialist paediatric care for children and young people
12. High quality diabetes care in hospital
13. Specialist care before, during, and after pregnancy
14. Access to specialist to help you manage your diabetes
15. Emotional and psychological support

Summary

- The aim should be for a person with diabetes to enjoy life to the full without their diabetes or its care causing problems now or in the future.
- Everyone with diabetes should be taught about their condition and what they and others need to do to ensure optimal care.
- Diabetes care should be appropriate, accessible, high standard, and evidence based.
- Tailor the care to the individual.
- Diabetes care should be practical.
- Evidence-based care should be used where available.
- Targets for risk reduction are smoking, BP, glucose, cholesterol, weight, and microalbuminuria
- Tissue damage should be detected and treated.
- Every patient should have an annual review.
- Practices and clinics should have a diabetes register with a call and recall system.
- Diabetes services should audit their care.
- Clinical services should make optimal use of resources.
- Care in England should conform to the NSF standards—which are in line with international evidence-based care.

Further reading

A detailed analysis of multiple diabetes studies is outside the scope of this book. Some are listed.

The American Diabetes Association (ADA) produces an annual summary and extensive reference list: 'ADA Standards of Medical Care in Diabetes 2014' (*Diabetes Care* 2014; **37** suppl 1 S1-80. doi: 10.2337/dc14-S014).

Joint British Societies' Consensus recommendations for the prevention of cardiovascular disease (JBS3). *Heart* 2014; **100**:ii1–ii67. doi:10.1136/heartjnl-2014-305693.

A H Barnett (ed.) 2006 Diabetes; best practice and research compendium. Amsterdam: Elsevier.

K McBrien et al. Intensive and standard BP targets in patients with type 2 diabetes mellitus. Systematic review and meta-analysis. (*Arch Intern Med.* 2012; **172**(17):1296–303; doi:10.1001/archinternmed.2012.3147).

Position Statement of the ADA and European Association for the Study of Diabetes (EASD) Management of hyperglycemia in Type 2 diabetes: a Patient-centred approach. (*Diab Care* 2012; **35**:1364–79; doi: 10.2337/dc12-0413) (update in press).

UK National Bariatric Surgical Registry first national report to March 2010. ♒ <http://nbsr.e-dendrite.com>.

References

ABCD	*N Engl Med* 1998; **338**:645–52 doi: 10.1056/NEJM199803053381003
ACCORD	*N Eng J Med* 2008;**358**:2545–59 doi: 10.1056/NEJMoa0802743 *N Eng J Med* 2010;**363**:233–44 doi: 10.1056/NEJMoa1001288 *Lancet* 2010;**376**:419–30 doi: 10.1016/S0140-6736(10)60576-4 *Diabetes Care* 2010;**33**:983–90 doi: 10.2337/dc09-1278
ACCORD/ ADVANCE/VADT	*Diabetes Care* 2009;**32**:187–92 doi: 10.2337/dc08-9026
ADVANCE	*N Engl J Med* 2008; **358**; 2560–72 doi: 10.1056/NEJMoa0802987 *Lancet 2007*; **370**: 829–40 doi:10.1016/S0140-6736(07)61303-8 *Diabetologia* 2012:**55**:636–643 doi: 10.1007/s00125-011-2404-1
AFCAPS/TexCAPS	*JAMA* 1998; **279**:1615–22
ALLHAT	*JAMA* 2002; **288**:2981–97 doi:10.1001/jama.288.23.2981
ASCOT	*Lancet* 2005; **366**:895–906 doi:10.1016/S0140-6736(05)67185-1
BENEDICT	*N Engl J Med* 2004; **351**:1941–51 doi: 10.1056/NEJMoa042167
Canadian Task Force on Preventive Health Care	*Can Med Assoc J* 1999; **160**:513–25
CARDS	*Lancet* 2004; **364**:685–96 doi:10.1016/S0140-6736(04)16895-5
CARE	*N Engl J Med* 1996: **335**:1001–9 doi: 10.1056/NEJM199610033351401
CTT	*Lancet* 2008; **371**:117–25 doi:10.1016/S0140-6736(08)60104-X *Lancet. 2010*;**376** :1670–81 doi: 10.1016/S0140-6736(10)61350-5

DAIS	*Lancet* 2001; **357**:905–10 doi:10.1016/S0140-6736(00)04209-4
DCCT	*N Engl J Med* 1993, **329**:977–86 doi: 10.1056/NEJM200002103420603 *Am J Cardiol* 1995; **75**:894–903 *JAMA* 1996; **276**:1409–15 doi:10.1001/jama.1996.03540170053032 *N Engl J Med* 2000; **342**:381–9 doi: 10.1056/NEJM200002103420603
DCCT/EDIC	*N Engl J Med* 2005; **353**:2643–53 doi: 10.1056/NEJMoa052187 *Diabetes Care* 2006; **29**:340–44 doi:10.2337/diacare.29.02.06.dc05-1549
FACET	*Diabetes Care* 1998; **21**:597–603 doi:10.2337/diacare.21.4.597
FIELD	*Diabetes Care* 2009 **32**:493–98 doi:10.2337/dc08-1543
Helsinki	*Diabetes Care* 1992; **15**:820–5 doi:10.2337/diacare.15.7.820
HOPE/MICRO-HOPE	*Lancet* 2000; **355**:253–9 doi:10.1016/S0140-6736(99)12323-7
HOT	*Lancet* 1998; **351**:1755–62 doi:10.1016/S0140-6736(98)04311-6
HPS	*Lancet* 2003; **361**:2005–16 doi:10.1016/S0140-6736(03)13636-7
IDNT	*N Engl J Med* 2001; **345**:851–60 doi: 10.1056/NEJMoa011303
IRMA-2	*N Engl J Med* 2001; **345**: 870–8 doi: 10.1056/NEJMoa011489
JBS3	*Heart* 2014;**100**:ii1–ii67. doi:10.1136/heartjnl-2014-305693
LIPID	*N Engl J Med* 1998; 339:1349–57 doi: 10.1056/NEJM199811053391902
LIFE	*Lancet* 2002; **359**:995–1003 doi:10.1016/S0140-6736(02)08089-3 *Lancet* 2002; **359**:1004–10 doi:10.1016/S0140-6736(02)08090-X *Hypertension* 2004; **22**:1805–11
MARVAL	*Circulation* 2002; **106**:672–8 doi: 10.1161/01.CIR.0000024416.33113.0A
NICE	℅ <http://www.nice.org.uk> CG15 (2004) CG66 (2008) and 87 (2009)
ONTARGET	*N Engl J Med* 2008; **358**:1547-59 doi: 10.1056/NEJMoa0801317
RENAAL	*N Engl J Med* 2001; **345**:861–9 doi: 10.1056/NEJMoa011161
SENDCAP	*Diabetes Care* 1998; **21**:641–8 doi:10.2337/diacare.21.4.641
4S	*Diabetes Care* 1997; **20**:614–20 doi:10.2337/diacare.20.4.614
Syst–EUR	*Arch Int Med*;1998; **158**:1681–91
UKPDS	℅ <http://www.dtu.ox.ac.uk/index.php?maindoc=/ukpds/> UKPDS 33 *Lancet* 1998; **352**:837–53 doi:10.1016/S0140-6736(98)07019-6

UKPDS 34 *Lancet* 1998; **352**:854–65
doi:10.1016/S0140-6736(98)07037-8
UKPDS 38. *BMJ* 1998; **317**:703–13
UKPDS 39 *BMJ* 1998; **317**:713–20
UKPDS 41 *BMJ* 2000; **320**:1373–8
doi: http://dx.doi.org/10.1136/bmj.320.7246.1373
UKPDS 80 *N Eng J Med* 2008; **359**:1577–89
doi: 10.1056/NEJMoa0806470

VADT   *N Eng J Med* 2009; **360**:129–39
doi: 10.1056/NEJMoa0808431
Diabetes 2009; **58**:2642–8
doi:10.2337/db09-0618
J Diabetes Complications 2011; **25**:355–61
doi:10.1016/j.jdiacomp.2011.10.003

For more papers, see:
🐾 <http://www.diabetespublications.co.uk/study.html>

Diabetes education

Essential to survival

Diabetes information and education are essential to patient survival. It is the person who has the condition who determines his or her own outcome. The patient needs to know*:

- What is diabetes
- How may it affect you (your health, family, work, leisure)
- How the relevant body systems work
- Healthy eating
- Health exercise
- What treatment to take, how, and when, with hazard warnings
- How to adjust treatment and things that could affect glucose
- Self-monitoring of blood glucose by finger-prick (SMBG)—if appropriate—how, when, and why, and what to do about results
- Carry diabetic card and glucose if taking drugs that may cause hypoglycaemia
- About free prescriptions (UK)
- Where and how to get supplies of medication or equipment
- Complications of the diabetes
- How to stay well (reduce risk factors, spot potential problems)
- How to avoid problems
- How to manage problems if they occur
- How to include all the above in everyday life in a practical, acceptable way
- Need for annual review and eye photograph (free)
- What the annual review should include
- How to revise and learn more
- Name of place where future diabetes care will occur
- Names of healthcare professionals who will deliver diabetes care and their roles (update as required)
- ⚠ When to seek help with phone numbers 24/7

*Adapted from the Hillingdon Consensus Care Guidelines 2001.

It is particularly important to equip patients with the knowledge to work things out for themselves. Problems may arise which require a logical extension of the instructions given by the doctor or nurse. The situation may deteriorate and the patient has to know when to seek help, and how urgently. N.B. Very low or very high blood glucose levels impair thinking.

The two stages are information and education for self-care (diabetes self-management education (DSME)).

Factors influencing learning

- Emotions: how the patient feels on the day
- Motivation
- Circumstances of teaching session
- Support from family or friends sharing learning
- Personal experiences of diabetes (e.g. diabetes in a relative or friend, past gestational diabetes)
- Media portrayal of diabetes (TV, newspapers, Internet—entering 'diabetes' into Google™ produced > 400 million results)
- Personal health beliefs
- Influences of family and friends (supportiveness or attitudes)
- Anxiety
- Attitudes to health professionals
- Age
- Educational background and abilities
- Reading abilities (if leaflets, etc. used)
- Visual or hearing loss
- Memory problems
- Social factors
- Cultural and religious factors
- Ethnic and language factors—are healthcare staff and patient both using the same language in the same way?

N.B. People with diabetes are more likely than the general population to have visual or hearing problems, memory problems, learning disability, anxiety, and depression.

Agendas

The patient's agenda

'Teach me what I want to know, when I want to know it.' Start with this. People won't take in what they are being told until their concerns have been addressed. No question is ever stupid if it has to be a question. The patient will not have a tidy checklist in his/her head. The heart will be pounding and the head will be whirling with confused thoughts and anxieties.

The teacher's agenda

The standard lesson must be tailored to individual need. Patients see many members of the multidisciplinary diabetes team, in both primary and secondary care, as well as other healthcare professionals not specializing in diabetes care. Train staff involved in treating diabetic patients elsewhere. Ensure consistency of information.

A woman stumbled into a diabetic clinic in tears having been informed by a midwife that she had miscarried because she was injecting her insulin into the subcutaneous tissue of her abdomen. Even people who should have good understanding of human physiology and anatomy may harbour gross misconceptions.

Some patient anxieties

- Is it serious? Am I going to die? 'Die–abetes'!
- Why me?
- Will I get better?
- Am I going to lose my legs like that man in the waiting room?
- Will I go blind?
- Will I lose my job?
- Am I going to lose my driving licence?
- Will I lose my boyfriend?
- What are you going to do to me now?
- Will I need to have injections?
- Will it hurt?
- Will people think I'm a junkie? Will I get addicted to insulin?
- Will I embarrass myself?
- Will I go into a coma?
- Can I eat chocolate?
- Can I go out for a meal?
- Do I have to buy special food?
- Will I have to use complicated machines?
- Something awful will go wrong if I don't do it properly!

'What is diabetes?' may be a long way down the patient's list. Once the shock of diagnosis is over, other questions relating to living with diabetes emerge—what exactly the diagnosis means, what diet and other treatment are needed, how to use the appropriate technology (e.g. finger-prick blood glucose testing, needles, syringes), self-care, the prevention of short- and long-term complications, and how to manage diabetes under different circumstances. Practicalities such as where to get supplies of medication and equipment, clinic/surgery arrangements, and whom to call for help also need to be covered.

'We can't afford a formal programme'

Structured diabetes education programmes (➜ p. 63) have been demonstrated to improve some outcomes, and the concept is supported by NICE. However, such programmes may be expensive in terms of finance and/ or staff resource, despite proven long-term savings. The next section provides some practical suggestions for practices and clinics but is not a formal evidence-based programme.

What patients should know

Three-stage programme
- Newly diagnosed—a survival kit (Table 4.1)
- Main body of knowledge—the full package
- Revision and update

The details of each of these three stages are covered in subsequent chapters. Extend the patient's knowledge in several sessions. Most importantly, in each session give the patient time to talk. Listen a lot, and answer the patient's questions. Until you have done this the patient may not listen to the information you wish to pass on.

Table 4.1 The survival kit: vital points to be discussed following diagnosis

The diagnosis	Diabetes:
	is long term but controllable
	has symptoms that will be relieved rapidly
	is not catching
	is not immediately fatal!
Diet	Know what and how much to eat—in simple terms
Treatment	Medication if needed; if injectable, know the basic technology
	Hazard warnings
	Free prescriptions for those on tablets or insulin
Monitoring	SMBG if on drugs that can cause hypoglycaemia
Carry	Diabetes card, and glucose everywhere (unless diet alone)
Drivers	If a driver, tell DVLA and motor insurance company immediately if rules require
Implications	Immediate implications for work, family, or leisure activities
Contact	Provide details of whom to contact for help
Concerns	Any questions or concerns
Appointments	With whom, where, when. Contact details

Full package
- What is happening in your body
  - Causes of diabetes
  - Why this person has diabetes (if known)
  - How the pancreas works
  - Basic biochemistry of glucose, insulin, and fat
- The implications of diabetes

- Food and drink
  - What happens to the food you eat
  - What to eat; how much to eat
  - CHO counting and glycaemic index, as appropriate
  - Give more detailed personalized dietary information
  - Achieving and maintaining desirable weight
  - Alcohol
- Exercise
  - Personalized targets
  - Forms of exercise
  - Glucose control and treatment adjustment
  - Safety (hypoglycaemia, issues around tissue damage)
- Treatment
  - Tablets for glucose control: their name(s), what is the dose, how to take them, how they work, side effects, self-adjustment, what to do if you miss a dose, how to get supplies. Other tablets—same details.
  - Insulin: the name(s), what is the dose, how to inject (ask patient to demonstrate), how insulins work, how injection devices work (ask patient to demonstrate), side effects, injection site problems, self-adjustment, what to do if you miss a dose, how to get supplies, help-lines.
  - Injectable incretin-effect enhancers as for insulin
- Finger-prick blood glucose testing
  - How to do it, lancets, finger-pricking devices, strips, meter; how it all works; what to do if it goes wrong
  - Personalized glucose targets
  - Controlling the blood glucose—what to do if it is too low or too high
  - Glucose emergencies—hypoglycaemia, diabetic ketoacidosis
  - Use of more sophisticated monitoring techniques as required
- Can the patient produce his or her diabetic card and emergency glucose?
- Sick-day rules
- Preventive care
  - Blood pressure—personal target, treatment if appropriate
  - Cholesterol—personal target, treatment if appropriate
  - Glucose and HbA_{1c} personal targets
  - Microalbuminuria
  - Tests—what tests are for and what the results mean
  - Personal hygiene
  - Dental care
  - Immunizations—influenza annually, pneumococcus once, tetanus every 10 yrs if doing finger pricks, hepatitis B course.
- Annual review
  - Weight, abdominal circumference
  - Height until fully grown
  - HbA_{1c}
  - Eye check with digital eye photography in a screening programme
  - Foot check, including skin, shape, pulses, sensation

- Blood pressure
- Kidneys: eGFR, microalbumin-to-creatinine ratio (ACR)
- Cholesterol and triglyceride
- Thyroid function in type 1 diabetes
- Coeliac test once if type 1 diabetes < 20 yrs old
- Diabetic complications
  - Eyes
  - Kidneys
  - Nerves
  - Feet
  - Heart
  - Circulation
  - Stroke
  - Skin
  - Dental
- Driving
  - Personal, work-related (LGV, PCV)
  - Confirm licensing agency (e.g. DVLA) and insurance company have been told.
  - Safety—hypoglycaemia avoidance; problems from tissue damage; e.g. cannot feel pedals if severe neuropathy
- Work
  - Telling employers and colleagues
  - Safety issues
  - Legal issues
  - Practical issues, e.g. shift work, ability to access food, privacy for injections if desired
- Family
  - Avoiding pregnancy
  - Planning pregnancy—preconception, antenatal care, post-partum care
  - Inheritance of diabetes
  - Sexual dysfunction
- Leisure
  - Practical issues—sports, hobbies
  - Glucose balance and treatment adjustment
  - Safety (hypoglycaemia, issues around tissue damage)
  - Travel
- Smoking—don't
- Street drugs—don't
- Who's who in the diabetes system—primary, community, and secondary care. How the diabetes system works in your district. How to make the best use of this resource
- How to get help—urgent, non-urgent. Where and how to get supplies
- Local and national self-help or support groups
- Useful websites
- How to get help/advice locally
- The next meeting

Revision and update

Skills and knowledge decline rapidly after training, especially if unused. They need updating regularly, perhaps every 6 months. Even the most experienced patient (or diabetes care professional) should have their insulin administration and blood glucose monitoring techniques checked regularly. Information gaps occur. One may discover people who have not told the DVLA about their insulin-treated diabetes, many years after diagnosis. And why is their diabetes card and glucose always in the other coat? Misconceptions may persist. Patients and relatives (or friends) may need updating too.

Jo, an intelligent young woman with insulin-treated diabetes, was recorded as injecting fast-acting Actrapid® three times a day and long-acting Ultratard® (now unavailable) at night. Her blood glucose diary showed gross glucose fluctuations. After several years a doctor discovered that she was taking both Actrapid® and Ultratard® three times a day.

Mavis was losing weight. She often showed urinary ketones. 'My friend's grandfather was diabetic. She said I should never touch starch. Fatal, you see, for a diabetic. Makes sugar. So I'm always very strict. No bread, no biscuits, no potato ever.'

John was admitted to hospital with severe hypoglycaemia. He had collapsed from hypoglycaemia. His neighbour, an ardent first aider, rushed in and diagnosed a 'diabetic coma'. Surrounded by admiring relatives, he injected a large amount of insulin into John's leg.

Speak with one voice

Patients become confused if different staff members provide contradictory advice. The diabetes team should get together and agree a consistent approach to all aspects of diabetes education. This consistency should extend to everyone involved in patient care—GPs, hospital staff, school teachers. Use the national consensus where possible.

Coordinating diabetes education

The best person to coordinate diabetes education is the diabetes specialist nurse. Every person with diabetes should have access to a nurse with this special training. A chart in the patient's record, preferably the one the patient holds, can be used to check off items and name who has taught them.

Every team member should be able to provide basic diabetes advice—the podiatrist should know about healthy eating, and the dietitian about good foot care. The podiatrist can ask how the blood glucose control is going.

Diabetes education programmes

Studies of diabetes education have shown reduction in HbA_{1c} in the intervention groups in type 1 and type 2 diabetes, but have not been large or long enough to show that education alone produces major differences in patient outcomes in the long term. However, NICE (TA60, April 2003), stated that 'the Committee was convinced of the importance of patient education in improving glycaemic control and quality of life, while reducing the rate of complications associated with diabetes . . . all individuals with diabetes should be offered structured patient education at the time of diagnosis and ongoing patient education as required based on a formal, regular assessment of need, recognising that needs change over time.' The appraisal advised the following.

- The use of established principles of adult education
- A multidisciplinary approach, with teams including—as a minimum—a diabetes specialist nurse (or a practice nurse with experience in diabetes) and a dietitian, with appropriate training provided to educators
- Use of group education sessions
- Provision of educational opportunities that are accessible to the broadest range of people, taking into account culture, ethnicity, disability, and geographical issues
- Educational programmes based on a variety of learning techniques, adapted to meet varying needs, and integrated into routine diabetes care over the longer term

Structured patient education in diabetes

See ℘ <http://www.dh.gov.uk/en/Publicationsandstatistics/Publications/PublicationsPolicyAndGuidance/DH_4113195>
- Use a structured education programme
- Use trained educators
- Be quality assured
- Be audited

DAFNE (Dose Adjustment for Normal Eating): Type 1

Dr Michael Berger developed this programme which teaches patients to adjust their insulin to ordinary eating habits. It does not advocate unhealthy eating. Published benefits include improved glycaemic balance and quality of life. Participants report greater enjoyment of food and flexibility. Participants should have had diabetes for at least six months, be on multiple insulin injections daily, and be prepared to adjust their insulin according to multiple finger-prick glucose tests daily. Eight self-selected participants attend a five-day course taught by the multidisciplinary team. One year after completing a DAFNE course, 939 attendees were reviewed. Diabetic ketoacidosis (DKA) was reduced from 0.07 to 0.03 epsodes/patient/year. Emergency treatments for DKA and severe hypoglycaemia were reduced with costs falling from £119,470 to £42,948. (*Diab Med* 2014; **31**:847–53; doi:10.1111/dme.12441). ℘ <http://www.dafne.uk.com>

DESMOND (Diabetes Education and Self-Management for On-going and Newly Diagnosed): Type 2

DESMOND assesses educational and psychological factors, and then provides structured education for groups of patients with type 2 diabetes. Participants showed improvements in weight loss, smoking cessation, and beliefs about illness, but not in HbA_{1c} compared with non-participants (Br Med J 2008; **336**:491; http://dx.doi.org/10.1136/bmj.39474.922025). See ℘ <http://www.desmond-project.org.uk/>

X-pert (Expert Patient Education): Type 1 and Type 2

This is a structured education programme for patients that meets NICE criteria. An audit of 35,123 participants in 4314 X-pert programmes followed for 2 years showed a fall of HbA_{1c} from 61 to 54.6 mmol/mol (7.7 to 7.1 %); fall in weight from 89.8 to 88.6 kg; total cholesterol 4.5 to 4.1 mmol/l; LDL cholesterol from 2.5 to 2.2 mmol/l; diastolic BP from 77.5 to 75 mm Hg. See ℘ <http://www.xperthealth.org.uk/>

EPP (Expert Patients Programme) Chronic disease

The Expert Patients Programme (EPP) is an NHS-based training programme that provides opportunities to people who live with long-term chronic conditions to develop new skills to manage their condition better on a day-to-day basis. Patients attend sessions run by a trainer, looking at different aspects of personal health and well-being, and working with healthcare professionals. Patients reported more self-confidence and control in managing their condition(s) and their lives, healthier eating, and fewer visits to doctors. Most courses are not designed to make a patient an expert in a particular condition. See ℘ <http://www.expertpatients.co.uk/>

Local diabetes education programme

Check what is available locally. The local clinical commissioning group (CCG), community diabetes service, Diabetes Centre, diabetologists, and hospital diabetes service may provide an education programme for people with diabetes in your area.

Care planning

Work with the patient to agree his or her plan of care for the year. The education programmes will help, and care plan training is being developed (for patients and professionals). Patient support organizations can help inform people with diabetes about options. The Year of Care Diabetes project found that:

- People with diabetes report improved experience of care and real changes in self-care behaviour.
- Professionals report improved knowledge and skills, and greater job satisfaction.
- Practices report better organization and team work.
- Productivity is improved: care planning is cost-neutral at practice level: there are savings for some.
- Care planning takes time to embed: changes in clinical indicators across populations may be seen after two or three care planning cycles.

See ℘ <http://www.diabetes.org.uk/Professionals/Service-improvement/Year-of-Care/>.

Patient support

Patient support groups

Patients gain much from mutual support, but remember that it is often those most severely affected by a condition who attend meetings most often, and this can frighten new and less-affected members. Most areas have local patient support groups and everyone with diabetes can access the national organization Diabetes UK.

Diabetes UK

This is the main UK source of trusted patient information. It provides support and education for people with diabetes and health care professionals. It was one of the first patient self-help organizations in the world and was founded by a person with diabetes and a doctor specializing in the condition. Diabetes UK provides a wide range of educational resources and patient leaflets in a variety of languages. This includes their fifteen care essentials; see ✍ <http://www.diabetes.org.uk/15-essentials>. There is a website for patients and professionals: ✍ <http://www.diabetes.org.uk>. There are local branches of Diabetes UK in most districts.

Diabetes UK's careline provides information and support for those with diabetes, but it does not offer individual medical advice. Interpreters can be located so that non-English speakers can be helped. Telephone: 0345 123 2399

✍ <http://www.diabetes.org.uk/How_we_help/Careline/>.

Pharmaceutical company helplines

NovoNordisk customer care helpline
Tel: 0845 600 5055 ✍ <novonordisk.co.uk>

Saofi-Aventis Diabetes careline
For people using Sanofi-Aventis insulin or devices.
Tel: 08000 352525 ✍ <https://www.diabetesmatters.co.uk/>

Eli Lilly Diabetes Careline
For people using Eli Lilly insulin pens
Tel: 0800 783 6764
✍ <https://www.lillypro.co.uk/diabetes/patients>

Summary

- Diabetes education is essential to the patient's healthy survival.
- Many factors influence whether the patient absorbs what you think you have taught, and whether he or she applies what has been learnt appropriately or indeed at all.
- Help people with diabetes to understand what diabetes is and how it may affect him or her.
- Regard patient education as part of care (like measuring blood pressure).
- Regard care planning as part of care.
- The professionals must provide the patient with the knowledge and the tools to monitor his or her condition and to adjust treatment.
- Knowledge should be provided as and when the patient wants it, tailoring the professionals' agenda to the patient's individual needs.
- Knowledge should be consistent and teaching should be professional.
- Use the three-stage programme: the starter kit, the full package, and the revision and update sessions.
- Speak with one voice.
- Provide frequent revision sessions and support whenever it is required.
- Assess learning needs formally and use a structured education programme, developed either nationally or locally (see NICE guidelines).
- Structured education has proven benefits for patients and is cost-effective.
- Use the existing literature and professional support.
- Tell all patients about Diabetes UK and other patient support groups.

Healthy eating and drinking (including management of obesity)

Aims of a healthy diabetic diet

The two parts of the diet are what you eat and how much. A healthy diet provides energy for daily activity and maintains the right body weight for height (Box 5.1). It is a lifelong eating plan. It is important that people continue to enjoy their food and that the treatment of their diabetes is adjusted to their usual eating pattern and not vice versa. New patients start enthusiastically and then lapse, so weight may fall and then rise again within a year.

> **Box 5.1 Aims of a healthy diabetic diet**
> - Physically healthy
> - Feeling well
> - Energy for life and exercise
> - Well-balanced diet
> - Good day-to-day glucose control
> - HbA_{1c} 48–58 mmol/mol (6.5–7.5 %) without hypoglycaemia (tailor to patient)
> - Total cholesterol < 4 mmol/l
> - LDL cholesterol < 2 mmol/l
> - Triglyceride < 2.3 mmol/l
> - BMI* 18.5–24.9 kg/m^2
> - Waist circumference
>   - < 102 cm in men (< 92 cm in Asian men)
>   - < 88 cm in women (< 78 cm in Asian women)
> - Alcohol in moderation if desired
> - Low salt
>
> *BMI unhelpful in very muscular people.
> BMI upper limit in Asian/African-Caribbean or Chinese people = 23 kg/m^2

Dietitian

Every patient should see a dietitian on diagnosis of diabetes and annually thereafter. The diabetic diet is an integral part of treatment and medical staff must ensure that patients realize this. Patients may wrongly assume that there is no need to worry about diet if they are taking their diabetes tablets or insulin. All those caring for people with diabetes should be aware of dietary requirements and be able to answer questions about food. Advise patients to keep a week's food diary (using your local format) to help their discussions with the dietitian.

Which diet is best for glucose control in people with diabetes?

We don't know. Everyone should eat a generally healthy diet as described and have the right amount of calories to reach or maintain a healthy weight. There have been many dietary studies in diabetes. A review of literature from 2001–10 found that whether the diet had very low, low, moderate, or high carbohydrates (CHO), high or low glycemic index (GI) CHO, or had high- or low-fibre content did not produce consistent results on blood glucose levels compared with the relevant control group. (*Diabetes Care* 2012; **35**:434–45; doi: 10.2337/dc11-2216).

What to eat

A healthy balanced daily diet

People without diabetes should eat this way too. People's needs vary, so each person should have a personalized eating plan.

- Include:
  - Starchy CHO foods such as bread, potato, pasta, rice, cereals spread throughout the day. These should be high in fibre and not cooked or dressed in fat.
  - Five to seven portions of fruit or vegetables per day (which can include pulses, beans, or fruit juice, but each only once a day).
  - Two small portions of meat, fish, or pulses for protein. Remove skin and fat, and do not cook or dress in fat.
  - Three portions of low-fat dairy foods: milk (skimmed/semi-skimmed), cheese (matchbox size), yoghurt (small pot).
  - Alcohol in moderation.
- Exclude:
  - Most sugar and fat. Use low-sugar or low-fat options.
- Calorie content of foods is:
  - Fat: 9 kcal/g
  - Protein: 4 kcal/g
  - CHO: 3.8 kcal/g
  - Alcohol: 7 kcal/g
- The standard unit is a kilocalorie. This is expressed as calorie throughout this book as this is common usage. Food also contains water, fibre, micronutrients (e.g. vitamins and minerals), and inedible waste such as pips or pith.

Consider using the Food Standards Agency Eatwell plate: see ℘ <http://food.gov.uk/multimedia/pdfs/theeatwellplate.pdf>.
The segments on the plate occupy:

- Bread, rice, potatoes, pasta, and other starchy foods: 33 %
- Fruit and vegetables: 33 %
- Milk and dairy foods: 15 %
- Meat, fish, eggs, beans & non-dairy sources of protein: 12 %
- Foods and drinks high in fat and/or sugar: 8 % (try to reduce this segment in people with diabetes)

18 yr olds need more calories a day (3000 for a man, 2500 for a woman) than 45 year olds (2500 man, 2100 woman). Pregnancy (last trimester) adds about 200 calories a day, lactation about 300.

Prepared foods are often highly calorific. Fat and sugar make food taste good and act as cheap bulking agents in manufactured prepared foods. Home cooking can also be calorific; a roast lunch may contain over 1000 calories.

Food labels

In packaged foods, ingredients are listed by weight, with the first one listed contributing the biggest proportion to that food by weight. Beware manufacturers' values (e.g. calories 'per portion') as the portions are often small. Values are also shown per 100 g (Table 5.1).

Table 5.1 Quantities in a complete meal or 100 g snack

Food	A little	A lot
Fat	≤ 5 g	≥ 20 g
Saturated fat	≤ 1 g	≥ 5 g
Sugars	≤ 5 g	≥ 10 g
Fibre	≤ 0.5 g	≥ 3 g
Sodium (1 g sodium ≈ 2.5 g salt)	≤ 0.1 g	≥ 0.5 g

With thanks to Pat Smith, Dietitian, The Hillingdon Hospital.

What should I eat?

Most patients are concerned about what they are supposed to eat. Some are prepared to look at their food in detail (see CHO counting), but many are not. The calculations in Table 5.1 are rarely necessary. Suggested stages of education are:

- Different types of food (CHO, protein, fat)
- The healthy plate or Eatwell plate
- Personal portion sizes (use food diary)
- Personal eating for health, work, exercise, leisure
- CHO counting (for those injecting insulin)
- Glycaemic index

Carbohydrates (CHOs)—starchy sugary foods

The old, rigid division into simple and complex CHOs is not always helpful as many foods and most meals combine more than one sort of CHO.

Sugars

These provide rapidly absorbed CHO. When eaten alone, glucose produces an abrupt rise in blood glucose concentration, starting in minutes and lasting about 2 hours. Normally this stimulates pancreatic insulin release to parallel the blood glucose rise. The insulin or subcutaneous insulin of a diabetic patient may not match the glucose rise. Analogue insulins are designed to mimic natural insulin release (➔ p. 151).

- Monosaccharides: glucose, galactose, fructose
- Disaccharides:
  - Sucrose (glucose + fructose) from sugar cane or beet
  - Lactose (glucose + galactose) from milk
  - Maltose (glucose + glucose) from fermenting grain

When sucrose is eaten as part of a meal, the blood glucose rise following that meal is similar to that of a meal of the same caloric value without sucrose. The fat and fibre content of the meal slow glucose absorption. Better compliance may be achieved if patients can have a sweet/pudding during the meal within their total calorie intake.

In insulin-treated patients exercising vigorously, liver glucose release may not keep up with glucose uptake by muscles. The blood glucose can fall precipitously if the patient does not top up with sugar or glucose (➔ pp. 239–40). Thus insulin-treated patients can use sugar-containing foods when exercising; athletes may find they have to do so. Regular exercise may eventually be fuelled mainly by unrefined CHOs.

Glucose or sucrose ('sugar') is essential in the treatment of hypoglycaemia (➔ pp. 188–93). Obvious? Not necessarily. If you tell the patient 'no sugar', he or she may obey you to the letter, fighting off all attempts to treat hypoglycaemia with sugar lumps. Lactose digestion will be slowed by fat in milk products. The fat in chocolate slows digestion/absorption of glucose, sucrose, and lactose. Patients on acarbose, a disaccharidase inhibitor, must use glucose to treat hypoglycaemia. They cannot break down sucrose. Granular sugar substitutes such as sucralose (Splenda®) will not resolve hypoglycaemia! Plain glucose (e.g. glucose tablets/drink) is the best treatment for hypoglycaemia (➔ p. 188).

Complex CHOs—starchy foods

Each patient will have his/her staples: bread, cereals, corn (maize), legumes (e.g. beans), pasta, potatoes, and rice are the most common. Many of these are made more palatable with fat: bread and butter, cornflakes and milk, pasta with sauce. Some people count beans as protein, but they contain more CHO.

Complex CHOs have to be digested into simple CHOs before absorption. The rate at which this happens varies (➲ p. 71, pp. 73–4).

Fibre

Insoluble fibre (e.g. in wheat bran, vegetables) bulks out food and make it filling. Examples are wholemeal bread, wholemeal pasta, brown rice, potatoes in their jackets, celery, and cabbage. Soluble fibre in beans and pulses slows digestion and absorption of CHO. People with diabetes should eat some beans, lentils, chick peas, or other pulse every day (Box 5.2).

More people are used to a high-fibre diet. A patient unfamiliar with this should introduce the new foods slowly to reduce abdominal griping and flatulence.

Box 5.2 Examples of fibre content

White bread	2 g fibre/100 g
Baked beans	6 g fibre/100 g
Wholewheat bread	7 g fibre/100 g
Bran cereal	43 g fibre/100 g

CHO portions and CHO counting

CHO counting (Box 5.3) was popular for many years, went out of fashion, and is now back, particularly for type 1 diabetes. For many it makes it easier to balance insulin doses with food. The huge range of CHO foods, portion sizes, and presentations available can make this daunting. Patients should start with learning to count the CHO foods they usually eat.

Many books on the subject are American, creating problems for British readers as portions are usually quoted in cups (1 UK cup = 1.25 American cups):

One cup = 16 tablespoons (levelled off for solid foods)
One tablespoon = 3 teaspoons (levelled off for solid foods).

Getting started

A dietitian should advise on the total daily calories needed to achieve and maintain a healthy weight for that person.

- Total daily diet 2000 kcal/day includes about 240–320 g CHO, 24–32 × 10 g portions
- Total daily diet 1000 kcal/day includes about 120–160 g CHO, 12–16 × 10 g portions

Box 5.3 Example of CHO counting

Chicken sandwich:

Two slices white bread	2×12 g
Butter	0
Piece of chicken	0
One medium tomato	5 g
One large banana	30 g
Total	about 60 g CHO
	6×10 g CHO portions

NB: this takes no account of calories or fibre.
Source: USDA database (➲ p. 86).

Different centres use different 'portions' or 'exchanges'. The latter are familiar to many patients with long-standing diabetes. A portion of 10 g CHO is simplest (e.g. small slice of bread, small apple). Packaged food lists CHO content. Patients can use personal observation and detailed records to calculate their insulin dose in units per 10 g CHO portion. Dietitians can provide 10 g CHO portion lists or 'exchanges'. Beware confusion as American books often quote 15 g portions, as do some UK centres.

For insulin dose, divide 500 by the total daily dose (TDD), i.e. the total of all the insulin injected in 24 hours. Thus, if the TDD is 50 units, 500/50 =10, so the insulin-to-CHO ratio is 1 unit insulin to 10 g CHO. For a total daily dose of 25 units of insulin, the insulin-to-CHO ratio would be 1:20 g (Box 9.1, ➲ p. 165). Many people use experience to work out their ratio.

Patients are often advised to subtract the amount of fibre in the food if over 5 g to achieve the final CHO count upon which they base their insulin dose.

Glycaemic index

The glycaemic index is calculated by performing multiple blood glucose tests on people who have eaten the test food on its own after fasting overnight. It compares the area under the blood glucose curve after eating a particular food with that after eating an equivalent amount of CHO as glucose. With this technique, an apple has a glycaemic index of 39 %, baked beans 40 %, brown rice 66 %, wholemeal bread 72 %, honey 87 %, and Lucozade® 98 %, some cooked potatoes 111 %. Glucose is 100 %.

The major problem with the use of the glycaemic index is that foods are rarely eaten on their own. These are some of the factors which alter the rate of CHO absorption.

- Other foods—fats and fibre slow absorption
- Liquids
- Alcohol
- Total quantity of food eaten
- Patient at rest or exercising
- Emotional factors
- Gastric status, e.g. gastroparesis from autonomic neuropathy
- Nausea or vomiting

- Intestinal status, e.g. malabsorption or diarrhoea
- Cardiovascular factors
- Drugs, e.g. acarbose, metformin

Information about using glycaemic index for patients can be found on ℘ <http://www.rbch.nhs.uk/bdec2/advice/diet/pdf/gi.pdf>

Confused?

So are patients. Few patients will be prepared to do the complete complex calculations. However, a practical working knowledge of the CHO of their usual foods and how fast it is likely to be absorbed can significantly improve their use of insulin and may help tablet-treated patients. The most useful figure is the CHO count, and seeing food as 10 g portions of CHO allows this to be factored into insulin dose calculations.

The CHO foods should be spread out over three meals a day, convenient for the patient. If they are taking insulin, a coffee-time and tea-time snack may be desirable, and a bed-time snack is usually essential. Insulin may be needed to cover snacks > 10 g CHO. Overweight patients not on insulin should avoid snacks.

Diabetes UK has guidance that may help:

℘ <http://www.diabetes.org.uk/Guide-to-diabetes/Managing-your-diabetes/Carb-counting/>

Fruit and vegetables

We should eat five to seven portions of fruit or vegetables a day. Fruit tastes sweet because it contains sucrose and fructose. The sweeter it tastes (e.g. grapes), the more refined is the CHO it contains. Fruit is an important source of vitamin C. Large amounts of fruit will elevate blood glucose and weight. One portion at a time is best.

Vegetables can be divided into two groups: those which can be eaten in large amounts with little influence on weight or CHO, and those which have to be considered as an energy source. Leafy vegetables such as lettuce and cabbage, big watery containers of small seeds like cucumbers and courgettes, and swollen stalks such as celery can be eaten with impunity. Green leafy vegetables are particularly good. Starchy root vegetables, such as potatoes, and big seeds (e.g. beans, peas, lentils, and other pulses) contain a lot of CHO to fuel the growing plant after germination. All starchy root vegetables and big seeds need to be considered in the CHO total. Potatoes are not included in the 'five-a-day' totals. Nuts contain a lot of fat, absorption of which varies markedly with chewing.

Fats—greasy oily foods

All fats are fattening! Reduce fat intake. No more than about a third of dietary calories should come from fat. This is a tiny amount of visible fat because so much is concealed in other foods, especially manufactured foods. Fat makes food taste good and few people realize how calorific it is. The pat of butter may contain as many calories as the slice of bread on which it is spread.

Avoid visible fat. Spread butter thinly; better still, use a poly-unsaturated low-fat spread or go without. Eat lower-fat meats such as skinned chicken or turkey. Avoid hard cheese, cream cheeses, and lard or dripping. Avoid cream and use semi-skimmed or skimmed milk. Avoid fried foods. Do not use oil-based salad dressings.

Hidden fat can be avoided by self-catering. Do not add fat to cooking unless essential—use low-fat cookery books. Advise patients to read the label on ready-made meals. Warn that 'reduced-fat foods' may still be high in fat (and sugar)—e.g. half the calories in lower-fat crisps still come from fat. Meat products (sausages, salami, pork pies, beef burgers) are very high in fat.

Fat slows gastric emptying and hence food absorption.

Saturated, mono-unsaturated, poly-unsaturated, and transfats

- *Saturated* fats are usually found in animal-derived products and increase LDL cholesterol. Intake should be reduced. They are found in dairy and animal fats (e.g. cheese, cream, fat on meat).
- *Mono-unsaturated fats* (e.g. rapeseed oil, olive oil, avocado oil) and poly-unsaturated fats (e.g. sunflower oil, fish oils) have less effect on LDL cholesterol and may enhance HDL. The omega-3 fatty acids found in herring, mackerel, wild salmon, and sardines appear to be cardio-protective. Mono- and poly-unsaturated fats should form a greater proportion of the total fat intake (but should still be limited in weight-reducing diets).
- *Transfats* are found naturally, mainly in animal-derived products. Most are manufactured by hydrogenating vegetable oils to prolong shelf-life and flavour of foods. Many such products become solid at room temperature. Transfats are found in margarines and butter-substitute spreads, dressings, snack foods, biscuits, and some cooking fats. Transfats raise LDL cholesterol, and contain the same amount of calories as other fats. Most are eaten in manufactured biscuits and snacks. Transfat intake should be minimized.

Plant stanols or sterols

Products (e.g. spreads) fortified with plant stanols or sterols (2-3 g/day) reduce cholesterol (*Diabetes Res Clin Prac* 2009;**84**:e33-7; doi: 10.1016/j. diabres.2009.01.015).

Protein

Many proteins are closely associated with fat. Skinned white meat, fish, and vegetable protein (e.g. soya or pulses), some low-fat cheese, and one or two eggs a week, should be the main protein source. Red meat should be lean and grilled or casseroled rather than roasted or fried; eat one or two portions a week.

Salt

Sodium chloride is linked with hypertension and may worsen fluid retention in oedematous patients. Do not add salt at table and use it sparingly in cooking (unless exercising in hot weather or participating in endurance sports). Avoid too many manufactured foods as these tend to be higher in salt.

Vitamin D

People with diabetes are more likely to be vitamin D-deficient than the general population, even allowing for ethnicity (*Arch Int Med* 2007; **167**:1159–65; doi:10.1001/archinte.167.11.1159). All pregnant or breastfeeding women, and children aged < 5 years should routinely receive vitamin D supplementation of 10 micrograms/day, as should > 65 year olds who do not have regular sun exposure. Others at risk of vitamin D deficiency are darker skinned people and those who avoid sunlight or cover up out-of-doors. Supplement vitamin D in those with low levels. Ensure adequate calcium intake—usual in UK unless avoiding dairy foods. See:

℘ <http://www.gov.uk/government/publications/vitamin-d-advice-on-supplements-for-at-risk-groups> and ℘ <http://www.nos.org.uk/document.doc?id=1352>.

Haematinics—iron, folate, and vitamin B12

About one in five people with diabetes have anaemia (*Diabet Med* 2010; **27**:655–9; doi: 10.1111/j.1464-5491.2010.02987.x). Diabetic kidney disease accounts for some of the anaemia, and may require erythropoietin injections. However, haematinic deficiencies are common. Older people and vegetarians are likely to be iron-deficient. Encourage red meat (one or two portions weekly) or iron supplements if preferred.

Folic acid is found in green leafy vegetables and is added to some cereals and other foods. This is insufficient for pregnancy and diabetic women planning conception should take 5 mg folic acid daily.

One in five patients with type 2 diabetes is vitamin B12-deficient, especially if they are taking metformin (➽ pp. 120–2). Metformin appears to block calcium-dependent absorption in the ileum and can be reversed by calcium supplementation (*Diabetes Care* 2000; **23**:1227–231; doi:10.2337/diacare.23.9.1227). Pernicious anaemia is 3–5 times commoner in people with type 1 diabetes than the general population. Autoimmune B12 lack requires replacement by injection. Other people should ensure adequate dietary intake e.g. from meat. Vegans need B12 supplements.

B12 or folate lack can cause neuropathy and dementia.

Drinks

Aim for 6–8 cups of fluid a day. Tea and coffee may contain full-fat milk, cream, and sugar. Therefore 6–8 cups of tea a day can include a pint of milk and a lot of sugar. A coffee-shop 'tall latte' can include 200 calories. Introduce semi-skimmed milk and artificial sweeteners such as aspartame. Better still, use skimmed milk and no sweetener, or no milk.

Aerated 'diet' drinks containing artificial sweeteners can be drunk in moderation. Care is needed in reading the labels of some products marked 'sugar-free' which may contain other refined CHOs, e.g. glucose.

Fruit juices may contain a lot of sugars. Read the label. Fruit smoothies should be pure fruit. They will also contain some sucrose and will produce a rapid glucose rise as they are easily absorbed. Vegetable juices could be substituted. Other savoury drinks, such as Bovril, can be very salty and should be drunk only occasionally.

Alcohol

Moderation in all things. The recommended amount is 1–2 units a day—up to 14 units/wk for women and 21 units/wk for men. A unit is half a pint of beer, lager, or cider, a single pub measure of spirits, or a glass of wine. Alcohol is highly calorific, ranging from 285 kcal/unit for sweet cider to 50 kcal/unit for spirits.

Confusion is generated by the CHO content of alcoholic drinks. Very sweet drinks should be avoided, but otherwise there is no benefit in using low-CHO products as the CHO has been turned to alcohol by further brewing. The total calorie content should be considered if the patient needs to lose weight, but it is better to ignore the CHO contribution of alcoholic drinks.

Alcohol impedes glucose release from liver glycogen stores and may precipitate or worsen hypoglycaemia. It also reduces the growth hormone rise stimulated by hypoglycaemia and therefore lengthens the glucose recovery. People with diabetes should not drink alcohol on an empty stomach. A packet of crisps or preferably another lower-fat snack, if available, should be consumed if alcohol is drunk outside mealtimes.

Modified products—'Diabetic foods' and sweeteners

'Diabetic foods'

These are sweets, biscuits, and cakes in which glucose and sucrose have been replaced by fructose or sorbitol. There is no evidence that fructose is any better for diabetics than sucrose, and it may be metabolically worse. Sorbitol, the other commonly used sweetener, causes abdominal griping and diarrhoea when consumed in large amounts. It is a polyol compound and, although CHO is not absorbed to the same extent, 15 g of sorbitol should be counted as about 7 g of absorbable CHO. Many of these products contain fat and are highly calorific. Discourage patients from buying them.

Sweeteners

These include Aspartame (Nutrasweet®), saccharin, acesulfame potassium (acesulfame K), cyclamates, and sucralose. Stevia leaf extract or rebaudioside A—Truvia®) is a recent addition. There has been concern that aspartame may have adverse effects. The European Food Safety Authority has said that it is safe. The US Food and Drug Administration (FDA) states '[t]o date, FDA has not determined any consistent pattern of symptoms that can be attributed to the use of aspartame, nor is the agency aware of any recent studies that clearly show safety problems'.

Vary artificial sweeteners so that none is used in excess of advised daily intake.

How much to eat

Eat as much as is necessary to reach and maintain normal weight and fuel current physical activity:

calories in = calories out—weight stays the same.

calories in > Calories out—weight gain

calories in < Calories out—weight loss

Obesity and weight reduction

Obesity is common across the Western World. The Health Survey for England 2011 found that 89 % of men, and 84 % of women were either overweight or obese. Many patients with type 2 diabetes are obese. It is easy to gain weight and hard to lose it. Treat the patient with courtesy and respect. Listen to his or her story (Box 5.4).

Different methods of calorie restriction suit different people. Some prefer general restriction, others low fat, or low CHO, others meal replacements (e.g. with shakes or bars for some meals, others very low calorie diets (expert supervision essential). Once weight loss has been achieved the main problem is sustaining the new, lower BMI. Most patients regain weight.

Recognize patients' difficulties in finding the willpower to lose weight, and their need to have the occasional forbidden food. Discuss the overall goal but set a reasonable interim goal in agreement with the patient. Aim for a loss of 0.5–1 kg per week (1–2 lb per week). Praise success, however slight. Success breeds success. Note difficulties reaching the goal. Encourage further efforts. Group support may help as may paying for support, as in Weight Watchers. Enlisting a family member to watch the diet and give encouragement may help for some people.

Ask the patient to monitor his or her own progress. Advise weekly weigh-ins, preferably by someone else, at the same time of day and in the same clothes, with the result written on a graph.

There is no easy formula to help people lose weight—the one constant factor of most studies is that continued interest and support is helpful.

Box 5.4 Assessing an overweight patient
- Is the patient worried about his/her weight?
- Does he/she have any weight-related symptoms?
- Will losing weight help this particular patient?
- Is this a good time for him/her to try to lose weight?
- Willingness and motivation to change?
- What is the usual eating pattern? How does he/she use food?
- Conditions contributing to the obesity
- Medical problems
- Psychological factors
- Medication
- Non-drug treatments
- Previous dietary efforts or weight-reducing treatments or surgery
- Family history, especially of obesity
- Lifestyle, exercise, work, and leisure
- Family and social aspects—e.g. support

Diet diary

Most people do not realize how much they eat (Box 5.5). A diet diary (underline the importance of honesty) for a week is helpful guide if the patient wishes to comply. Otherwise take a dietary history.

Modify the type of foods eaten

- Reduce fat
- Reduce alcohol
- Reduce manufactured foods and take-aways
- Increase green leafy vegetables; reduce solid starchy vegetables
- Increase large watery fruits or high-fibre crunchy fruits; reduce small sweet fruits or starchy fruits
- Avoid sauces or dressings unless low-calorie

Reduce the quantities eaten

Obese people often choose larger portions than slim people. Use a small spoon and a small plate. Eating out often presents larger portions. Ask for a smaller helping, or leave some. Eat more slowly so that the food lasts.

Box 5.5 Factors influencing food intake

- Hunger
- Appetite (not the same as hunger)
- Emotion
- Motivation
- Health beliefs
- Previous dietary advice/experience of dieting
- Cultural factors
- Family pressure: 'eat up, clean your plate'
- Outside pressure: friends, healthcare professionals, other 'advisers'
- Courtesy: don't want to upset the hostess
- Attractiveness or otherwise of food
- Exercise
- Ambient temperature
- Boredom
- Habit (popcorn in the cinema)
- Portion size (self-selected, served at home, served in restaurant, etc.)
- Comfort eating (distress or stress)
- A 'treat'—'naughty but nice'
- Alone or in company
- Because it's there
- To keep up with glucose-lowering treatment, e.g. insulin
- To treat a hypoglycaemic episode
- Drugs, e.g. insulin, steroids
- Hormonal conditions, e.g. Cushing's syndrome, polycystic ovary syndrome
- Intracranial and hypothalamic disorders
- Psychiatric illness

Slow down

Rapid eaters consume more than slower eaters and speedy eating is linked with obesity (*J Am Diet Assoc.* 2011; **111**:1192–7; doi: 10.1016/j. jada.2011.05.012).

When is the food eaten?

Eat at mealtimes and not in between. Enjoy the food. Avoid habit eating, e.g. while watching television, while driving (dangerous, illegal), while working at a desk, while serving behind the counter, while chatting. This food is chewed but not savoured. Substitute calorie-free chewing gum or a minimum calorie drink.

Why do people eat?

Overweight people need to eat very little to survive. Appetite can overcome satiety—we can be completely full of meat and vegetables but still fancy a piece of chocolate gateau. Food is a great comforter. It is an excuse for a social or family gathering. It is an expression of welcome, a thank-you present, a sign that you care, a religious symbol. It is sometimes used as a weapon, especially by children. Eating may simply be something to do with your hands. Find out why your patient is eating the foods he or she eats and suggest substitution of another activity or lower-calorie foods as appropriate.

Where is the food eaten and with whom?

Eating alone allows unwitnessed greed. Eating with a bad influence can encourage dietary sinning. No-one actually likes being good all the time. What food is available at work? Could a packed lunch be taken?

Home-cooked meals may prove difficult if the cook is not the person with diabetes and does not understand dietary requirements. Wives usually change their diet to suit their husband's diabetic diet. A husband rarely changes his diet if his wife has diabetes.

Binge eating and night eating ('midnight snacks') are commoner among obese people than those who are slim.

Read the label

Most foods now have detailed content and calorie lists. However, few packs weigh exactly 100 g. And what is a gram? Many British cooks still think in pounds and ounces: 100 g is 3.5 oz; 1 ounce is about 30 g.

Increase exercise

Advise at least 30 min of moderate intensity physical activity on at least 5 days a week (➲ pp. 233–43). Continue this regardless of weight lost. Any exercise is better than none—just walking round the garden, for example.

Avoid hypoglycaemia

As people exercise more and eat less, less glucose-lowering treatment will be needed. Warn patients of the risk of hypoglycaemia and take steps to avoid this, especially during or after exercise.

Weight-reducing drugs

NICE CG43 states that '[d]rug treatment should be considered for patients who have not reached their target weight loss or have reached a plateau on dietary, activity and behavioural changes alone'. Weight-reducing drugs should be prescribed only as part of a weight-reducing plan which includes psychological support, dietetic support for healthy eating, and exercise—and a plan for post-drug care. Do not prescribe more than one weight-reducing drug at a time.

The drugs available act either within the gastrointestinal tract or centrally. Those acting within the gut are orlistat and methylcellulose. The latter is a high-fibre bulking agent aimed to induce satiety and it is rarely used. Centrally acting drugs have been withdrawn because of adverse effects.

Orlistat

Mechanism of action of orlistat
Inhibition of lipase which reduces absorption of fat.

Beneficial effects of orlistat
Weight loss when used with a low-fat weight-reducing diet.

Indications for orlistat
Criterion for use in diabetic patients is a BMI of 28.0 kg/m^2.

Contraindications and cautions for orlistat
- Do not prescribe orlistat to patients who refuse to reduce their fat intake
- Chronic malabsorption (avoid)
- Cholestasis (avoid)
- Breastfeeding (avoid)
- Pregnancy (caution)
- Gastrointestinal problems or diarrhoea for any reason (caution)
- Known faecal continence problems or anal problems (caution)

Dosage of orlistat
- 120 mg orally immediately before, during, or up to 1 hour after each main meal (up to a maximum of 360 mg daily). Gradual increase advised.
- Therapy should be continued beyond 3 months only if the person has lost weight since starting drug treatment.

Side effects of orlistat
Gastrointestinal side effects are common and may lead the patient to stop taking orlistat. They are usually due to excessive fat intake. As the fat is not absorbed, it passes through the bowel causing oily diarrhoea and rectal leakage or incontinence. Specifically warn patients of this risk.
- Gastrointestinal: rectal oil leak, oily diarrhoea, faecal urgency, faecal incontinence, flatulence, abdominal distension, abdominal pain; rarely rectal bleeding; very rarely diverticulitis, cholelithiasis, hepatitis
- Impaired absorption of fat-soluble vitamins (if supplement needed take at least 2 hours after orlistat or at bed-time, whichever is the longest)
- Tooth and gum problems

- Respiratory and urinary tract infections
- Tiredness
- Anxiety
- Headache
- Menstrual problems
- Hypoglycaemia
- Very rarely, skin problems and blisters
- Withdrawal: weight may rise
- Renal impairment (avoid if severe)

Bariatric surgery

See (pp. 21, 42)

The IDF position statement 2011 states that: '[b]ariatric surgery is an appropriate treatment for people with type 2 diabetes and obesity not achieving recommended treatment targets with medical therapies, especially when there are other major co-morbidities. Surgery should be an accepted option in people who have type 2 diabetes and a BMI of 35 or more. Surgery should be considered as an alternative treatment option in patients with a BMI between 30 and 35 when diabetes cannot be adequately controlled by optimal medical regimen, especially in the presence of other major cardiovascular disease risk factors.'

NICE CG189 (2014) states:

'Bariatric surgery is a treatment option for people with obesity if all of the following criteria are fulfilled:

- They have a BMI of 40 kg/m^2 or more, or between 35 kg/m^2 and 40 kg/m^2 and other significant disease (for example, type 2 diabetes or high blood pressure) that could be improved if they lost weight.
- All appropriate non-surgical measures have been tried but the person has not achieved or maintained adequate, clinically beneficial weight loss.
- The person has been receiving or will receive intensive management in a tier 3* service.
- The person is generally fit for anaesthesia and surgery.
- The person commits to the need for long-term follow-up . . .

Bariatric surgery for people with recent-onset type 2 diabetes:

- Offer an expedited assessment for bariatric surgery to people with a BMI of 35 or over who have recent-onset type 2 diabetes as long as they are also receiving or will receive assessment in a tier 3 service (or equivalent).
- Consider an assessment for bariatric surgery for people with a BMI of 30–34.9 who have recent-onset type 2 diabetes as long as they are also receiving or will receive assessment in a tier 3 service (or equivalent).
- Consider an assessment for bariatric surgery for people of Asian family origin who have recent-onset type 2 diabetes at a lower BMI than other populations . . . as long as they are also receiving or will receive assessment in a tier 3 service (or equivalent).'

Many obese patients are not fit for surgery and/or have not shown commitment to long-term therapy.

---

* Tier 3 obesity service: a primary/community care based multi-disciplinary team to provide an intensive level of input to patients.

Different diets

Vegetarians often find a healthy diet easy. They may well be following it anyway. Vegans can obtain protein from vegetable sources (such as quorn, pulses, nuts) but may become deficient in vitamin B12, requiring replacement therapy. Lacto-vegetarians should use lower-fat dairy products. A Mediterranean diet reduces cardiovascular risk.

Be sensitive to religious dietary requirements (➔ pp. 375–7, 379–80). Limitations on meats are rarely a problem in working out the diabetic diet, but some traditional ways of cooking may use a lot of fat (e.g. ghee). Brown rice or wholemeal flour can be substituted for lower-fibre products (but remember that eating white rice may reflect higher status). Rural diets of peoples in South Asia and Africa are high in fibre and low in sugar, but urban diets in those countries or in emigrants to the West may not be. Unless the person who actually cooks the patient's food sees the dietitian or diabetes team it is unlikely that dietary advice will succeed (➔ p. 80).

Fast days or periods of denial occur in many religions, both Eastern and Western. Ramadan places particular demands on insulin-treated patients. Most religious leaders will exempt a diabetic person from this religious observance, but the patient may feel participation to be essential for spiritual well-being. Sometimes meals are eaten during the hours of darkness, and attention should be given to long-lasting CHO with plenty of fibre in the last meal before dawn. Insulin doses must be adjusted to cope with the long period without food (➔ pp. 379–80).

Never underestimate the strength of a person's belief in the rightness of his/her usual diet. Many hours of explanation may be needed to convince the patient that a new diet is better for them.

Eating out and abroad

People with diabetes need not avoid other people's cooking. The occasional non-diet meal can be included. However, if they eat out often, care is needed. A reasonable meal could be a starter of melon or consommé, a main course of grilled fish or steak, or skinless chicken, with baked or boiled potatoes and vegetables or salad, followed by fruit. Avoid sauces and roast dishes, limit alcohol, and limit the sweet trolley.

When abroad, identify the local staple CHO. The patient should ensure regular clean meals. He or she can enjoy trying local foods. Some homework beforehand may make CHO counting easier.

Emergency foods

Everyone taking insulin injections or other glucose-lowering medication should carry glucose to treat hypoglycaemia and keep a store of emergency food to substitute for a missed meal. It should be durable, conveniently packaged, and easy to carry around. The wide range of muesli and high-fibre bars contain some starchy CHO and some sucrose mixed with fibre, but watch the fat content. They fit in a pocket, handbag, or workbox, and keep for months. Small boxes of fruit juice, nuts and raisins, and packs of savoury snacks are useful.

Eating disorders in diabetes

Eating disorders are more common in people with diabetes than in non-diabetics. The constant emphasis on food and diet in diabetes may encourage unusual eating behaviours, whether or not they can be formally defined as eating disorders. Eating problems associated with diabetes range from restriction of CHO or omitting meals to reduce the blood glucose to a more sinister severe CHO restriction to reduce the insulin dose and reduce weight. Some anorexic patients deliberately induce insulin deficiency and hyperglycaemia to lose weight. They tend to be admitted in biochemical chaos and ketoacidosis. Laxative abuse and insulin deficiency cause danger-ous hypokalaemia. Anorexia nervosa may alternate with bulimia. Bulimia produces gross fluctuations in glucose balance as the overeating may need large insulin doses, but the self-induced vomiting then precipitates hypo-glycaemia. Such patients should be referred to a specialist diabetes service and should be seen in conjunction with psychiatric and psychological sup-port. Abnormal eating patterns may persist for many years before being detected, and some people with diabetes never again have a normal atti-tude to food (➡ p. 414).

Among people with type 2 diabetes, both binge eating, and night eating are commoner than in the general population, and may occur in up to one in four people.

Summary

- A diet is what you eat. Teach patients about the types of food and the amounts of food to eat.
- A healthy diet should be high in CHO, high in fibre, low in sugar, low in fat, and low in salt, with alcohol in moderation.
- Weight reduction is the most important part of treatment for the obese type 2 patient.
- All patients should achieve normal weight for their height.
- Try to strike a balance between practicality and theory. Use common sense and do not forget that patients are people.
- Adapt the treatment to the patient, not the patient to the treatment.

Further information

Diabetes UK. Diabetes UK evidence-based nutrition guidelines for the prevention and manage-ment of diabetes *Diabet Med.* 2011; **28**:1282–8. ℳ <http://www.diabetes.org.uk/Documents/Reports/Nutritional_guidelines200911.pdf>

Department of Health, 2012, Manual of Nutrition. The Stationery Office ℳ <http://www.tso.co.uk>

Glycaemic index ℳ <http://www.glycemicindex.com>

NICE Clinical guideline CG 43.

The USDA National Nutrient Database for Standard Reference ℳ <http://www.nal.usda.gov/fnic/foodcomp/search/> gives full nutritional information for a wide range of foods including CHO values by weight or portion size.

Virtual supermarket tour for patients: ℳ <http://www.storetour.co.uk/Store.aspx>

Patient leaflets for healthy eating:

British Dietetic Association. ℳ <http://www.bda.uk.com/foodfacts/>

Diabetes UK ℳ <http://www.diabetes.org.uk>

Urine testing

Introduction

Urine has been studied for thousands of years. Nowadays, patients may feel embarrassed about providing a sample and they often fail to comply, or do not follow instructions. Provide discreet facilities, an opaque bag to put the bottle in, and clear explanations. Beware the shy patient who repeatedly fails to provide urine for testing—he or she may have hidden nephropathy.

Uses of urine testing

- Annual review for urinary microalbumin:creatinine ratio
- Patients with micro- or macroalbuminuria—to confirm this and monitor
- Symptoms of urinary tract infection
- Unwell diabetic patient with no obvious cause
- Hyperglycaemia: ?ketones, ?infection
- Unstable glucose control: ?ketones, ?infection
- Impaired renal function for cells, casts, blood, protein, and infection
- Patient glucose self-monitoring (rare nowadays)
- But NOT to diagnose diabetes

Unexpected glycosuria in a non-diabetic should be followed by blood tests (➜ p. 9) but cannot be used to diagnose diabetes. Non-diabetic patients with a low renal threshold will have glycosuria (renal glycosuria). Because of the variation in renal threshold, absence of glycosuria does not exclude diabetes. Post-prandial testing is more likely to detect diabetes than fasting samples. Up to 15 % of pregnant women show glycosuria, but most of these do not have diabetes. Patients on SGLT2 inhibitors will always have glycosuria (➜ pp. 139–40).

Home urine glucose monitoring can be used for some patients, as can urine ketone assessment at times of hyperglycaemia.

Practical points

- Teach all patients how to do a clean midstream urine specimen suitable for microbiological testing.
- Always use this method for spot urine samples, whether done at home or in the clinic.
- Encourage them to produce an early morning sample at home on the day of clinic.
- Keep all samples until the end of clinic/surgery.
- Send off those requiring microbiological testing at the end as this avoids the need for repeat urine samples.
- Give patients a urine sample bottle for next time as they leave.
- Ask all female patients of childbearing age if they are menstruating.
- Keep urine pregnancy testing kits in clinic.

Urine glucose monitoring

The person testing the urine must:
- understand why they are doing the test
- be capable of following instructions
- follow the instructions
- not be colour blind
- not suffer visual impairment
- not have impeding upper-limb disabilities

Home urine glucose monitoring is not precise and results can be misleading. It will not detect hypoglycaemia and the variability of renal threshold (blood glucose level at which glucose 'spills over' from blood to urine) from person to person and over time, makes results hard to interpret. Urine glucose testing can be a first step to learning about self-monitoring, or be the only means of self-monitoring in needle-phobic patients or in those whose renal threshold allows consistency.

Ideally, urine glucose monitoring should be used only after urinalyses during an oral glucose tolerance test or blood glucose series have demonstrated the renal threshold. The threshold is usually about 10 mmol/l. Urine glucose monitoring is too imprecise for insulin-treated patients. Do not use it as the sole means of testing in any patient capable and willing to measure finger-prick blood glucose. Some physicians advocate urine testing for well-controlled type 2 patients and blood testing for type 1 patients. While there may be less rapid fluctuations in blood glucose concentration in type 2 diabetes, it is helpful for patients to have an accurate knowledge of their blood glucose status. Some patients like to use both blood and urine testing.

When to test for glycosuria

To monitor the overnight blood glucose, test the first urine passed on rising in the morning. For a fasting pre-breakfast test, empty the bladder on rising, and then test a specimen voided 30–60 min later, but before eating. Remind patients that the concentration of glucose in the urine depends upon the height of the blood glucose above the renal threshold during the period since last voiding (often many hours) and the volumes of fluid passed. Many patients think that the urine glucose at the time of testing reflects the blood glucose at the time of testing. The results should be written down, with an indication of the period covered.

Urine vs blood glucose testing

In the UK it is now unusual to monitor glucose control using urine testing.

For
- No needles, no finger-pricks
- No risk of infection to the tested and minimal risk of infection to testers
- Simple equipment—just a bottle of strips—which is easy to use

Against
- The method is dependent upon renal threshold which varies from person to person and over time in one individual
- Needs a lavatory or other appropriate place
- It is retrospective
- If there is no glucose in the urine the patient does not know whether his/her blood glucose is normal, or whether he or she is hypoglycaemic—hence the old advice to keep a trace of glucose in the urine (which, in practice, meant keeping the blood glucose > 10 mmol/l, hardly normoglycaemia)
- Aspirin and vitamin C interfere with urine glucose testing, giving false-negative results

Urine ketones

Ketones are a product of fat breakdown. Their presence in urine is a sign of insulin deficiency. However, anything which causes major fat breakdown, such as a strict weight-reducing diet (e.g. Atkins) produces ketonuria, as can alcohol excess or rare inborn errors of metabolism. Some patients have been alarmed by the teaching that ketonuria always means impending coma.

The strips measure acetone, but the predominant ketone in diabetic ketoacidosis is β-hydroxybutyrate which can now be measured by finger-prick testing (➔ p. 110). Patients with type 1 diabetes should be given blood ketone test strips (➔ p. 110).

Urine ketone testing strips are available in bottles and also individually foil-wrapped. The latter are most suitable for patient use as they keep well and most patients need them infrequently. Urine ketones levels above ++ require immediate action (?DKA ➔ pp. 216–19). Type 1 patients with any ketonuria require review of their clinical condition (?developing DKA) and insulin treatment unless they are well and are deliberately reducing calorie intake to lose weight.

When to test for ketones

New patients

Always test newly diagnosed diabetic patients for ketones. If present in large amounts they indicate the need for insulin treatment.

Unwell insulin-treated patients

⚠ May have relative insulin deficiency and should be encouraged to test for ketones. This is especially important if they are vomiting or are short of breath. Such patients who present to their doctor must have a urine or blood ketone test and require emergency admission.

Very high blood glucose

⚠ Type 1 patients should test for ketones if their blood glucose concentration is > 15 mmol/l, even if they are otherwise well.

Urine vs blood ketone testing

For

- Widely available
- Cheap
- Can be combined with other tests on a single strip

Against

- Measure acetone, but the main ketone in DKA is β-hydroxybutyrate
- Must wait for patient to urinate
- Cannot be used in anuric patients
- Need lavatory or suitable place
- Measures acetone
- False positives—levodopa (e.g. Sinemet®), valproic acid, vitamin C, phenazopyrazine

Urine albumin

Which test?

- A spot urine test, preferably first passed in morning.
- Do not request 24-hr urine tests (bothersome for patients, rarely correctly performed or timed)
- Measure albumin, not total protein. Some nephrologists may monitor patients with established nephropathy with protein:creatinine ratios (PCR)
- Measure laboratory albumin:creatinine ratio (ACR)
- Do not use point of care tests to determine need for treatment

The Renal Association (2011 guidance) states: '[s]everal studies have shown good correlations between the total protein or albumin to creatinine ratio on early morning spot urine sample and 24-hr urinary protein excretion. Furthermore urine protein to creatinine ratio on a spot morning specimen has been shown to predict the risk of progression at least as reliably as 24-hr urinary protein excretion in CKD patients without diabetes and urine albumin to creatinine ratio has been shown to predict renal outcomes better than 24h urinary protein or albumin excretion in diabetic patients with CKD'. ℘ <http://www.renal.org/Clinical/GuidelinesSection/Detection-Monitoring-and-Care-of-Patients-with-CKD.aspx>.

ACR test results

Everyone loses some albumin in their urine—in fit adults, the loss ranges from 2.5 mg to 11 mg per 24 hrs. Send all samples for laboratory analysis. Do not use ACR point-of-care tests e.g. dipsticks.

- *Early morning urine ACR.* Sample from first urine passed on waking. Normal < 3.5 mg/mmol in women and < 2.5mg/mmol in men.
- *Urine ACR on sample passed in clinic.* Normal taken as < 3.5 mg/mmol in women and < 2.5mg/mmol in men, but less reproducible because of exercise and posture.

False positives

- Cetrimide (e.g. Savlon®)
- Chlorhexidine (e.g. Hibitane®)
- Concentrated urine (hence correction for urinary creatinine concentration)

When to test for albumin

All newly diagnosed patients

Should have a urine ACR test.

All patients

Should have their urine laboratory ACR checked annually, including those who are known to have CKD. (NICE Type 2 diabetes pathway 'Identifying and managing kidney damage'.)

Patients with microalbuminuria

Exclude/treat urinary tract infection (UTI). If microalbuminuria is confirmed on two further tests during the next month, prescribe ACE inhibitor treatment. Repeat tests at least annually after intervention to monitor progress. (➲ pp. 276–9).

Overt proteinuria

See Renal Association guidance and discuss with your local renal team. Use spot ACR or PCR to monitor overt proteinuria rather than performing 24 hr urine collections.

Multiple test analysis

UTIs are common in men and women with diabetes. Some clinics use multiple dipstick urine checks at every clinic visit. This often detects unsuspected UTIs.

Test for UTIs

- Check blood, protein, nitrite, and leucocytes in:
  - patients with symptoms of UTI
  - pregnant diabetic women every visit (risk of premature labour with UTI)
  - patients with renal disease every visit
  - unwell patients
  - patients with high glucose or erratic glucose control
  - patients on pioglitazone before prescribing it, and on each visit thereafter (possible risk of bladder cancer)
- False positives:
  - failure to close bottle of strips between tests
  - contamination during urination (especially in women)

Proteinuria on these strips should be confirmed by laboratory ACR, assuming contamination and UTI have been excluded.

Summary

- Patients may find providing urine samples embarrassing. Respect their dignity and privacy.
- Patients may not follow instructions for collection, or may not provide the sample at all. Beware repeat lack of samples and hence hidden early nephropathy.
- Beware false negatives and false positives in all forms of urine testing.
- Do not use urine glucose testing to diagnose diabetes. Glycosuria in post-prandial samples in a person without known diabetes requires laboratory venous glucose or HbA_{1c} testing for diagnosis.
- Urine glucose testing is occasionally used to monitor glycaemic balance but is less reliable than blood glucose testing.
- Urine ketone (acetone) testing should be used to detect the need for insulin therapy in newly diagnosed patients. It may indicate the need for increased insulin dosage in those who are ill or markedly hyperglycaemic. Finger-prick blood ketone (β-hydroxybutyrate) testing is much better.
- Annually test spot laboratory albumin-to-creatinine ratio (ACR) to detect or monitor microalbuminuria, or tests for albuminuria. Urine microalbumin testing detects patients at risk of worsening nephropathy at a stage when intervention may slow the rate of progression. It also warns of increased risk of cardiovascular mortality in type 2 patients. There is rarely any need for 24-hr urinary albumin testing nowadays.
- Protein:creatinine ratio (PCR) is sometimes used to monitor patients with known chronic kidney disease.

- General multiple test dipstick urinalysis can detect urinary tract infections which are common in men and women with diabetes and may not have typical symptoms.
- Monitor patients on pioglitazone before and during treatment for haematuria.

Chapter 7

Blood glucose and ketone testing

Blood glucose

Blood glucose assessment includes capillary blood glucose monitoring from finger-prick samples, laboratory estimation of venous plasma (or whole blood) glucose, or retrospective measures using glycosylated proteins (fructosamine and HbA_{1c}).

Blood glucose results from separate but simultaneously taken samples in the same person may vary for the following reasons.

- Whether arterial, venous, or capillary sample
- Whether whole blood or plasma used in assay
- Fasting or post-prandial
- Level of blood glucose (more variation at higher readings)
- Patient's central and peripheral temperature
- State of the patient's circulation
- Amount of interstitial fluid at the finger-prick site
- Laboratory or hand-held meter (point of care) assay
- Which meter is used
- Length of delay from venesection to analysis in laboratory compared with instant analysis of finger-prick blood

Laboratory venous plasma glucose is the international gold standard (WHO). Finger-prick glucose is usually higher than venous plasma glucose with greater variation at higher levels (*Diabetes Technol Ther* 2011; **13**:586–91; doi:10.1089/dia.2010.0218). Because this is a complex topic, in this book it is assumed that, for practical purposes, venous plasma glucose and capillary glucose targets are approximately the same (except in the diagnosis of diabetes where laboratory venous plasma glucose levels must be used).

Blood glucose targets

Whenever possible the target should be to have a glucose level close to the non-diabetic range, provided that this is safe and practical for that individual. Increasing concerns about over-rigorous application of glucose targets causing hypoglycaemia have led to a trend to avoid general blood glucose targets. The aim should be to return the blood glucose towards ranges found in people without diabetes in a safe and practical way for each patient and to adjust this as necessary to reflect changes in the patient's health and circumstances.

Laboratory blood glucose measurement

This is the gold standard against which other methods are compared. When taking venous blood, record the time. Note that after venesection plasma glucose level in the sample tube falls by 5–7% per hour so a value of 7 may fall to 6.1 mmol/l in 2 hrs at room temperature even in fluoride (➔ p. 8). Prompt analysis is best. Even so, most results will arrive after the patient has left. Record the results, tell the patient, and act as outlined. Temper these guidelines with your knowledge of the individual patient (Table 7.1, Box 7.1).

Table 7.1 Published blood glucose targets (laboratory or capillary)
Use these as a starting point for discussion when personalizing glucose aims which will differ in different patients. Take care to avoid hypoglycaemia

Situation adults	Blood glucose target mmol/l	
	Before meals	2 hrs after food*
Not diabetic	3.5–5.5	< 7.8
Type 1 diabetes NICE 2004	4–7	< 9
Type 2 diabetes NICE 2008	4–7	< 8.5
Pregnant women NICE 2008	3.5–5.9	< 7.8 1 hr after food

*without hypoglycaemia.

Box 7.1 Acting on results of laboratory venous plasma glucose tests

3.9 mmol/l or less ⚠
Telephone patients on medication that could cause hypoglycaemia to make sure that they are not still hypoglycaemic. Did you or the patient realize that they were hypoglycaemic at the time? If not, warn the patient that they have hypoglycaemic unawareness. And you need to sharpen your clinical observation. Reduce glucose-lowering treatment unless it was a one-off low with a one-off explanation.

4.0–6.9 mmol/l
Within normal limits; no action need be taken.

7.0–10.9 mmol/l
OK if post-prandial. Too high before food. Discuss eating less or increasing glucose-lowering treatment.

11.0–19.9 mmol/l
Too high. Review diet, self-adjustment of treatment, exercise. Increase treatment if necessary.

20 mmol/l or more ⚠
Much too high. Many patients tolerate blood glucose levels like this much of the time. Others will be symptomatic or ill. Telephone the patient that day and check that they are all right. If the level is ≥ 30 mmol/l the patient should be seen by a doctor that day. They may need insulin and many need hospital admission (➔ pp. 205–7).

Capillary blood glucose testing

This is a much more direct and precise way of monitoring blood glucose concentration than urine testing. Urine testing should not be used by professionals in hospitals or surgeries to monitor glycaemia in known diabetes. The Medicines and Healthcare Products Regulatory Agency (MHRA) ♙ <http://www.mhra.gov.uk> highlights capillary glucose testing issues: ♙ <http://www.mhra.gov.uk/SearchHelp/GoogleSearch/index. htm?q=glucose%20testing>

Diabetes UK's position is 'that people with diabetes should have access to home blood glucose monitoring based on individual clinical need, informed consent and not on ability to pay. Home monitoring is essential in the context of diabetes education for self-management in order to enable the person to make appropriate treatment or lifestyle choices'.

Self-monitoring of blood glucose (SMBG) is expensive and thus causes concern for those with financial responsibilities for healthcare who may put pressure on prescribers to reduce glucose test strip prescriptions. SMBG can be painful, and is a waste of time and money without appropriate patient education about what results mean and what to do about them. Preventing access to SMBG in well-trained patients who need it is dangerous and could even prove fatal.

Who may use capillary glucose testing?

People with diabetes or their relatives or carers

SMBG has taken the guesswork out of life with diabetes. Patients no longer have to rely on urine tests and symptoms to manage their diabetes. SMBG allows patients to adjust their treatment and eating, and to monitor their own condition. It should not be a ritual just to produce numbers for the doctor. People with diabetes for whom SMBG helps to improve health and well-being should be helped to use this technology in the best possible way for them. People with diabetes for whom it is not helpful should not be asked to do finger-prick tests.

The person testing the blood must:
- understand why they are doing the test
- understand when the test is or is not appropriate
- learn how to obtain an appropriate blood sample
- be aware of health and safety issues of blood testing and safe disposal of sharps
- be aware of normal and abnormal results—and what to do about them
- have had a formal training session with the device and be able to demonstrate its use
- be aware of potential technical problems and what to do about them
- know how to seek help
- take part in a quality assurance system (e.g. using manufacturer's test samples)
- use a meter if colour blind (most people use meters nowadays)
- use a talking meter if visually impaired
- not have severe impeding upper-limb disabilities

A patient produced her home glucose-testing diary. Every day for a month her glucose was 9.6 mmol/l. When asked to demonstrate the test she pricked her finger, ignored the blood, and looked at the meter, which was set on memory and showed the result of 9.6 produced when the diabetic nurse had originally demonstrated blood glucose testing.

Professionals

Assisted monitoring of blood glucose (AMBG) provides point-of-care measurement of blood glucose. If the test is performed properly, the results are comparable with those obtained in the laboratory. If the user and the meter participate in a quality assurance scheme and the user has regular retraining, the results can be used for most diabetes management. All hospitals and clinics using this technique should participate in a quality assurance scheme. Record the results on a hospital-wide chart. Many insulin prescription charts now include glucose monitoring records to show the effects of dosage changes. Finger-prick glucose tests should not be done on cold, 'shut-down', or oedematous hands. Problems may arise when inexperienced personnel are asked to test blood glucose without any training. Every finger-prick glucose-testing problem investigated in one busy district general hospital was found to be due to user error. Many hospitals now use meters that require user and patient barcode identification, that will not work if not calibrated regularly, and results are downloaded to part of the laboratory system.

How to do a finger-prick blood glucose test

Like all laboratory techniques performed outside the laboratory, finger-prick blood glucose measurement is a waste of time unless it is done properly. Important factors are as follows.

- *The finger* should be warm, clean, and dry. Wash with water and then dry. Do not use alcohol swabs, which may interfere with the test. Sticky fingers give falsely high blood glucose levels. The sides of the finger are less sensitive than the tip. The ear lobe can be used, as can upper arm or thigh with some meters.
- *Making the hole*. Finger-pricking lancets are for single use only. Spring-loaded devices are less painful. Lancets are of different gauges—the higher the gauge, the smaller the hole. Some devices have platforms to press on to the finger. Platforms of different thickness allow deeper or shallower finger-prick. In hospitals or clinics use individual spring-loaded lancets for each patient to avoid transmission of blood-borne infection which is a risk with devices with platforms.
- *The blood drop* should be allowed to form naturally. If necessary 'milk' up blood from the base of the finger. Squeezing the fingertip may dilute the blood with serum and may cause soreness. Drop the blood onto the strip without smearing. Some systems wick up the blood from the end of the strip.
- *The electrode strips* must be in date and dry. Never handle the pad onto which the blood will be dropped—your sticky fingers might influence the result.

- *Read the result*. Use a meter. Visually read strips are rarely used nowadays. Each bottle of strips has a colour chart against which to match the colour changes of the strips in that bottle. (The dyes in each batch may differ so strips must not be matched against a bottle from a different batch.) The person reading the result must have normal colour vision. People with diabetic retinopathy, especially those who have had laser treatment, may not have normal colour vision.

People may not always understand instructions.

One elderly couple tried to make words out of the numbers on the meter. A nurse read a meter upside-down—07 instead of LO.

Warning messages may be misinterpreted—a nurse said a patient had ketones in her blood. When asked how she had measured this, she said, 'Came up on the meter'. What the biosensor actually indicated was 'Check ketones'. Some meters do measure ketones but only if a specific ketone strip is used.

Factors affecting capillary glucose results

Different meters may be affected in different ways by the patient's age, condition, or treatment (Box 7.2). Check that the meter you are using is right for the job, especially in a neonatal or maternity unit.

Box 7.2 Factors affecting capillary glucose results*

- Variation in haematocrit—neonates, pregnancy
- Peripheral shut-down, e.g. hypotension, dehydration, shock, peripheral arterial disease
- Over-squeezing finger (dilutes with tissue fluids)
- Water on finger
- Glucose on finger
- Oedema of finger
- Dialysis treatments: some peritoneal dialysis fluids may contain maltose which interferes with some strips
- Variations in oxygenation, e.g. intensive oxygen therapy
- Non-glucose reducing substances, e.g. ascorbic acid infusions
- Jaundice
- Hypertriglyceridaemia
- Total parenteral nutrition

*See MHRA website ℐ <http://www.mhra.gov.uk>

Record the result

Many patients do not record their results. While a one-off test may be of use at the time it was done, without a record neither the patient nor his or her carer can assess overall glucose balance and the need or otherwise for intervention. There may be other problems.

There is a human tendency to under-read or to fail to record unpalatable results. A few patients make up their results to please their doctor. A sophisticated faker may be detected only by repeated marked disparity between the HbA$_{1c}$ and SMBG. Most modern meters have memories making it possible to review, with the patient, what the results actually were. Many patients use smart-phone apps or download the results onto a computer. Nowadays, diabetes clinics should have the software to view such results, with patient consent. Some people use apps, e.g.

🔗 <http://www.diabetes.org.uk/How_we_help/Diabetes-iPhone-Tracker-app/>

> A teenage patient produced a tidy glucose diary with lots of tests for the past month. Unfortunately she had been seen making-up the results in the waiting room!

Acting on the result

It is no use noting an abnormal result and doing nothing about it. In one district general hospital audit, only one in four markedly abnormal blood glucose results recorded by nursing staff was acted upon. Patients frequently record high or low results for weeks without taking action.

Strips and meters

Today, most people use meters. They have increasingly sophisticated data management systems and most will, with appropriate leads and software (obtainable from the manufacturers), download results to computers. Lifescan has developed Bluetooth® technology and others are likely to do so. DSNs will help patients find the most appropriate meter. These are not currently available at NHS expense although many diabetes services can give some out free of charge, as do some manufacturers at times. Keep them clean, handle them gently, follow the instructions, and obey calibration rules. Ask the manufacturing company's trainer to visit the surgery, clinic, or ward each year to update staff. Use the test solutions provided and share in any quality assurance scheme for meters. Many patients buy meters off the shelf. Check that they are using them properly. The Monthly Index of Medical Specialties' (MIMS) website has an up-to-date list of meters, strips, finger-prickers, and lancets.

🔗 <http://www.mims.co.uk/Tables/1096963/Finger-Prickers-Compatible-Lancets/> 🔗 <http://www.mims.co.uk/Tables/882434/Blood-Glucose-Testing-Strips-Meters >

There are talking blood glucose meters for visually impaired patients e.g.: 🔗 http://www.supercheck2.co.uk/bloodglucosemeter.htm

Protecting patients and staff

Each patient should have his or her own personal finger pricker and meter which are not to be shared by anyone else. Patients can use their own spring-loaded lancet holders for new lancets each test. They should follow manufacturers' instructions for cleaning their equipment.

When staff do finger-prick tests (AMBG) there is an obvious risk of acquiring or transmitting infection for both staff and patients. AMBG has been implicated in hepatitis B outbreaks in health and long-term care facilities. Wear disposable gloves. Use single-use lancing devices which permanently retract the needle into a safety cover for each patient. Never use multiple-test lancet holders. Assign a blood glucose meter to each individual patient if possible. Clean and disinfect meters according to manufacturers' instructions. Do not share a meter that cannot be cleaned/disinfected. Do not store used meters with unused ones. See ℘ <http://www.cdc.gov/injectionsafety/blood-glucose-monitoring.html> (*J Diabetes Sci Technol* 2010; **4**(5):1027–31); ℘ http://www.rcn.org.uk/__data/assets/pdf_file/0008/418490/004135.pdf.

SMBG in insulin-treated diabetes

It is essential that these patients learn how to use SMBG for insulin dose adjustment and for safety checks. Diabetes UK states: '[s]elf-monitoring of blood glucose levels should be regarded as an integral part of treatment of everyone with Type 1 diabetes and access to blood glucose testing strips and meters should not be restricted. SMBG is an effective tool in the self-management of glucose levels in people with. . .Type 2 diabetes using insulin therapy. It helps people with diabetes using insulin achieve tight control and to identify low blood glucose levels before development of severe hypoglycaemia.'

SMBG in non-insulin-treated type 2 diabetes

A report published by NHS Diabetes in 2010 based on a Health Technology Appraisal states: '[t]he data from clinical trials show that in patients treated by lifestyle modification or oral agents, SMBG with appropriate education and clear objectives leads to improvement in blood glucose control. The improvements in blood glucose control when SMBG is used without education and clear objectives are so small as to be of doubtful clinical benefit. There is also evidence that some psychosocial outcomes deteriorate. Pricking one's finger is painful and some people find it distressing. There is a strong case for stopping blood glucose monitoring activity in people who derive no benefit from it, particularly where it is damaging their quality of life.

SMBG should be available to people receiving sulfonylurea treatment because of the risk of hypoglycaemia with this treatment.

Some newly diagnosed individuals and others with diabetes of longer duration but not taking insulin clearly benefit from measuring their blood glucose. In those individuals who find modern technology essential to managing their diabetes, arbitrary withdrawal of treatment should not occur. It would limit patient choice and may lead to a deterioration in blood glucose control.'

♒ <http://webarchive.nationalarchives.gov.uk/20130513172055/ http://www.diabetes.nhs.uk/our_publications/reports_and_guidance/ diagnosis_and_ongoing_care/#>
Health Technol Assess. 2010;**14**(12):1–140. doi: 10.3310/hta14120.

When to test

Test whenever you want to know the blood glucose so that action can be taken if required. Tell patients that SMBG allows them to check their glucose at any time, virtually anywhere, to ensure that they are safe and comfortable, and that any changes in treatment, eating, or exercise can be made on a day-to-day basis. Use local SMBG guidelines if available. On most occasions when you see someone with diabetes, measure his or her finger-prick blood glucose. HbA$_{1c}$ provides good long-term information about glycaemia, but an HbA$_{1c}$ of 53 mmol/mol (7.0 %) can be achieved by the blood glucose oscillating between 1 mmol/l and 20 mmol/l. Also, some patients may have unrecognized problems with accurate measurement (or they are simply not checking). If this is the case, SMBG is unlikely to helpful. A small but significant number of insulin-treated patients will be hypoglycaemic while talking with you.

HbA$_{1c}$ is usually the better measure to use to assess overall glucose control. SMBG or AMBG is useful when glucose changes may be expected (e.g. illness, strong emotion, new treatment, etc.) (Table 7.2).

Insulin-treated patients

These patients should test before each meal and before bed until their blood glucose levels are stable. Patients using short-acting insulins or insulin pumps should continue to test at least four times a day for optimum flexibility in insulin dosage adjustment and glucose control. If the number of tests is being reduced, the one that should always remain is the pre-bed-time test to ensure that patients go to bed with a safe glucose concentration.

Non-insulin-treated patients

These individuals can test two to four times a day when treatment has just started, if their treatment regimen has been changed (to see if the new treatment is working and to check for hypoglycaemia); or if they are unwell. In type 2 diabetes the pre-breakfast, fasting test is a useful indicator of overall glucose balance. It should be 4–7 mmol/l in most patients. These patients can learn how to adjust their tablets (over weeks) according to blood glucose levels. Patients with good fasting glucose but high HbA$_{1c}$ should test post-prandially. There is usually no need to continue routine testing if the HbA$_{1c}$ is within target for that patient unless the patient wishes. However, patients who find it helpful (e.g. those who are on repaglinide or nateglinide) and adjust their treatment for meals and exercise, should continue to test.

Illness, pregnancy, or exercise

More frequent finger-prick glucose tests may be needed in illness or pregnancy, or when undergoing new, hazardous, or vigorous exercise.

Table 7.2 Suggested indications for SMBG

Which patients?	Frequency of testing
What is my glucose? (all patients)	Any time
Illness (all patients)	4–6 times daily until well
Unusual circumstances/exertion (all patients)	Any time
Planned exercise (all patients unless on diet alone or diet and metformin alone)	Pre/post-exercise until stable
Unstable glucose (all patients)	2–4 times daily
Change in treatment (all patients)	2–4 times daily
Pre-pregnancy	4–6 times daily
Pregnancy (type 1/2, gestational diabetes)	4–6 times daily
Insulin pump patients	4–6 times daily + for driving
Type 1 or 2 diabetes (basal-bolus insulin)	4 times daily + for driving
Type 1 or 2 diabetes (twice daily insulin)	2 (vary times) to 4 times daily + for driving
Type 2 on basal insulin	Fasting daily; post-prandial 1–7 times a week + for driving
Type 2 on sulfonylureas (initial/change dose)	Fasting + a post-prandial daily until stable, then weekly / Drivers twice daily + for driving
Type 2 on meglitinides	Fasting + post-prandially as required for dose adjustment / Drivers twice daily + for driving
Type 2 on glitazones or incretin-effect enhancers (initial/change dose)	Fasting + a post-prandial daily until stable, then weekly
Type 2 on diet or metformin alone	Not routinely unless patient wishes or as above; use HbA_{1c} every 2–6 mths

Post-prandial tests

Post-prandial hyperglycaemia contributes considerably to overall glycaemia. Test results 1–2 hrs after a meal should be within the patient's personal limits (e.g. Table 7.1) without hypoglycaemia at any time.

Night-time tests

If under intensive control (e.g. when pregnant), waking hypoglycaemia after reduction in overnight insulin, waking high glucose.

Safety checks

Drivers, especially PCV and LGV drivers, on glucose-lowering treatment which could cause hypoglycaemia, and others involved in hazardous work or sports activities should test regularly to avoid hypoglycaemia and danger to themselves or others. Their access to test strips must not be restricted. The DVLA rules (➲ pp. 395–9) state:

Table 7.3 Indications for finger-prick capillary glucose monitoring in hospital/clinic/practice

Situation	Frequency of testing
Hospital	
ICU/HDU/resuscitation area	Hourly
In theatre and recovery area	Hourly
Very sick patient anywhere	Hourly
IV Insulin infusion	Hourly
Acute ward	6 hourly (pre-meals, pre-bed)
Nocturnal hypoglycaemia? Or risk of this	2 a.m.
Not ill but awaiting care package	As for Table 7.2
Clinic/practice	
Annual check	
Each visit	

Meters should conform to current ISO standards:
<http://www.iso.org/iso/catalogue_detail?csnumber=54976>

Group 1 (cars, motorcycles):
Insulin-treated people
There must be appropriate blood glucose monitoring. This has been defined by the Secretary of State's Honorary Medical Advisory Panel on Driving and Diabetes as no more than 2 hours before the start of the first journey and every 2 hours while driving.

Group 2. PCV, LGV (lorry, bus):
Insulin-treated people
Regularly monitors blood glucose at least twice daily and at times relevant to driving, (no more than 2 hours before the start of the first journey and every 2 hours while driving), using a glucose meter with a memory function to measure and record blood glucose levels. At the annual examination by an independent Consultant Diabetologist, 3 months of blood glucose readings must be available.

Those on sulfonylureas or glinides:
Regularly monitors blood glucose at least twice daily and at times relevant to driving.
<https://www.gov.uk/government/publications/at-a-glance>

Continuous blood glucose monitoring

Continuous glucose monitoring system (CGM)

A fine needle sensor is inserted into the subcutaneous tissue to record interstitial fluid glucose levels very frequently e.g. every few mins, transmitting these wirelessly to be viewed on a receiver within 3–6 metres. CGM can be linked to an insulin pump and it has been used successfully in closed-loop algorithms for automatic control of nocturnal insulin infusion. Closed-loop systems ('artificial pancreas') are still at the research stage.

Because CGM measures glucose in interstitial fluid it needs to be calibrated against blood glucose, thus the accuracy of the SMBG affects the accuracy of the CGM. There is a very complex relationship between glucose dynamics in blood and interstitial fluid. There has been concern about accuracy of CGM, especially in recognizing hypoglycaemia. Time taken for glucose to diffuse into the interstitial fluid may vary from 0–45 mins (usually the lag is about 5–15 mins). (*Sensors (Basel)* 2010;**10**:10936-52).

Provided users and clinicians are aware of the concerns, CGM can help in day-to-day management of diabetes. It can show glucose excursions, and, assuming accurate timing is set up, what happens to glucose with food, exercise, and insulin. A meta-analysis of non-pregnant adults with type 1 diabetes showed that CGM use was associated with a significant reduction in HbA_{1c}, especially in those with high HbA_{1c} at baseline and those who most frequently used CGM. Exposure to hypoglycaemia was also reduced. The authors concluded that '[t]he most cost effective or appropriate use of CGM is likely to be when targeted at people with type 1 diabetes who have continued poor control during intensified insulin therapy and who frequently use continuous glucose monitoring.' (*Br Med J* 2011; **343**:d3805; doi: http://dx.doi.org/10.1136/bmj.d3805). ABCD's position statement describes the use of CGM to lower HbA_{1c} safely, especially in pregnancy, and in the management of suspected (e.g. nocturnal or unaware) or actual hypoglycaemia (*Pract Diab Int* 2010; **27**:66–8; doi: 10.1002/pdi.1448).

Abbott, Dexcom, and Medtronic all manufacture CGM. These technologies have not yet been reviewed by NICE. Most studies have been in type 1 diabetes and more data are needed in type 2.

Glycosylated haemoglobin (HbA$_{1c}$)

Glucose binds with many proteins—glycosylation. Glycosylated haemoglobin A$_{1c}$ (HbA$_{1c}$) is used to monitor glucose balance because it is a marker for the risk of diabetic tissue damage—the higher the HbA$_{1c}$, the greater is the risk. HbA$_{1c}$ is related to glycaemia over the life of the red cell, which is about 120 days.

HbA$_{1c}$ looks at the past, and reflects mean blood glucose concentration. A finger-prick blood glucose relates to 'now', and fluctuates during the day. Glucose in the preceding

- 30 days contributes to ≈50 % of the HbA$_{1c}$
- 30–90 days contributes to ≈40 % of the HbA$_{1c}$
- > 90 days contributes to ≈10 % of the HbA$_{1c}$

Patients often ask what HbA$_{1c}$ means in terms of blood glucose levels. The estimated average glucose (EAG) has been calculated in an international group of patients, 84 % of whom were of non-Hispanic White ethnicity (*Diabetes Care* 2008; **31**(8):1473–8; doi:10.2337/dc08-0545). It is not widely used in the UK. For example:

- HbA$_{1c}$ 53 mmol/mol (7 %), EAG 8.6 (6.8–10.3) mmol/l
- HbA$_{1c}$ 86 mmol/mol (10 %), EAG 13.4 (10.7–15.7) mmol/l

There are several different methods for measuring HbA$_{1c}$. The method used may mean that abnormal haemoglobins (e.g. HbS in sickle cell disease) interfere with analysis. The National Glycohemoglobin Standardization Program (NGSP) has a list of HbA$_{1c}$ assay interference and analysers, at: ℘ <http://www.ngsp.org/interf.asp>. Modern methods in the UK are standardized to the international reference measurement procedure advocated by the International Federation of Clinical Chemists (IFCC). These results are reported as mmol/mol. Previously, UK results were reported as a percentage aligned to the DCCT study (*New Engl J Med* 1993; **329**: 977–86; doi: 10.1056/NEJM199309303291401). Some countries still report this way. An international consensus statement (*Diabetologia* 2007; **50**: 2042–3; doi: 10.1007/s00125-007-0789-7) agreed that:

- HbA$_{1c}$ test results should be standardized worldwide
- The IFCC reference system should be used
- HbA$_{1c}$ should be reported worldwide in IFCC units (mmol/mol) and derived NGSP units (%) using an IFCC–NGSP master equation
- An HbA$_{1c}$-derived average glucose will also be reported to make it easier for patients to understand HbA$_{1c}$ (A1c-Derived Average Glucose is more usually known as EAG).

HbA$_{1c}$ should be measured in the laboratory unless using a near-patient finger-prick capillary system with quality assurance that performs to laboratory standards. This does not apply to some point-of-care systems so check before use or purchase.

Check HbA$_{1c}$ twice a year in stable patients, and preferably on every visit more than 2 months since the last test. Patients can attend the laboratory for a blood test 1–2 weeks before clinic so that the result is available for discussion. Some units estimate this in blood-spots on filter paper or little finger-prick collector bottles sent in by the patient a week or two in advance.

Non-glucose factors influencing HbA$_{1c}$

These include factors that affect red cell production or destruction, hae-moglobinopathies or abnormal haemoglobins, factors affecting glycation, and assay factors.

- Increased HbA$_{1c}$: iron or B12 deficiency anaemia; reduced erythropoesis, alcoholism, chronic liver disease, splenectomy, hyperbilirubinaemia, chronic opiate use.
- Decreased HbA$_{1c}$: iron, B12, or erythropoeitin therapy; frequent blood transfusions, aspirin, vitamin C or E, and antiretroviral therapy, rheumatoid arthritis, and hypertriglyceridaemia.
- Variable effects on HbA$_{1c}$: haemoglobinopathies and genetic abnormalities.

(*Journal of Diabetes* 2009; **1**:9–17; doi: 10.1111/j.1753-0407.2009.00009.x).

Fructosamine

Fructosamine measures glycosylation of several plasma proteins, espe-cially albumin. Therefore it reflects glucose balance 1 or 2 weeks before the sample is taken. Fructosamine is affected by anything which influences plasma protein levels and should be corrected for plasma protein level. It is not regarded as such a reliable test as HbA$_{1c}$ but does reflect a shorter time span. Fructosamine should be used in some of the situations listed (e.g. thalassaemia with frequent blood transfusions). Seek advice from your laboratory.

HbA$_{1c}$ targets

HbA$_{1c}$ in a person with diabetes should be close to that for a non-diabetic person provided that treatment does not induce hypoglycaemia (Table 7.4). The higher the HbA$_{1c}$, the greater is the risk of diabetic tissue damage (Table 7.5).

Table 7.4 HbA₁c Targets to start the discussion about personalized glucose control

Treatment	HbA₁c target
	TAILOR THE TARGET TO THE PATIENT Avoid hypoglycaemia
Non-diabetic	< 48 mmol/mol (6.5 %)
Diet alone	< 48 mmol/mol (6.5 %)
Metformin alone	< 48 mmol/mol (6.5 %)
Other non-insulin drugs + insulin	42–58 mmol/mol (6.0–7.4 %) if safe and practical* ⚠ danger of hypoglycaemia with insulin and sulfonylureas
Planning pregnancy**	< 43 mmol/mol (< 6.1 %) if safe ⚠ danger of hypoglycaemia in Type 1 patients

*Type 1 diabetes, see NICE CG15.
*Type 2 diabetes, see *Diabetes Care* 2012; 35:1364–79; doi: 10.2337/dc12-0413.
**Preconception NICE CG63.

Table 7.5 HbA₁c DCCT aligned vs IFCC units

DCCT aligned (%)	IFCC (mmol/mol)
4.0	20
5.0	31
6.0	42
7.0	53
8.0	64
9.0	75
10.0	86
11.0	97
12.0	108

Diabetes UK ☞ <http://www.diabetes.org.uk> has a converter.

Blood ketone testing

Ketones rise with fasting, insulin deficiency, and alcohol excess. Management of hyperglycaemia and DKA has been revolutionized by finger-prick capillary ketone testing (Tables 7.6 and 7.7) (Abbott Optium Xceed™ or Glucomen® LX plus). This measures β-hydroxybutyrate, the main ketone in ketoacidosis. The urine test measures acetone (➔ p. 91). Blood ketone measurement is a better predictor of DKA than urine ketones (*Diabetes Metab* 2007; **33**:135–9; <http://dx.doi.org/10.1016/j.diabet.2006.11.006>). Blood ketones can be used in A&E departments to identify which hyperglycaemic patients have DKA or compensated DKA (*Diabet Med* 2005; **22**:221–4; doi : 10.1111/j.1464-5491.2004.01374.x). Blood ketones also reflect metabolic recovery from DKA better than urine ketones.

Table 7.6 Indications for finger-prick blood ketone testing

Situation	Frequency of testing
Patients/carers	
Vomiting, insulin-treated	Daily. If ketones present, 6 hourly until gone
Ill, insulin-treated	Daily. If ketones present, 6 hourly until gone
Glucose > 15 mmol/l	Once. If ketones present, 6 hourly until gone
Insulin pump patients	Meter and blood ketone strips at home
Patients with frequent DKA	Meter and blood ketone strips at home
Healthcare professionals	
Vomiting, insulin-treated	Once
Ill, glucose >11 mmol/l	Once
All emergency attenders	
Glucose > 11 mmol/l	Once
'Well', glucose > 15 mmol/l	Once
Ketones ≥ 1 mmol/l	6 hourly until < 1 mmol/l
Ketones ≥ 3 mmol/l	⚠ DKA. Admit
	2 hourly until 1 mmol/l

Table 7.7 Act on finger-prick blood ketone results

Ketones (mmol/l)	Action
<1 mmol/l	Good glucose balance + nutrition
1–2.9 mmol/l	Risk of DKA. Increase insulin, check nutrition
≥3 mmol/l	⚠ DKA. Extra insulin preferably IM. 999 to A&E Admit
	IV fluids, IV insulin infusion
≥ 6 mmol/l	⚠ DKA. Risk of death. Admit HDU/ICU

Summary

- Hyperglycaemia is one manifestation of diabetes, which is a multisystem disorder.
- Laboratory venous glucose (or HbA_{1c}) is the only criterion for formal diagnosis of diabetes. Laboratory glucose levels should be checked from time to time in patients in whom other glycaemic monitoring techniques are in use.
- For everyday use, SMBG provides instant assessment of blood glucose concentration anytime, anywhere. It can be used by professionals and patients or their carers.
- Finger-prick blood glucose testing is a laboratory method carried out away from the laboratory. The results are of use only if the test is performed accurately, according to instructions.
- Pay attention to each stage of the testing technique, whether performed by doctor, nurse, or patient.
- Use all meters and sensors according to instructions: the result is only as good as the user's technique.
- Ensure robust cross-infection prevention.
- Anyone with diabetes can use finger-prick blood glucose measurement provided that they can understand what they are doing and why, and are properly taught with regular revision sessions.
- Finger-prick blood glucose testing has replaced urine glucose testing.
- Blood glucose goals should be tailored to individuals.
- HbA_{1c} provides a longer-term view of glycaemia. The higher the HbA_{1c} the greater is the risk of diabetic tissue damage.
- HbA_{1c} goals should be tailored to individuals.
- Only use point-of-care HbA_{1c} devices that conform to laboratory quality assurance standards.
- Finger-prick blood ketone measurement allows prompt recognition of ketosis and can be used to help manage DKA. It is better than urine ketone testing.
- Patients at risk of DKA should have ketone strips with meter at home.

Non-insulin medications

Treat each patient according to his or her individual condition.

Always check drug information in a current edition of the British National Formulary (BNF) ✍ <http://www.bnf.org> before prescribing any medications described in this book.

Be alert for warnings from the MHRA (✍ <http://www.mhra.gov.uk>).

To review the Summary of Product Characteristics (SPC) and Patient Information Leaflet (PIL), see ✍ <http://www.emc.medicines.org.uk>

Introduction

Type 2 diabetes treatment is a major growth area for pharmaceutical companies. It is hard to keep up to date with the drugs that are available. New agents have yet to find their full place in patient care. Multiple drug combinations are now possible. These drugs may be for life and early studies rarely last long enough to discover all the adverse effects. Concerns have been raised about potential risks of some drugs, particularly CVD and cancer risk. There has been much debate about this. However, remember that untreated diabetes has known, frequent, and severe adverse effects. Consider benefit vs risk when prescribing. Pursue personalized, non-drug measures (diet and exercise) vigorously to reduce the need for medication. Readers are strongly advised to keep an eye on NICE and MHRA guidance, check local prescribing policy, and discuss any questions with a local consultant diabetologist.

When to use non-insulin medication

Non-insulin drugs are mainly used in type 2 diabetes. These agents work only if the patient is producing or taking insulin. By the time diabetes has been diagnosed about half the insulin production has failed in most patients, and ~ 4 % is lost every year thereafter. Many patients with type 2 diabetes will need insulin.

Immediate insulin treatment is essential in type 1 diabetes. Adding metformin to insulin may reduce insulin requirement in type 1 patients, especially if they are overweight.

Provide education about diabetes and lifestyle advice for all patients—healthy eating, regular exercise, not smoking, alcohol in moderation. Previous advice was to try diet and exercise in all before adding glucose-lowering medication. Most patients find it hard to keep to a new diet. Each month of high glucose increases the risk of tissue damage.

Practical suggestions for patients with type 2 diabetes are as follows:

- Glucose levels > 11 mmol/l, especially if symptomatic and/or complications present:
  - check for concurrent illness (e.g. infection) and treat it
  - dietary advice
  - exercise advice as appropriate
  - add glucose-lowering medication at diagnosis, especially if glucose > 15 mmol/l
  - see frequently and adjust glucose-lowering medication according to glucose level
  - reduce or stop medication if hypoglycaemic symptoms, glucose < 4 mmol/l, or HbA$_{1c}$ below target range (➔ p. 109)
- Glucose ≤ 11 mmol/l or asymptomatic, uncomplicated patient: start with diet and exercise alone
  - if, after 2 months, HbA$_{1c}$ is not within patient's target range (➔ p. 109) start anti-diabetic drugs while continuing diet/exercise advice
  - at any time, if glucose ≥ 11 mmol/l and patients become symptomatic, glucose rises, or infections, complications, or problems appear, start glucose-lowering medication (and treat additional problems)

Studies of adherence to glucose-lowering medication have shown that up to half the patients do not take it as prescribed. Check concordance before increasing the dose.

Patient education

- These medicines work only if you are making or taking insulin. They help control the blood sugar levels.
- These medicines are not insulin. They help control your glucose in other ways.
- They must be taken in the dose prescribed, at the right time every day.
- If the dose is to be adjusted to finger-prick glucose levels, explain how to do this and what the target glucose range is.
- They are for long-term treatment, not a short course.
- Warn about hypoglycaemia if relevant.
- Double-check for contraindications, including previous intolerance or hypersensitivity.
- Warn about relevant side effects and the need to report these to staff.
- Warn about interacting medications—there are a lot (most just require some SMBG).

Non-insulin glucose-lowering medications

- Biguanide: metformin
- Sulfonylureas: glibenclamide, gliclazide, glimepiride, glipizide, tolbutamide
- Thiazolidinedione: pioglitazone
- Meglitinides (prandial glucose regulators): repaglinide, nateglinide
- Incretin-effect enhancers:
  - Dipeptidylpeptidase-4 (DPP-4) inhibitors: alogliptin, linagliptin, saxagliptin, sitagliptin, vildagliptin
  - Glucagon-like peptide-1 receptor (GLP-1) agonists: exenatide, liraglutide, lixisenatide injections
- Sodium-glucose co-transporter 2 (SGLT2) inhibitors: canagliflozin, dapagliflozin, empagliflozin
- α-Glucosidase inhibitor: acarbose

Which drug? How stringent?

Set individual targets for blood glucose or HbA_{1c}, taking the patient's overall clinical state, mental state, and personal circumstances into consideration (Box 8.1). Strict glucose balance may not be appropriate in an elderly person living alone, for example.

Start with metformin, especially in overweight patients. In patients for whom metformin is inappropriate or not tolerated, use generic sulfonylureas. In those in whom it would be helpful to adjust tablet dose to food or exercise use meglitinides. Consider pioglitazone in patients in whom metformin is inappropriate or not tolerated (but check safety concerns).

Use long-acting or combined preparations where available if concordance is an issue.

Box 8.1 Factors that might require less stringent glucose-lowering treatment

Patient wishes
Lack of motivation
Less likely to take medication as prescribed
Less able to look after himself or herself
Less likely to look after himself or herself
Frail (whether young or old)
Less able to recognize hypoglycaemia
Less able to self-treat hypoglycaemia
Previous problems with hypoglycaemia
Previous problems with adverse reactions to other medications
Lives alone
Lacks support
Long duration of diabetes
Complications of diabetes, e.g. cardiovascular disease, dementia, renal or liver disease
Some comorbidities
Life expectancy short
Receiving palliative care

Metformin and glibenclamide (and glipizide in fewer patients) were used in UKPDS (➲ pp. 40–1). Gliclazide (modified release) was the sulfonylurea used (with additional agents as required) in ADVANCE (➲ pp. 40–1). Gliclazide is the commonest sulfonylurea used in the UK.

If glycaemic targets are not met, check that the patient understands how to take the medication, and is actually taking it, and then increase the dose according to licensed guidance, rechecking HbA$_{1c}$ every 2–3 months until the target is achieved and stable. Encourage healthy diet and exercise.

Combined therapy (see specific sections for individual drugs)

If patients on sulfonylureas or metformin fail to achieve acceptable blood glucose levels, add the other agent. The combination of a sulfonylurea and metformin produces significant glucose lowering and may stave off insulin therapy. Some doctors give small doses of each together early in treatment because each potentiates the effect of the other.

In UKPDS 34: '[w]hen metformin was prescribed in the trial in both non-overweight and overweight patients already treated with sulfonylurea there was a significant increase in the risk of diabetes-related death and all-cause mortality.' The authors point out that the patients on sulfonylurea were older, more hyperglycaemic, and followed up for 5 yrs less than other patients. They concluded: '[t]he epidemiological analysis did not corroborate an association of diabetes-related deaths with combined sulfonylurea and metformin therapy although the confidence intervals were wide.' Check the patient every 2–3 months until glycaemic targets are met.

Pioglitazone may be added to either metformin or sulfonylurea, or to both for triple therapy.

Incretin-effect enhancers can also be used as the second drug if either metformin or sulfonylurea is insufficient, not tolerated, or not appropriate, or as the third drug with a combination of metformin and sulfonylurea. GLP-1 mimetics are particularly helpful in overweight patients, or in those in whom weight gain is an issue. SGLT2 inhibitors can be added to metformin or insulin in type 2 diabetes, or used as triple therapy.

Do not continue treatment that is not working despite the patient taking it regularly. If an appropriately adjusted anti-diabetic drug is not achieving desired glucose-lowering by 6 months, stop it.

See international guidance: Diab Care 2012;**35**:1364–79; DOI: 10.2337/dc12-0413. Check BNF and see the following sections. There is a risk of hypoglycaemia every time another glucose lowering drug is added.

Right drug, right patient

- *Overweight* Metformin, incretin-effect enhancers
- *Very symptomatic* Sulfonylureas, then add others
- *Need short-acting preparation* Meglitinides, tolbutamide
- *Need flexible dose for variable meals* Meglitinides
- *Drives for a living, dangerous job or leisure activity:* Metformin, consider incretin-effect enhancer (see DVLA guidance, ➲ pp. 395–9)
- *Gastrointestinal problems* Sulfonylureas
- *Problems remembering medication* Once-daily preparations, e.g. modified release, combined preparations

- *Hypoglycaemia* Metformin or SGLT inhibitor as monotherapy, incretin-effect enhancer
- *Fasting hypoglycaemia on sulfonylureas* Metformin, pioglitazone, meglitinides, incretin-effect enhancer, SGLT inhibitor

High-risk patients

This list is not exhaustive.

- *Problems learning about, recognizing, or treating hypoglycaemia* Any patient with these problems should be given metformin if possible. Add incretin-effect enhancer or SGLT inhibitor if needed. Use other agents with care to avoid hypoglycaemia.
- *Old age* Start on a small dose and increase it cautiously. Start with metformin. If sulfonylurea is needed, tolbutamide or glipizide are short-acting and perhaps safer. Gliclazide may also be used but is longer-acting. Emphasize the need for regular meals. Newer agents generally lack prolonged experience in older people and most SPCs advise caution ➲ pp. 362–3.
- *Cardiac disease* Metformin may rarely cause lactic acidosis in severe cardiac failure or hypotension. Pioglitazone contraindicated. β-Blockers can reduce symptoms of hypoglycaemia. Diuretics reduce the glucose-lowering effect. ACE inhibitors may cause hypoglycaemia. Avoid SGLT2 inhibitors in cardiac failure. Use insulin in patients with acute myocardial infarction (➲ pp. 428–9).
- *Renal disease* Most glucose-lowering agents are potentially hazardous in patients with renal impairment. Long-acting versions should rarely be used. Metformin is contraindicated in severe renal impairment. Sulfonylureas (or active metabolites) such as glibenclamide or glimepiride can accumulate in renal failure. Glipizide and gliclazide are metabolised in the liver, with little urinary excretion of active compounds, so are safer. Linagliptin does not require dose adjustment in renal disease. The dose should be reduced in chronic kidney disease (CKD) stage ≥ 3 for the other DPP-4 inhibitors. Exenatide and lixisenatide should be used with care for CKD 3 and not used in CKD ≥ 4. Liraglutide should not be used in CKD stage ≥ 3. Pioglitazone can be used in renal failure, although not in dialysis patients. Do not start SGLT2 inhibitors if eGFR is < 60. Insulin is excreted in urine—reduce the dose substantially as renal failure worsens.
- *Hepatic disease* The liver is involved in the metabolism and/or excretion of all sulfonylureas, so these are usually avoided. Pioglitazone can worsen liver function (although some diabetologists have been using it in patients with fatty liver–non-alcoholic steatohepatitis (NASH) (➲ p. 290). Metformin is contraindicated as lactic acid accumulation can occur in hepatic decompensation. Alcohol excess can predispose to lactic acidosis. Reduce the dose of dapagliflozin, and avoid canagliflozin and empagliflozin in severe liver disease. SPCs do not warn against GLP-1 agonists in liver disease; these drugs have been shown to improve non-alcoholic fatty liver disease (NAFLD) (➲ p. 290) although are not licensed for this. DPP-4 inhibitors should be reduced in mild/moderate liver disease and avoided in severe liver impairment. Patients with

severe hepatic disease are usually treated with insulin and great care (in an alcoholic, for example, this can be difficult and risks hypoglycaemia).

- *Gastrointestinal disease* Any condition which could seriously impair absorption of oral medication is an indication for insulin therapy. Avoid metformin and incretin-effect enhancers as they have gastrointestinal side effects. Avoid acarbose in patients with gastrointestinal disease. Cimetidine interacts with both metformin and sulfonylureas.
- *Arthritis* Anti-inflammatory drugs, including aspirin, can also potentiate the hypoglycaemic effect of sulfonylureas.
- *Anticoagulant treatment* May displace sulfonylureas from protein binding and potentiate their action, and vice versa.
- **Allergy to sulfonamides** Precludes the use of sulfonylureas.
- *Porphyria* Do not give sulfonylureas.
- *Galactose intolerance* Avoid all tablets which contain lactose.

⚠ Drug Interactions

Many drugs can increase or decrease the hypoglycaemic effects of diabetes medications; e.g. the hypoglycaemic effect of repaglinide may be enhanced by trimethoprim. Manufacturers advise avoid concomitant use (Table 8.2). Diabetes drugs may interfere with the effects of other medication; e.g. exenatide may enhance the effect of warfarin, SGLT2 inhibitors may increase the diuretic effects of diuretics. Check the BNF list before prescribing.

Biguanide—metformin

See Box 8.2.

Suggested mechanisms of action
- Reduces gluconeogenesis and hence liver glucose release
- Enhances glucose uptake and utilization by tissues
- Reduces appetite
- Reduces glucose absorption from the gut
- Does not enhance pancreatic insulin production

Beneficial effects
- Lowers the blood glucose towards normal but is very unlikely to cause hypoglycaemia as monotherapy
- Prevents/delays onset of diabetes in patients with impaired glucose tolerance (evidence-based but unlicensed use)
- May prevent weight gain or even help reduce weight
- In polycystic ovary syndrome (unlicensed use unless patient also diabetic) may improve ovulation and hirsutism—but probably will not
- May improve NASH
- Possible lipid-lowering effect

Indications
- Uncontrolled glucose in type 2 diabetes alone or in combination.
- Consider metformin as the initial treatment for any type 2 diabetic patient, but particularly:
  - *obese patients* because metformin may reduce appetite and may be less likely to cause weight gain than sulfonylureas.
  - *vocational drivers* of large goods vehicles, passenger-carrying vehicles, and trains should be started on metformin because of the minimal risk of hypoglycaemia.
  - *those who operate hazardous machinery, or others in whom hypoglycaemia would be especially dangerous.*
  - *older patients*: consider metformin because of the reduced risk of hypoglycaemia, but beware the rare risk of lactic acidosis in those with cardiac, renal, or hepatic disease.
  - *Polycystic ovary disease with diabetes* (→ pp. 334–5); used but not licensed for polycystic ovary disease without diabetes).
  - Metformin may also be added to the usual insulin treatment in type 1 diabetic patients whose glucose is high, especially if they are overweight.
  - Metformin has been used in children (see BNF for children).

Pregnancy: metformin has been shown to be as safe as insulin in gestational diabetes and metformin was preferred by patients. (*N Engl J Med* 2008; **358**:2003–15; doi: 10.1056/NEJMoa0707193); and has been used to stimulate ovulation in polycystic ovarian disease. NICE CG 63 states: 'Metformin is used in UK clinical practice in the management of diabetes in pregnancy and lactation. There is strong evidence for its effectiveness and safety. This evidence is not currently reflected in the SPC . . . The SPC advises that when a patient plans to become pregnant and during pregnancy, diabetes should not be treated with metformin but insulin should be used to maintain blood glucose levels. Informed consent on the use of metformin in these situations should be obtained and documented.' (➲ pp. 339–40)

Breastfeeding: NICE CG 63 states: '[m]etformin is used in UK clinical practice in the management of diabetes in pregnancy and lactation. There is strong evidence for its effectiveness and safety. This evidence is not currently reflected in the SPC . . . The SPC advises that metformin is contraindicated in lactation. Informed consent on the use of metformin during lactation should be obtained and documented.'

Contraindications

- Type 1 diabetes unless on insulin; DKA
- Kidney disease: contraindicated if creatinine > 130 micromol (NICE) or creatinine clearance < 60 ml/min (SPCs). Metformin is increasingly used off licence in patients with kidney disease. The NICE pathway 'Blood glucose-lowering therapy for Type 2 diabetes' advises reviewing the dose if estimated glomerular filtration rate (eGFR) < 45 and avoiding metformin if eGFR < 30 (see also BNF). A recent US review (*Diabetes Care*, 2011; **34**: 1431–7; doi: 10.2337/dc10-2361) recommended the following:
  - eGFR ≥ 60—continue metformin, annual eGFR
  - eGFR < 60 and ≥ 45—continue metformin, eGFR every 3–6 mths
  - eGFR < 45 and ≥ 30—prescribe metformin with caution, reduce dose, e.g. by 50 % or half maximal dose; do not start new patients on metformin; monitor eGFR every 3 mths
  - eGFR < 30—stop metformin
  - additional caution is required in patients at risk of acute kidney injury or fluctuations in renal function
- Conditions risking acidosis, e.g. low blood pressure, hypoxia, shock, dehydration, severe cardiac or respiratory disease. However, an observational study showed that 'metformin, alone or in combination, in subjects with heart failure and type 2 diabetes was associated with lower morbidity and mortality compared with sulfonylurea monotherapy.' (*Diabetes Care* 2005; **28**:2345–51; doi:10.2337/diacare.28.10.2345) (➲ pp. 255–6)
- Alcohol excess or alcoholism
- Liver dysfunction
- Radiological investigations using injected contrast media which could cause kidney dysfunction—stop the metformin before the procedure and restart 48 hrs later after checking renal function
- Gastrointestinal disease (e.g. ulcerative colitis) where it could precipitate or worsen symptoms
- Warfarin dose may need to be adjusted
- Cimetidine reduces renal clearance of metformin

Dosage

Standard release (non-proprietary metformin)

- 500 mg or 850 mg tablets.
- Start gradually to reduce likelihood of gastrointestinal side effects.
- Gastrointestinal side effects may settle if a low dose is continued for a few weeks.
- Prescribe metformin 500 mg daily with breakfast, increased by 500 mg every 10–15 days according to fasting blood glucose (SMBG or laboratory).
- Usual dosage range is 500–2000 mg/day in divided doses *after meals.*
- The manufacturers state a maximum dose of 3000 mg daily.
- Metformin is also available as a sugar-free oral solution 500 mg/5 ml.

Modified-release

- 500 mg daily, increased every 10–15 days if required.
- Maximum 2 g once daily with evening meal, or 1 g twice daily.
- Change to standard release if target glucose not reached.
- May have fewer gastrointestinal side effects than standard-release metformin.

Tests

- Before starting check renal function.
- On treatment check:
  - vitamin B12 and folate levels annually in patients on ≥ 1500 mg/day
  - plasma creatinine or eGFR annually in patients without renal impairment, and at least 6-monthly in those with impairment (see test described)

Side effects

- Poor appetite
- Nausea and vomiting
- Diarrhoea (which may be severe)
- Abdominal discomfort, cramp, or pain
- Unpleasant or metallic taste
- Extremely rare: lactic acidosis (in alcohol excess, or elderly with renal impairment, hypotension, or hypoxia); requires immediate admission, often to intensive care unit (ICU) or high dependency unit (HDU). Stop metformin and avoid in future. Doubt has been cast on whether metformin actually causes lactic acidosis ℘ <http://www.bibliotecacochrane.com/pdf/CD002967.pdf>
- Decreased vitamin B12 absorption (up to 30 % of patients on high-dose or long-term treatment (*Arch Intern Med.* 2006; **166**:1975–9; doi:10.1001/archinte.166.18.1975)
- Decreased folate absorption
- Skin: erythema, pruritus, and urticaria
- Liver: hepatitis

Interactions

- The following drugs may interact with metformin: ACE inhibitors, alcohol, cimetidine, disopyramide, ketotifen (avoid concomitant use), MAOIs, rilpivirine, topiramate.

Box 8.2 Information for patients on metformin

Your diabetes tablets are called metformin.

    Take. . . . . mg (. . . tablet) with or after breakfast;

    Take. . . . . mg (. . . tablet) with or after lunch;

    Take. . . . . mg (. . . tablet) with or after main evening meal.

Metformin will help your diabetes diet to control your blood glucose level. It will only help you to lose weight if you stick to a weight-reducing diet.

The tablets will work only if you take them regularly as prescribed!

If you are too unwell to take your tablets for any reason contact your doctor or diabetes nurse immediately.

If you cannot eat, or are vomiting, do not take your tablets but contact your doctor or diabetes nurse immediately.

Occasionally metformin can cause stomach and bowel upsets, but these are often temporary and less likely if treatment is started gradually. Never exceed your alcohol limit (ask your doctor what this should be)—excess alcohol could make you very ill. Large doses of metformin may cause anaemia by reducing vitamin B12 and folate absorption. If you take 1500 g or more a day have an annual blood count and B12 and folate check. Patients with severe kidney trouble should not take metformin. Ensure that your doctor checks your kidney function regularly.

Over the years your diabetes may slowly progress. As your pancreas 'wears out', the tablets may become less effective. Some people may need insulin injections eventually. You may also need insulin temporarily if you are ill or have an operation.

Although your diabetes does not need insulin treatment at present you must take just as much care of yourself in general as someone on insulin injections. There is no such thing as mild diabetes. Your doctor will help you to stay well.

Carry a diabetes card with you.

Sulfonylureas

See Box 8.3.

Names
- Glibenclamide, gliclazide, glimepiride, glipizide, tolbutamide

Mechanisms of action
- Enhancement of glucose-stimulated pancreatic insulin release
- May reduce glucagon release
- May reduce liver glucose release and increase glucose uptake in peripheral tissues

Beneficial actions
- Reduces glucose and improves HbA$_{1c}$
- Long-term outcome data, e.g. for glibenclamide (UKPDS (➲ pp. 40–1) and gliclazide modified-release (ADVANCE (➲ pp. 40–1)

The drugs, their dosage, and approximate duration of action are shown in Table 8.1. Start with a small dose. Adjust the dose of sulfonylurea every 2 weeks according to SMBG.

Indications
Uncontrolled glucose in type 2 diabetes—alone or in combination. Sulfonylureas are used to treat monogenic diabetes (MODY) associated with HNF1–α (➲ p. 17).

Table 8.1 Dosage for sulfonylureas

Name	Dosage range per 24 hrs	Dosage frequency
Glibenclamide*	2.5–15 mg	Once daily after breakfast
Gliclazide*	40–160 mg	Once daily with breakfast
	160–320 mg	Divided doses with meal
Gliclazide* m/r	30–120 mg	Once daily with breakfast
Glimepiride	1–4 mg (rarely 6 mg)	Once daily before/with 1st main meal
Glipizide*	2.5–15 mg	Once daily pre breakfast or lunch
	15–20 mg	Divided doses pre meals
Tolbutamide	500–2000 mg	Once to three times daily with or immediately after meal

*Non-proprietary version available.
UK names shown, names vary world-wide.

Which sulfonylurea?

The one you are used to.

- *Gliclazide* is widely used. There is good long-term efficacy and long-term safety evidence.
- *Glibenclamide* is still commonly used worldwide, although less so in the UK. The glucose-lowering effect may last > 24 hrs, especially in renal impairment. Glibenclamide may cause profound or prolonged hypoglycaemia even at low dose. It is the commonest cause of hypoglycaemia due to oral agents and 83 % more likely to do so than other sulfonylureas (*Diabetes Care* 2007; **30**:389–94; doi: 10.2337/dc06-1789. One in three patients taking glibenclamide experiences hypoglycaemia.
- *Tolbutamide* is short-acting and can be linked to meals to allow some patients flexibility in dosage—small meal, small dose; big meal, big dose. Tolbutamide treatment was linked to cardiac events in a 1970s study, but these conclusions have been questioned since.
- *Glipizide* can also be linked to meals.
- *Glimepiride* can cause hypoglycaemia but is less likely to do so than other sulfonylureas (see *Diabetes Care* 2007 reference above).

Contraindications and cautions

- Type 1 diabetes or DKA
- Pregnancy (except glibenclamide in 2nd and 3rd trimester (➲ pp. 339–40))
- Avoid in women of childbearing potential unless using contraception
- Breastfeeding
- Allergy to sulfonamides
- During surgery (➲ p. 434)
- Serious infections
- Caution in renal dysfunction
- Caution in hepatic dysfunction
- Some drug interactions with sulfonylureas are outlined in Table 8.2
- Manufacturers state that these drugs should not be used in children, but with increasing type 2 diabetes in the under-18s, sulfonylureas are being used off-licence in this age group
- Porphyria
- G6PD deficiency

Tests

Before starting and on treatment, check:

- Renal function
- Liver function
- Cardiovascular disease?

Side effects

- Hypoglycaemia
- Weight gain
- Allergic rashes
- Gastrointestinal disturbances (usually mild) such as anorexia, nausea and vomiting, altered bowel habit
- Reduction in platelets and white cells, or aplastic anaemia (rare)

- Alcohol flushing
- Hepatic dysfunction, rarely severe
- Hyponatraemia (especially with glimepiride and glipizide)

A review and meta-analysis in 2013 suggested that sulfonylureas may increase the risk of CVD, both cardiovascular events and mortality. The study included different sulfonylureas. In studies where different hypo-glycaemic therapies were compared, the overall cardiovascular risk with sulfonylureas was greater than that of patients taking metformin although similar to those on thiazolidinediones. The studies included patients with and without known CVD. It would seem sensible to optimize metformin use wherever possible and to consider avoiding sulfonylureas in patients with significant cardiovascular disease if there are other options (*Diab Med* 2013; **30**:1160–71; doi: 10.1111/dme.12232).

Table 8.2 Some possible drug interactions with sulfonylureas

	Lower blood glucose	Raise blood glucose
General	Alcohol	
Antimicrobials	Chloramphenicol Co-trimoxazole Miconazole Fluconazole Posaconazole Voriconazole Sulfonamides Ciprofloxacin Norfloxacin Ritonavir Tetracyclines	Rifampicin
Cardiovascular	β-Blockers (+ reduce hypo warning) ACE inhibitors Fibrates Fluvastatin Disopyramide	Diazoxide Loop diuretics Thiazides (risk of low sodium) Nifedipine
Anticoagulant	Warfarin	
Gastrointestinal	H_2 antagonists	Aprepitant Colesevelam
Endocrine/ metabolic	Octreotide Lanreotide Pasireotide Testosterone	Corticosteroids Oestrogens Progestogens Contraceptives
Joints	Aspirin Phenylbutazone NSAIDs Sulfinpyrazone Azapropazone Leflunomide	
Psychiatric or Neurological	MAOIs	Lithium Phenobarbital Tricyclics (+ postural ↓BP) Phenothiazines Topiramate

This list changes–see the British National Formulary for an up-to-date list.

Tolbutamide increases phenytoin blood levels.

Box 8.3　Information for patients on sulfonylurea tablets

Your diabetes tablets are called...

They belong to a family of medicines called sulfonylureas.

Take. . . . . .mg (. . . . . .tablet(s)) with breakfast;

Take. . . . . .mg (. . . . . .tablet(s)) with lunch;

Take. . . . . .mg (. . . . . .tablet(s)) with main evening meal.

The tablets will help your diabetic diet to control your blood glucose level.

The tablets will work only if you take them regularly as prescribed!

If you are too unwell to take your tablets for any reason contact your doctor or diabetes nurse immediately.

If you cannot eat, or are vomiting, do not take your tablets but contact your doctor or diabetes nurse immediately.

Side effects are usually mild and infrequent, and include stomach or bowel upset and headache. Allergic rashes, jaundice, and blood problems occur rarely.

These tablets work by reducing the blood glucose. Sometimes the blood glucose may fall too low (i.e. below 4 mmol/l). This is called hypoglycaemia and may happen if you are taking too big a dose, eat too little, or exercise more than you expect. If you feel muddled, slow-thinking, tingly, unduly emotional or cross, sweaty, or shaky, or notice your heart thumping fast, eat some glucose, then have a big snack. Contact your doctor or diabetes nurse. You may need to reduce your dose of tablets.

Over the years your diabetes may slowly progress. As your pancreas 'wears out' the tablets may become less effective. Some people may need insulin injections eventually. You may also need insulin temporarily if you are ill or have an operation.

Although your diabetes does not need insulin treatment at present you must take just as much care of yourself in general as someone on insulin injections. There is no such thing as mild diabetes. Your doctor will help you to stay well.

Always carry a diabetes card and some glucose with you.

Meglitinides (prandial glucose regulators)

Names
Nateglinide, repaglinide.

Mechanism of action
Also known as prandial glucose regulators. Stimulate insulin release from pancreas by acting on β-cell receptors.

Beneficial effects
- Glucose-lowering
- Rapid absorption from gut with rapid action and duration
- Reduced likelihood of hypoglycaemia especially overnight

Indications
- Uncontrolled glucose in type 2 diabetes
- Repaglinide—alone or combined with metformin
- Nateglinide only in combination with metformin

Contraindications
- Pregnancy
- Avoid in women of child-bearing potential unless using contraception
- Breastfeeding
- < 18 yrs of age
- > 75 yrs of age
- Debilitated or malnourished patients
- Severe renal impairment
- Severe hepatic impairment
- During surgery—stop that morning, restart with normal eating.
- Do not combine with sulfonylureas

Interactions
Repaglinide may interact with gemfibrozil, causing severe hypoglycaemia. Avoid the combination. Repaglinide may also interact with ciclosporin, clarithromycin, itraconazole, trimethoprim, octreotide, lanreotide, and rifampicin. See Table 8.2—many interactions are similar.

Interactions for nateglinide include fluconazole, gemfibrozil, rifampicin, ACE inhibitors, and drugs which inhibit cytochrome P450.

Dosage
Repaglinide
- Start with 500 mcg within 30 min before main meals
- If transferring from another glucose-lowering drug, start with 1 mg of repaglinide before each main meal; adjust the dose every 1–2 weeks according to SMBG
- Maximum single dose, 4 mg
- Maximum total dose in 24 hrs, 16 mg

Nateglinide
- Start with 60 mg, within 30 min before breakfast, lunch, and evening meal
- Adjust the dose every 1–2 weeks according to SMBG
- Maximum dose 180 mg three times daily

Tests

Before starting and on treatment check:
- Renal function
- Liver function

Side-effects

- Hypoglycaemia can occur (glucose will stimulate further insulin release so continue monitoring; further glucose and food as necessary for 6 hrs)
- Gastrointestinal: nausea and vomiting, abdominal pain, altered bowel habit
- Rash, pruritus, urticaria
- Vasculitis
- Visual disturbance
- Transient elevation in liver enzymes; it would seem prudent to stop the drug if liver enzymes rise > 3 x ULN (upper limit of normal)

Thiazolidinedione—pioglitazone

Mechanisms of action

Peroxisome-proliferator-activated receptor-gamma (PPAR-γ) agonists like pioglitazone reduce the body's resistance to insulin action. PPAR-γ has multiple effects on the body, including influencing production of osteoblasts in the bone marrow. Troglitazone and rosiglitazone were withdrawn because of adverse effects.

The CVD effects of pioglitazone vs placebo were studied in PROactive. Pioglitazone did not reduce primary CVD endpoints but did reduce secondary endpoints (total mortality, myocardial infarct, stroke) despite increasing heart failure. (*Lancet* 2005; **366**:1279–89; doi:10.1016/S0140-6736(05)67528-9). It was suggested that this was not solely due to improving blood pressure, lipids and glycaemia; this theory was questioned (*Lancet* 2006; **367**:25–6; doi:10.1016/S0140-6736(06)67914-2).

There has been increasing concern about the non-glucose effects of pioglitazone particularly the increased risk of heart failure, bladder cancer, and in women, fracture. In 2011 the European Medicines Agency stated: '[p]ioglitazone remains a valid treatment option for certain patients with type 2 diabetes, but only when certain other treatments (metformin) have not been suitable or have failed to work adequately.'

Beneficial effects

- Reduction in glucose and HbA$_{1c}$

Indications

- Uncontrolled type 2 diabetes only
- Alone only if metformin is inappropriate, especially if patient is overweight
- With metformin if sulfonylureas inappropriate
- With a sulfonylurea if metformin inappropriate
- With both metformin and a sulfonylurea as triple therapy
- With insulin in metformin-inappropriate patients (with care)

Contraindications and cautions

- Elderly patients—caution
- Pregnancy—avoid
- Avoid in women of child-bearing potential unless using contraception
- Women with polycystic ovarian disease not using contraception (may stimulate ovulation)
- Breastfeeding—avoid
- Ischaemic heart disease or other heart condition—caution
- Cardiac failure past or present—avoid
- Insulin treatment—greater risk of heart failure—caution
- Hepatic impairment—**alanine aminotransferase** (ALT) > 2.5 × ULN—avoid
- Severe renal impairment—risk of fluid retention
- Bladder cancer past or present—avoid
- Uninvestigated haematuria—avoid

- Risk factors for bladder cancer—e.g. elderly, smoker, family history of bladder cancer, occupational, pelvic irradiation—caution ℜ <http://www.cancerresearchuk.org/cancer-info/cancerstats/types/bladder/riskfactors/bladder-cancer-risk-factors>
- Macular oedema—caution
- Surgery—stop that morning
- Osteoporosis—caution
- May interact with sulfonylureas, meglitinides, NSAIDs, paclitaxel, gemfibrozil, rifampicin, and other inducers or inhibitors of cytochrome P450 2C8 (e.g. cerivastatin, repaglinide, carbamazepine, cyclophosphamide, montelukast, omeprazole, phenytoin, trimethoprim, warfarin)
- Do not combine with dapagliflozin (➲ pp. 139–40)

Dosage

- Pioglitazone 15–30 mg once daily, increasing to 45 mg once daily if necessary (use lowest dose with slow increments in elderly)
- Combination preparations with metformin are available

Tests

- Before starting check:
  - history or risk of bladder cancer
  - weight
  - cardiac function (for risk of failure or ischaemic event)—caution
  - liver function
  - full blood count
  - renal function (avoid if eGFR < 10)
  - calcium and vitamin D or presence of osteoporosis
  - urine—for haematuria
  - Warn patients to report jaundice, abdominal pain, nausea, vomiting, urinary symptoms including dark urine or blood in urine, breathlessness, oedema, blurred vision, rapid weight gain
- On treatment check patient at ≤ 3 mths, 6 mths, and regularly thereafter
  - weight
  - heart failure—signs and symptoms
  - liver function (stop if ALT > 3× ULN)
  - urine for blood

N.B. Stop pioglitazone if HbA$_{1c}$ has not fallen by at least 5 mmol/l (0.5 %) within 6 mths (NICE CG87).

Side effects

- Hypoglycaemia (in combination therapy)
- Oedema, especially when used with insulin
- Myocardial infarction (under debate at time of writing)
- Cardiac failure (especially when combined with insulin)
- Fractures
- Anaemia
- Weight gain
- Headache
- Gastrointestinal symptoms

- Upper respiratory symptoms
- Abnormal vision—macular oedema
- Arthralgia
- Dizziness or vertigo
- Fatigue, insomnia
- Altered sensation
- Sweating
- Erectile dysfunction
- Altered lipids
- Lactic acidosis
- Women with polycystic ovary syndrome may ovulate as insulin resistance is reduced—risk of pregnancy. Pioglitazone is contraindicated in pregnancy.
- Hepatic dysfunction: stop if liver enzymes are > 3× ULN.

Incretin-effect enhancers

Incretins enhance glucose-induced insulin secretion. GLP-1 is an incretin which is broken down within minutes by DPP-4. GLP-1 receptor agonists are similar to human GLP-1 but last longer. DPP-4 inhibitors block the breakdown of human GLP-1. Thus, both types of drug increase insulin secretion in response to raised glucose levels.

There has been concern that these drugs may have adverse pancreatic effects. The FDA and EMA 'agree that assertions concerning a causal association between incretin-based drugs and pancreatitis or pancreatic cancer ... are inconsistent with the current data. The FDA and EMA have not reached a final conclusion at this time regarding such a causal relationship. Although the totality of the data that have been reviewed provides reassurance, pancreatitis will continue to be considered a risk associated with these drugs until more data are available'. (N Eng J Med 2014; **370** (9):794–6. DOI: 10.1056/NEJMp1314078) Patients should be warned of this rare risk and told to report severe abdominal pain ± vomiting immediately. Check the BNF before prescribing these drugs as it is updated regularly.

The dose of sulfonlyurea or insulin may need to be reduced on starting an incretin-effect enhancer.

Glucagon-like peptide-1 receptor agonists
Names
Exenatide, liraglutide, lixisenatide

Mechanism of action
- Injectable incretin peptide mimetic. Acts like GLP-1 to enhance glucose-dependent insulin secretion by the pancreatic beta cells
- Reduces glucagon production
- Slows gastric emptying
- Satiety

Beneficial effects
- Improves glycaemic control when added to metformin ± sulfonylurea
- When used alone is unlikely to cause hypoglycaemia
- Weight loss—particularly suitable for seriously overweight patients otherwise requiring insulin

Indications
- Combined with metformin ± sulfonylureas—not alone
- In patients with type 2 diabetes whose glucose is not controlled on maximally tolerated doses of metformin ± sulfonylureas

Contraindications
- Pregnancy
- Avoid in women of child-bearing potential unless using contraception
- Breastfeeding
- < 18 yrs old
- Severe renal impairment (eGFR < 30)
- Severe gastrointestinal disease, gastroparesis

- Previous pancreatitis
- Gallstones
- Very high triglycerides

Cautions

- Caution in > 75-yr-olds
- eGFR 30–50
- Caution in underweight patients
- Interactions—warfarin, statins

Dosage

Table 8.3 shows the dosages of a number of incretin-effect enhancers.

Side effects
Check BNF or SPC for individual drugs

- Hypoglycaemia is increased in patients on sulfonylureas or insulin
- Nausea and vomiting
- Gastrointestinal symptoms: anorexia, dyspepsia, reflux, abdominal pain, abdominal distension, diarrhoea, constipation, flatulence, burping, impaired taste
- Weight loss

Table 8.3 Incretin-effect enhancers: GLP-1 receptor agonists (check BNF for details)

Drug	Dosage range	Dose frequency	Licensed combinations	Comments
Exenatide*	5–10 micrograms	Twice daily**	Metformin Insulin Pioglitazone Sulfonylurea	1 hr before meals, at least 6 hrs apart Never after food Increase dose after 1 mth
Exenatide modified release	2 mg	Once a week**	Metformin Pioglitazone Sulfonylurea	Effect may last 10 wks after stopping
Liraglutide*	0.6–1.8 mg daily	Once daily**	Metformin Pioglitazone Sulfonylurea	Increase dose after 1 wk NICE TA203 does not recommend 1.8 mg
Lixisenatide*	10–20 micrograms	Once daily**	Metformin Insulin Pioglitazone Sulfonylurea	1 hr before breakfast or evening meal Never after food Increase dose after 2 wks

* Do not give drugs whose action depends on gastric emptying within 1 hr of injection. Wait until >4 hrs after.

**All injected subcutaneously via a pre-filled pen.

- Slowed gastric emptying may delay absorption of other drugs—this may affect lipid levels.
- Dizziness
- Drowsiness
- Headache
- Pancreatitis
- Anaphylaxis
- Injection site reaction, rash, urticaria, pruritus, angioneurotic oedema
- Agitation (exenatide)
- Sweating (exenatide)
- Renal impairment (exenatide)
- Fever (liraglutide)
- Bronchitis, nasopharyngitis (liraglutide)
- Thyroid neoplasm, goitre, increased calcitonin (liraglutide)
- Palpitation, tachycardia (lixisenatide)

Dipeptidylpeptidase-4 (DPP-4) inhibitors

Names
Alogliptin, linagliptin, saxagliptin, sitagliptin, vildagliptin

Mechanism of action
- Inhibits clearance of the incretin GLP-1, thus increasing the amount available to stimulate glucose-stimulated insulin secretion
- Reduces glucagon release
- May slow gastric emptying

Beneficial effects
- Improves glycaemic control when added to metformin, pioglitazone or sulfonylurea
- Used alone are unlikely to cause hypoglycaemia

Indications
- Combined with metformin, pioglitazone or sulfonylurea
- Type 2 diabetic patients whose glucose is not controlled on metformin, pioglitazone or sulfonylurea alone
- Patients intolerant of metformin, pioglitazone or sulfonylurea

Contraindications
Check specific drug in BNF.
- Type 1 diabetes
- Pregnancy
- Breastfeeding
- < 18 yrs of age
- > 75 years of age—care—evidence needed
- Cardiac failure
- Renal impairment—adjust dose (Table 8.4)—except linagliptin
- Liver impairment (reduce in mild impairment, avoid in severe impairment)
- Previous pancreatitis
- Gallstones
- Very high triglycerides

Table 8.4 Incretin-effect enhancers: DPP-4 inhibitors (check BNF for details)

Drug	Dosage range	Dose frequency	Licensed combinations	Comments
Alogliptin	6.25–25 mg	Once daily	Metformin Insulin Pioglitazone Sulfonylurea[1]	eGFR 30–50 reduce to 12.5 mg daily eGFR < 30 reduce dose to 6.25 mg daily with caution Monitor LFTs
Linagliptin	5 mg	Once daily	Metformin Insulin Sulfonylurea	No dose adjustment in renal impairment
Saxagliptin	2.5–5 mg	Once daily	Metformin Insulin Pioglitazone Sulfonylurea	Moderate renal impairment reduce dose to 2.5 mg daily Severe renal impairment use with caution
Sitagliptin	25–100 mg	Once daily	Metformin Insulin Pioglitazone Sulfonylurea	eGFR 30–50 reduce to 50 mg daily eGFR < 30 reduce dose to 25 mg daily
Vildagliptin	50 mg	Twice daily	Metformin Insulin Pioglitazone Sulfonylurea	Monitor LFTs. Warn patients of liver disease symptoms to report. If eGFR < 50 reduce to 50 mg once daily

[1]not in triple therapy.

Dosage

Dose of sulfonylurea or insulin may need to be reduced to avoid hypoglycaemia.

Side effects

- Nausea, vomiting, anorexia, dyspepsia, gastritis, abdominal pain, altered bowel habit
- Weight loss
- Pancreatitis
- Nasopharyngitis, upper respiratory tract infection, sinusitis, cough
- Headache
- Oedema
- Dizziness
- Rash or skin reactions, hypersensitivity, angio-oedema, urticaria, anaphylaxis
- Myalgia, arthralgia
- Hepatic dysfunction; monitor liver function tests (LFTs) (alogliptin, vildagliptin)
- Tremor (vildagliptin)
- Drowsiness (sitagliptin)
- UTI (saxagliptin)
- Raised triglycerides or dyslipidaemia (saxagliptin)
- Erectile dysfunction (saxagliptin)

SGLT2 inhibitors

SGLT2 inhibitors are a relatively new class of drugs still finding their place in the management of type 2 diabetes. Large-scale long-term study results are awaited.

Names

Canagliflozin, dapagliflozin, empagliflozin

Mechanism of action

Reduce glucose reabsorption in the proximal renal tubule thus increasing urinary glucose excretion. Also reduce gut glucose absorption.

Beneficial effects

- Glucose-lowering
- Weight loss (removes some glucose calories)
- May lower BP
- Hypoglycaemia unlikely unless combined with sulfonylurea or insulin

Indications

Canagliflozin, dapagliflozin, and empagliflozin are licensed for monotherapy or added to other glucose-lowering agents including insulin. Large scale studies of every possible combination are not available. All three SGLT2 inhibitors have been studied with metformin, sulfonylureas, and insulin; canagliflozin and empagliflozin have been studied with pioglitazone; canagliflozin and dapagliflozin have been studied with DPP-4 inhibitors (check for updates).

NICE TA 288 (dapagliflozin) advises, for type 2 diabetes, if glucose control is inadequate:

- adding to metformin if significant risk of hypoglycaemia or sulfonylurea inappropriate or;
- add to insulin, with or without other antidiabetic drugs
- do not give with pioglitazone (might theoretically increase bladder cancer risk)

A NICE technology appraisal is in progress for canagliflozin, dapagliflozin, and empagliflozin.

Contraindications

- Pregnancy
- Breastfeeding
- < 18 yrs of age
- > 75 yrs of age (dapagliflozin), >85 yrs of age empagliflozin
- ≥ 65 yrs of age consider renal function and risk of volume depletion (canagliflozin, empagliflozin)
- Severe liver impairment
- Renal impairment eGFR <60 (patients already on canagliflozin may continue at 100 mg daily; stop the drug if eGFR <45)
- Cardiac failure (limited experience)
- Volume-depleted or dehydrated patients (correct this first)
- Patients on loop diuretics
- Patients at risk of hypotension

- Patients with current or recurrent urinary tract infections
- Patients with active bladder cancer (FDA)
- Patients with elevated haematocrit

Dosage

- Consider reducing insulin or other antidiabetic drug doses to avoid hypoglycaemia
- Dapagliflozin 10 mg once daily (any time)
- Canagliflozin:
  - 100 mg once daily before the first meal of the day
  - If eGFR is ≥ 60 and glucose control is inadequate increase dose gradually to 300 mg daily
  - Take care when increasing the dose in patients ≥ 75 yrs old or those with CVD
- Empagliflozin
  - 10 mg once daily
  - If eGFR is ≥60 and glucose control is inadequage increase dose to 25 mg daily

Side effects (See SPCs)

- May be more likely in patients > 75 yrs of age
- Hypoglycaemia (especially when combined with insulin or sulfonylurea)
- Glycosuria (mechanism of action)
- Genital infections e.g. vulvovaginal candidiasis
- Urinary tract infections
- Thirst, polyuria, nocturia, dysuria
- Back pain
- Dyslipidaemia
- Increased haematocrit
- Nausea
- Dizziness, postural hypotension (may need to adjust hypotensives)
- Rash, pruritus
- Constipation
- Sweating
- Increased urea and creatinine (stop if eGFR < 60)

Interactions

- Enzyme inducers (such as St John's wort, rifampicin, barbiturates, phenytoin, carbamazepine, ritonavir, efavirenz) may reduce canagliflozin effect, as may colestyramine.
- Levels of digoxin, dabigatran, simvastatin and rosuvastatin may increase with canagliflozin although these effects may be small. This may also affect some anticancer drugs—see SPC.
- Similar interactions are possible with dapagliflozin but appear less of an issue (see SPC).
- There appear to be fewer interactions with empagliflozin but see SPC.

Acarbose

Mechanism of action

Acarbose is an α-glucosidase inhibitor which reduces the rate of sucrose digestion in the small intestine so that less glucose is absorbed after a carbohydrate meal. It is little used in the UK.

Beneficial effects

- Glucose-lowering
- Encourages reduced intake of sucrose
- Used alone does not cause hypoglycaemia

Indications

- Alone or in combination in type 2 diabetic patients in whom glucose is not controlled.
- Patients must adhere to a low-sugar (sucrose) diet.

Contraindications

- Pregnancy
- Breastfeeding
- < 18 yrs of age
- Past or present gastrointestinal disorders, e.g. intestinal obstruction, inflammatory bowel disease, colonic ulceration, hernias, any chronic gastrointestinal problem
- Malabsorption
- Patients prone to flatulence or in whom increased flatulence would be problematic
- Liver impairment
- Renal impairment
- Interactions—pancreatic enzymes, neomycin, colestyramine, digoxin
- May interfere with absorption of other drugs

Dosage

- Dose is 50 mg initially, increased to twice a day either chewed with the first mouthful of the meal, or before food with a drink of water. Increase gradually to 50 mg three times a day. The dose can be increased after 6–8 weeks to 100 mg three times daily if necessary. Gradual increase is best.
- Maximum dose 200 mg three times daily. Larger doses should be used with care (see SPC).
- ⚠ Warn patients on drugs which may cause hypoglycaemia (e.g. sulfonylureas) that they may become hypoglycaemic, and that hypoglycaemia must be treated with glucose and not sucrose because the latter will not be digested.

Side effects
- Side effects often preclude long-term use
- Gastrointestinal side effects are common. Most patients experience flatulence, also bloating, flatulence, diarrhoea, and nausea. Because acarbose interferes with carbohydrate metabolism, fermentation is increased. Symptoms are worse if patients eat sugar
- Liver—elevated liver enzymes, jaundice, hepatitis—monitor LFTs
- Skin rashes

Combining glucose-lowering medications
⚠ Adding a new class of glucose-lowering drug can cause hypoglycaemia. Doses of sulfonylurea or insulin should be reduced when a new drug is added.
- Check concordance with existing medication before adding more. More drugs or multiple doses = greater risk of non-concordance. Up to one in two patients do not take their diabetes medication as prescribed.
- Follow NICE guidance—check for updates
- Extra care is required with triple therapy; not all combinations are licensed—check (Table 8.5)
- Licensing may change
- Metformin can usually be combined with any other glucose-lowering drug
- Sulfonylureas can usually be combined with other glucose-lowering drugs except repaglinide or nateglinide
- Repaglinide and nateglinide can only be combined with metformin
- Pioglitazone can be combined with metformin, sulfonylureas; and insulin (⚠ danger of heart failure)
- DPP-4 inhibitors ('gliptins') can be usually combined with metformin, sulfonylureas, insulin, and (except linagliptin) with pioglitazone. Do not combine DPP-4 inhibitors with GLP-1 agonists
- GLP1 agonists ('-atides') can usually be combined with metformin, sulfonylurea, pioglitazone (not lixisenatide), and insulin. Do not combine GLP1 agonists with DPP-4 inhibitors
- SGLT2 inhibitors can be combined with metformin, or sulfonylurea, or insulin. NICE does not recommend combining dapagliflozin with both metformin and sulfonylurea. Check SPCs and NICE updates
- Acarbose can usually be combined with metformin, sulfonylurea or insulin
- Traditionally drugs are added one at a time. Recent research suggests triple therapy from the outset may achieve better glucose lowering. More studies are needed before adopting this approach generally.
- Seek specialist advice if triple therapy does not work

Table 8.5 Licensed combinations in triple therapy
When adding drugs, reduce doses to avoid hypoglycaemia

Metformin	Sulfonylurea	Pioglitazone
Metformin	Sulfonylurea	Saxagliptin
Metformin	Sulfonylurea	Sitagliptin
Metformin	Sulfonylurea	Vildagliptin
Metformin	Sulfonylurea	Exenatide
Metformin	Sulfonylurea	Liraglutide
Metformin	Sulfonylurea	Lixisenatide
Metformin	Sulfonylurea	Insulin
Metformin	Pioglitazone*	Alogliptin
Metformin	Pioglitazone*	Sitagliptin
Metformin	Pioglitazone*	Exenatide
Metformin	Pioglitazone*	Liraglutide
Metformin	Pioglitazone*	Lixisenatide
Metformin	Insulin	Alogliptin
Metformin	Insulin	Sitagliptin
Metformin	Insulin	Vildagliptin
Metformin	Insulin	Exenatide (not SR)
Metformin	Insulin	Lixisenatide
Insulin	Pioglitazone*	Exenatide (not SR)

*These combinations are not in the pioglitazone licence.

SGLT2 inhibitors have been less widely tested in all possible combinations. Their SPCs state that they can be added to other glucose-lowering drugs including insulin. (➲ pp. 139–40).

Monitoring non-insulin therapy

Patient knowledge
- Ask patients to bring their medication to their appointment and show you
- Does the patient know what and how much he/she is taking?
- When should he/she take the medication?
- What is it for?
- What should he/she do if he/she becomes ill?
- What precautions should he/she take?
- Is he/she aware of potential side effects?
- Is the patient on sulfonylureas aware of the risk and symptoms of hypoglycaemia?

Diabetes card? Carrying glucose?
Ask the patient to show it to you.

Hypoglycaemia
Always ask if patients have experienced this.

Blood glucose balance
Check this every 2–3 mths until stable (more frequently in unwell patients or those in whom new treatment has been started for other conditions) and then every 6 mths. A common reason for treatment failure is failing to take the medication. If the blood glucose is persistently above targets for that patient, check adherence to diet, exercise, and medication, and increase or augment hypoglycaemic therapy. If the glucose remains uncontrolled despite maximal non-insulin therapy in an appropriate combination, the patient needs insulin.

⚠ Do not delay insulin injections in a mistaken attempt to be kind. Diabetic tissue damage is not kind.

Clinical state
- Apart from usual tissue damage monitoring, have any conditions arisen which make it inadvisable to continue non-insulin hypoglycaemics?
- Is there any evidence of side effects of treatment?
- Does the medication need changing?
- Check weight in all before and during treatment
- Check cardiac function before starting pioglitazone or metformin, and during treatment

Laboratory monitoring
Continue usual diabetes monitoring. These tests are for specific reasons with all or some hypoglycaemic drugs.
- Before starting hypoglycaemic drugs check the following in everyone unless specified:
  - HbA_{1c}
  - urea and electrolytes

- creatinine (eGFR)
- LFTs (more often on vildagliptin)
- full blood count (metformin, pioglitazone, sulfonylureas)
- lipids (pioglitazone)
- calcium (pioglitazone)
- During treatment:
  - HbA_{1c}
  - urea and electrolytes
  - creatinine (eGFR)
  - liver function (or at least ALT)
  - lipids (pioglitazone)
  - full blood count (pioglitazone, metformin ≥ 1500 mg daily)
  - vitamin B12 + folate (annually in metformin ≥ 1500 mg daily)
  - calcium (pioglitazone, and in metformin with low B12)

Take home message

Write down the dose the patient should be taking and when he/she should be taking it. Remind the patient or rewrite it each visit. Make sure he/she has a copy of the sick day/missed medication rules.

Sick days and missed medication

If the patient misses a tablet he/she should not take double next time! Discuss each case individually. If the error is realized within 2 hrs of the correct time take the missed tablet(s) immediately. In someone on once-daily breakfast-time therapy, the missed tablet(s) could be taken within 4 hrs of the correct time.

If a dose of exenatide or lixisenatide is missed it should **not** be injected after the meal. Wait until the next dose is due and give the prescribed amount (not more).

If the patient has a vomiting illness or severe diarrhoea not only will he be unable to keep his tablets down (or fail to absorb them), but the illness is likely to push his blood glucose concentration up. The patient must contact his doctor immediately. Patients on metformin or incretin-effect enhancers should stop them. Monitor the blood glucose carefully and use insulin to control it. Diabetic patients on non-insulin glucose-lowering treatment who have illnesses severe enough to require hospital admission (e.g. cardiovascular diseases, infections, surgical emergencies) should be changed to insulin treatment until their condition has stabilized and they are eating normally. Some may require long-term insulin.

Keep a particularly careful eye on the blood glucose levels of elderly patients, as vague confusion may indicate hypoglycaemia. Non-specific symptoms can be accompanied by gross metabolic derangement and high glucose levels.

Summary

- Always check the BNF before prescribing medications. Even if the drugs are very familiar, review them when the new edition arrives as information changes.
- Check BNF, NICE, and MHRA websites regularly for updates and warnings.
- Non-insulin hypoglycaemics should be used early if dietary control fails or is unlikely to work.
- Non-insulin hypoglycaemics work only if the patient is making some of their own insulin.
- Non-insulin hypoglycaemics work only if the patient takes them!
- Eventually many patients taking oral hypoglycaemic agents will need insulin.
- Use the drug you are most familiar with, but consider the patient and his/her needs.
- Non-insulin hypoglycaemic drugs can cause hypoglycaemia. Be alert for this as the symptoms may be less clear cut than in insulin-treated patients.
- Use insulin if severe illness occurs.
- Patient education about therapy is as important as in insulin treatment.
- Non-insulin-treated diabetes is not mild. It can maim, blind, or kill.

Further information

Safe use of non-insulin medication e-learning
⟳ <http://www.healthcareea.co.uk/theinsulinsafetysuite>
British National Formulary (BNF) ⟳ <http://www.bnf.org>
Electronic Medicines Compendium (SPCs and PILs)
⟳ <http://www.emc.medicines.org.uk/>
Management of Hyperglycemia in Type 2 Diabetes: A Patient-Centered Approach. Position Statement of the American Diabetes Association (ADA) and the European Association for the Study of Diabetes (EASD) (update in press)
(*Diab Care* 2012;**35**:1364–79; DOI: 10.2337/dc12-0413)
Medicines and Healthcare Products Regulatory Agency (MHRA) ⟳ <http://www.mhra.gov.uk/>
Monthly Index of Medical Specialties (eMIMS) ⟳ <http://www.mims.co.uk/>
NICE is revising the diabetes guidelines: ⟳ <http://www.nice.org.uk>
UKPDS 34 *Lancet* 1998; **352**:854–65 ; doi:10.1016/S0140-6736(98)07037-8.

Insulin

Treat each patient according to his/her individual condition. Insulins should be prescribed by trade (proprietary) name and not the pharmacological generic name to avoid confusion. The trade names are used throughout this book. Always check drug information in a current edition of British National Formulary (BNF) ✍ <http://www.bnf.org> before prescribing any medications described in this book. Be alert for warnings from the MHRA ✍ <http://www.mhra.gov.uk>. To review the Summary of Product Characteristics (SPC) and Patient Information Leaflet (PIL) see ✍ <http://www.medicines.org.uk>.

Introduction

'I won't have to inject insulin, will I?'

For many people, having diabetes means insulin injections. They think that these injections will start on their first visit to the diabetic clinic. Sometimes this unexpressed anxiety can impede communication. This may be an unfounded fear, but unfortunately some people do need insulin, and, at present, this is usually given by injection.

Who needs insulin?

- Everyone with type 1 diabetes—such patients will die without insulin treatment (Table 9.1)
- Type 2 patients with hyperglycaemia uncontrolled on non-insulin treatments
- Patients with acute onset of severe symptoms

Intense thirst and polyuria can be devastating. Insulin cures these symptoms by reliably reducing the blood glucose towards normal levels. Thus, all such patients should be considered for insulin therapy, at least initially, to make them feel better. If the symptoms have arisen within weeks, or have progressed rapidly, it is likely that the patient requires long-term insulin therapy. If these symptoms are combined with ketosis and weight loss, insulin is mandatory.

Table 9.1 Type 1 diabetes. Potential blood glucose targets to be adjusted to suit each individual patient's situation

	Target finger-prick whole blood glucose level
Before meals	4.0–7.0 mmol/l
2 hrs after meals	6.0–8.9 mmol/l (10.0 mmol/l if hypoglycaemia prone)
Before bed	6.0–8.9 mmol/l*
HbA$_{1c}$ †	42–57 mmol/mol (6.0–7.4 %) without hypoglycaemia (personalize)
	Check every 2–6 mths

Non-diabetic ranges are:

Before meals 3.5–5.5 mmol/l

2 hrs after meals < 8 mmol/l

Set targets according to each individual's age, general health, and circumstances. For example, strict glucose balance is usually inappropriate in an elderly person living alone. Take great care to avoid hypoglycaemia and always reduce the blood glucose gradually. Many authors do not put a lower limit on post-prandial glucose levels, but of course readings should be above the hypoglycaemic range and readings < 6 mmol/l may be followed by hypoglycaemia with exertion.

*This is to reduce the risk of nocturnal hypoglycaemia and assumes that bedtime is 4–6 hrs after the last meal. Patients on insulin should have a bedtime snack.

† In DCCT (➲ pp. 40–1) the mean HbA$_{1c}$ of the intensively treated group, which showed a dramatic reduction in tissue damage, was 53 mmol/mol (7%). This was accompanied by frequent hypoglycaemia which is likely to be worse at lower HbA$_{1c}$ levels. Some patients will be safer with an HbA$_{1c}$ >57 mmol/mol (7.4%). Intensive glucose-lowering regimens need intensive specialist support to succeed safely.

Ketone producers

In someone with diabetes whose blood glucose concentration is > 11 mmol/l, moderate to high ketonuria or blood ketone levels > 1 mmol/l suggests the need for insulin therapy unless they are on strict weight-reducing or an 'Atkins style' diet. (Lower ketone levels do not definitely exclude the need for insulin.)

Insulin treatment is life-saving in acute DKA. Any patient who has had an episode of proven DKA in the past is likely to need lifelong insulin treatment. Rarely, patients subsequently produce enough of their own insulin to return to oral hypoglycaemic therapy. This decision should be made by a consultant diabetologist; however, patients should be encouraged to test their blood glucose particularly assiduously during intercurrent illness or stress. They should keep insulin in the refrigerator for immediate use if the blood glucose concentration rises to avert a further episode of ketoacidosis.

People who have lost weight unintentionally

Marked weight loss (e.g. > 3 kg) in anyone with newly diagnosed diabetes, especially those who have lost weight despite eating well, may indicate the need for insulin treatment.

Ill people

Insulin should be given to new or established patients with acute myocardial infarction if glucose control is required ($\bigodot$ pp. 254–5). People with diabetes who have an infection, an accident, or a surgical illness often need insulin until the additional illness is under control. The necessity of insulin treatment should be assessed in all diabetic patients urgently admitted to hospital.

Children and young people

The majority of people whose diabetes develops at < 30 yrs of age have type 1 diabetes with an absolute insulin requirement. Type 2 diabetes is increasing in this age group, but the decision not to use insulin should be taken very carefully by a consultant diabetologist or paediatric diabetologist.

Pregnant women

It is usual to give insulin to pregnant women with diabetes who cannot control their blood glucose by diet and metformin ($\bigodot$ pp. 339–40).

Type 2 patients who are hyperglycaemic despite non-insulin hypoglycaemic drugs, diet, and exercise

Consider insulin treatment in patients whose HbA_{1c} is persistently > 48 mmol/mol (6.5 %). In obese people or those who eat a lot of sugar it may be possible to improve matters by re-evaluation of the diet and exercise pattern.

Many patients who have declined insulin for years are astonished at how much better they feel on insulin and wish they had agreed to have it years before.

Patients with complicated diabetes

Insulin may help patients with severe painful diabetic neuropathy, even if their glycaemic balance is reasonably controlled on non-insulin therapy. The rationale is that aggressive normalization of the blood glucose with insulin may relieve the symptoms. Patients with other tissue damage may benefit.

Patients with severe hypertriglyceridaemia (i.e. ≥ 10 mmol/l) and diabetes are sometimes treated with insulin to achieve normoglycaemia and normotriglyceridaemia. A very low-fat diet and carefully balanced carbohydrate intake are needed, and lipid-lowering drugs may also be required ($\bigodot$ pp. 262–3).

Insulin preparations

There are many insulin preparations on the market (Table 9.2). Human insulin (e.g. Actrapid®, Humulin® S, Insuman® Rapid) is made using recombinant DNA technology. Novo Nordisk use the yeast *Saccharomyces cerevisae*, and Eli Lilly and Sanofi Aventis use the bacterium *Escherichia coli*. The human insulin is then modified to produce analogue insulins (e.g. Apidra®, Novorapid®, Humalog®) which do not form hexamers, thus speeding absorption. Porcine and beef insulins are produced from animal pancreas. Animal insulins are more antigenic than human insulin, but antibodies can be formed to all insulins.

When human insulin was introduced there was concern that its use might be associated with reduced warning of hypoglycaemia. Several careful studies have shown that this is not so. However, the issue highlighted the need to consider the effects of recent care improvements on patients' daily lives, and on the incidence of hypoglycaemia. If individual patients believe that they have experienced problems on human insulin, prescribe animal insulins if the patient prefers. It is the patient who is using the insulin, not you!

The patents will soon expire on some commonly used insulins. At the time of writing biosimilar insulins are not licensed in the UK but they are available in many other countries. Insulin is a biological compound and it is difficult to produce a copy that works in exactly the same way in patients as the original version. Biosimilars are not subjected to the extensive testing on large numbers of patients that the original drugs required. Insulin is expensive and the NHS is required to obtain value for money. Non-biological drugs are often subject to blanket changes to generic versions to produce local financial economies, but it should be remembered that insulin therapy is a very personal matter and each patient's situation should be carefully considered in discussion with the diabetes specialist team. NICE advises that biosimilars are prescribed by their proprietary name (as current insulins are).

Keep up-to-date about available insulins as manufacturers introduce new insulins and remove others from the market. Warn patients if their usual insulin will no longer be available and discuss other options with them. Ensure that they are taught how to use their new insulin. Changing insulin type is worrying for patients.

Whenever any patient's insulin is changed, whatever the make or species, he/she must be warned that he/she may experience unexpected hypoglycaemia, perhaps with different warning symptoms. He/she should check SMBG carefully.

Table 9.2 Insulin Preparations

Preparation	Manufacturer	Species	Form	Onset (approx)	Peak activity (approx)	Duration of action (approx)
Neutral Insulin Injection						
Actrapid®	Novo Nordisk		V	<30 min	1.5–3.5hr	7–8hr
Apidra® (insulin glulisine*)	Sanofi-aventis		V, P, C_4, C_5	10–20 min	55 min	1.5–4hr
Humalog® (insulin lispro*)	Lilly		V, P, C_2, C_3	15 min	1.5hr	2–5hr
Humulin® S	Lilly		V, C_2, C_3	30 min–1hr	1–6hr	6–12hr
Hypurin® Bovine Neutral	Wockhardt		V, C_2	30 min–1hr	1.5–4.5hr	6–8hr
Hypurin® Porcine Neutral	Wockhardt		V, C_2	30 min–1hr	1.5–4.5hr	6–8hr
Insuman® Rapid	Sanofi-aventis		P, C_4, C_5	<30 min	1–4hr	7–9h

Biphasic Insulin Injection**

NovoRapid® (insulin aspart**)	Novo Nordisk	V, P, C$_1$	10–20 min	1–3hr	3–5hr
Humalog® Mix25	Lilly	V, P, C$_2$, C$_3$	15 min	2hr	22hr
Humalog® Mix50	Lilly	P, C$_2$, C$_3$	15 min	2hr	22hr
Humulin M3®	Lilly	V, P, C$_2$, C$_3$	30 min–1hr	1–12hr	22hr
Hypurin® Porcine 30/70	Wockhardt	V, C$_1$	<2hr	4–12hr	24hr
Insuman® Comb 15	Sanofi-aventis	C$_4$, C$_5$	30 min–1hr	2–4hr	11–20hr
Insuman® Comb 25	Sanofi-aventis	V, P, C$_4$, C$_5$	30 min–1hr	2–4hr	12–19hr
Insuman® Comb 50	Sanofi-aventis	C$_4$, C$_5$	<30 min	1.5–4hr	12–16hr

(Continued)

Table 9.2 (Cont.)

Preparation	Manufacturer	Species	Form	Onset (approx)	Peakactivity (approx)	Duration of action (approx)
NovoMix® 30	Novo Nordisk		P, C_1	10–20 min	1–4hr	24hr
Isophane Insulin Injection						
Humulin I®	Lilly		V, P, C_2, C_3	30 min–1hr	1–8hr	22hr
Hypurin® Bovine Isophane	Wockhardt		V, C_3	<2hr	6–12hr	18–24hr
Hypurin® Porcine Isophane	Wockhardt		V, C_2	<2hr	6–12hr	18–24hr
Insulatard®	Novo Nordisk		V, C_3, D	<1.5hr	4–12hr	24hr
Insuman® Basal	Sanofi-aventis		V, P, C_4, C_5	<1hr	3–4hr	11–20hr
Insulin Zinc Suspension (Mixed)						
Hypurin® Bovine Lente	Wockhardt		V	2hr	8–12hr	30hr

Protamine Zinc Insulin Injection					
Hypurin® Bovine PZI	Wockhardt		V	4–6hr	10–20hr	24–36hr

Long-acting Insulin Analogues

Lantus® (insulin glargine)	Sanofi-aventis		V, P, C₁, C₅	30min–1hr	–	24hr
Levemir® (insulin detemir)	Novo Nordisk		P, C₁, D	30min–1hr	–	24hr
Tresiba® (insulin degludec)	Novo Nordisk		P, C₁	30min–1.5hr	-	>42hr

Reproduced from MIMS Monthly Index of Medical Specialties with permission. This table is updated monthly. Please see the current issue for up-to-date information: ℗ <http://www.mims.co.uk/Tables/1096962/Insulin-Preparations/>.

V = vial. P = preloaded pen. C = cartridge. C1 = compatible with NovoPen 4 and NovoPen Echo. C2 = compatible with Autopen Classic. C3 = compatible with Humapen Luxura HD, Humapen Memoir, Humapen Savvio. C4 = compatible with Autopen 24. C5 = compatible with ClikSTAR. D = InnoLet delivery device.

*Human insulin analogue

*Speed of onset is proportional to amount of soluble insulin

Pen needles: Microfine, Penfine and Unifine are compatible with all preloaded and reusable pens.

Problems with insulin injections

- Bleeding disorders such as thrombocytopaenia—risk of bleeding/bruising at injection site
- Major skin diseases affecting potential injection sites
- Severe needle-phobia (refer such patients to a clinical psychologist)
- Hypersensitivity to insulin or preservatives
- Hypersensitivity to syringe or pen components

Religious or ethical objections, e.g. to porcine insulin or recombinant DNA technology (➋ p. 151) can usually be resolved by offering another insulin variant.

If patients cannot inject their own insulin, family members (with appropriate training and support) may do so. Patients may need to be referred to community nurses who can rarely make more than two visits a day so the regimen may need to be simplified (➋ pp. 174, 176).

Side effects of insulin injections

Many of these effects relate to the rapid reduction of hyperglycaemia. It is best to decrease glucose gradually to reduce sudden changes in osmolality.

- Hypoglycaemia (➋ pp. 181–200)
- Injection site problems—bruising, bleeding, irritation, erythema
- Hypersensitivity reactions—local or generalized, itching, urticaria, including, rarely, anaphylaxis *(Diabet. Med.* 2005; **22**:102–6; doi: 10.1111/j.1464-5491.2004.01352.x; *Endocrine* 2010; **37**:33–9; doi: 10.1007/s12020-009-9256-1).
- Injection site infections
- Insulin lipohypertrophy (common) or lipoatrophy (uncommon) (➋ p. 173)
- Oedema—'insulin oedema' is uncommon but well-recognized and usually lasts days or weeks. Exclude cardiac or renal causes.
- Blurred vision as glucose falls, usually days or weeks—common. Ensure patient has had a full eye check including fundoscopy or digital retinal photography. Advise patient not to buy expensive spectacles but to use over-the-counter ones until the vision stabilizes.
- Rapid worsening of neuropathy which may be painful. This relates to rapid reduction of hyperglycaemia and gradually resolves but may take months to improve. Overall progression of neuropathy is reduced by improved glucose balance.
- Rapid worsening of retinopathy (as mentioned). Overall near-normalization of blood glucose reduces the likelihood of deterioration in retinopathy, but a few patients whose glucose is very high initially do show worsening at first.

Insulin safety

Right insulin, right dose, right time, right way.

From August 2003 to August 2009, the National Patient Safety Agency (NPSA) received over 15 000 insulin incident reports including 3881 reports involving wrong insulin doses, and other reports from the use of the wrong syringe. Some patients died. (*Br Med J* 2010; **341**:c5269; http://dx.doi.org/10.1136/bmj.c5269) In 2010 this led to a Rapid Response Alert requiring immediate action from all organizations in the NHS and independent sector in the UK. In particular, '[a]n executive director, nominated by the chief executive, working with the chief/lead pharmacist and relevant medical/nursing staff should ensure that . . . A training programme should be put in place for all healthcare staff (including medical staff) expected to prescribe, prepare and administer insulin.' ℘ <http://www.nrls.npsa.nhs.uk/alerts/?entryid45=74287>

Safe use of insulin e-learning modules for healthcare professionals are available at:

℘ <http://www.healthcareea.co.uk/theinsulinsafetysuite>

Two in five insulin-treated patients in the National Diabetes Inpatient Audit 2012 were found to have had a medication error in hospital, so training and care are essential.

℘ http://www.hscic.gov.uk/catalogue/PUB10506

Prescribing

Prescribing errors are common. A specific and separate insulin prescribing chart should be used in hospitals and residential accommodation which include the finger-prick blood glucose levels. The prescription should include the following.

- The word 'insulin' followed by the full proprietary name
- Full name of insulin(s) (e.g. Novomix® 30, not just Novomix®)
- Strength of insulin (in units/ml)
- The insulin vial/cartridge and/or the pen or injection device to be used
- The amount of each dose
- Write 'units' in full (otherwise the U may be seen as an 0 causing overdose). Thus '10 units', **not** '10U' or '10IU'
- Time of each injection and frequency
- Relationship to meals if relevant
- Start date
- Route—usually subcutaneous (SC) (if for intravenous (IV) infusion prescribe the carrier solution e.g. 0.9 % sodium chloride)
- Self-administering 'yes/no' if in hospital (➲ pp. 439–40)
- Name and signature of prescriber and date prescribed
- Then check it. Show the patient (he/she is usually more familiar with their insulin regimen than you are)

Concentration of insulin

Most insulin in the UK is provided as 100 units/ml (sometimes described as U100). Tresiba® is provided as either 100 units/ml or 200 units/ml in prefilled pens internally calibrated to show and deliver the dose as dialed in units. It is not available in any other way so no dose conversion is required if patients are transferred to the 200 unit/ml formulation. ℘ <http://www.mhra.gov.uk/home/groups/comms-ic/documents/websiteresources/con228797.pdf> Lantus® 300 units/ml may soon be available.

Insulin resistant patients may require 500 units/ml insulin, available on a named-patient basis only as vials of Humulin® R 500 units/ml from the US. All such patients should be under the care of a diabetes specialist team (DST). In this situation 1 unit as drawn up in a UK insulin syringe equals 5 units of 100 units/ml insulin. Great care is required in patient and staff education and Humulin® R 500 units/ml in use by inpatients must be very clearly labelled and kept completely separately from all other insulin (ideally in a lockable part of the patient's locker). ℘ <http://www.humulinhcp.com/Pages/index.aspx>

Other countries may not conform to this system and patients should be very careful if they obtain their insulin abroad.

Duration and peak action of different insulins

See Table 9.2.

Rapid-acting insulin analogues

The insulin made by the normal human pancreas is a clear, colourless fluid which, when released into the bloodstream via the portal vein, produces an effect upon the blood glucose within minutes and then clears within minutes

Rapid-acting analogues are modified so that active insulin is available almost immediately. They are clear and colourless. They are absorbed and start working within 5–20 mins of injection, peak at 30–90 mins and last 1—5 hrs. Rapid-acting insulins must be injected either immediately before eating (preferable), or during/immediately after food. If one is uncertain what food will be provided (e.g. in a restaurant) insulin can be injected as the meal finishes.

Apidra®, Humalog®, and NovoRapid® can be used in basal–bolus insulin patterns, or mixed with intermediate-acting insulins in twice-daily regimens. Because insulin levels peak with the glucose absorption from food, they produce an insulin effect similar to that of the normal pancreas and hypoglycaemia may be reduced. However, hypoglycaemia can still occur, and it may come on quickly and be severe. The insulin may 'run out' before the next injection and meal, thus there can be post-prandial normoglycaemia or hypoglycaemia, but pre-prandial hyperglycaemia.

Rapid-acting insulins are increasingly popular with patients as they allow more flexibility of lifestyle and enable more scope for fine-tuning glucose than older insulins.

Short-acting insulin

All short-acting insulins are clear and colourless. They include Actrapid®, Humulin® S (Humulin® R in USA), Insuman® Rapid, Hypurin® Porcine Neutral, and Hypurin® Bovine Neutral. The main difference between insulin in the non-diabetic person and insulin in the diabetic person is its route of delivery into the bloodstream and the lack of fine control. The effect of human insulin released by the pancreas in direct response to circulating blood glucose concentrations cannot be the same as the effect of subcutaneous insulin absorbed regardless of the blood glucose concentration. Even continuous intravenous insulin infusion cannot mimic the finely tuned glycaemia-appropriate response of the normal pancreas. Short-acting insulins are absorbed in < 30 mins to 1 hr and may last as long as 12 hrs.

Short-acting insulins can be used in basal—bolus regimens or mixed with intermediate-acting insulin in twice daily regimens.

Intermediate-acting

Isophane (NPH) insulin is produced by adding protamine and a small amount of zinc at the body's normal pH. This reduces solubility and hence prolongs absorption from the insulin injection site. Isophane insulins are cloudy. They start working in < 1–2hrs and last for up to 24 hrs (Table 9.2). Examples of isophane (NPH) insulins are Humulin® I, Hypurin® Bovine Isophane, Hypurin® Porcine Isophane, Insulatard®, and Insuman® Basal. Short-acting insulin can be mixed with isophane insulins and the mixture will remain stable. This is the basis of the fixed proportion mixtures, or of mixtures made by patients themselves.

Long-acting insulins

Zinc is used to precipitate insulin crystals thus slowing their absorption from the injection site to last > 24 hrs. Current versions Hypurin® Bovine Lente, and Hypurin® Bovine PZI. These are cloudy. Mixtures of these insulins with short-acting insulin are not stable.

Current long-acting analogue insulins include insulin Lantus® and Levemir® which both last about 24 hrs. Tresiba® lasts > 42 hrs. Do not mix these insulins with any other insulin. Long-acting analogue insulins are clear.

Combination or pre-mixed insulins

These are stable, cloudy mixtures containing varying proportions of short-acting insulin and isophane (NPH) insulin. These mixtures are inflexible—if the dose is increased, both the short-acting and the isophane insulin dose is increased. However, they gained popularity because of their simplicity and their avoidance of mixing errors (➲ p. 170). They include Humalog® Mix 25 and Mix 50, Humulin® M3, Hypurin® Porcine 30/70, Insuman® Comb 15, 25, and 50, and NovoMix® 30. The sole or first number refers to the proportion of fast-acting insulin as a percentage of total insulin.

⚠ *Risk of confusion with insulin names*

Many insulin names start with the manufacturer's brand name for their suite of insulins and then a number/letter/word defining the insulin properties. Both name and number/letter/word are essential.

- Humulin® S (Humulin® R in USA), Humulin® I, Humulin® M3
- Humalog®, Humalog® Mix25, Humalog® Mix50
- Hypurin® Bovine Isophane, Hypurin® Porcine Isophane, Hypurin® Porcine 30/70, Hypurin® Bovine PZI
- Insuman® Rapid, Insuman® Comb 15, Insuman® Comb 25, Insuman® Comb 50, Insuman® Basal

Be very, very careful.

Insulin in the user's hands

Checking and storing insulin

- Learn the name of insulins and the devices used to inject them.
- Do you have the correct insulin(s)? Patients and staff: check before you leave the pharmacist every time you collect an insulin prescription. Patients should check what healthcare staff are about to inject.
- If a patient has different insulins, are they labelled clearly (e.g. sticker on pen, different coloured pens)?
- Protect all insulin from light, heat (e.g. sun or heater), and vibration.
- Store unused insulin at 2–8 °C in a fridge, away from the freezing compartment.
- Insulin pen/vial in use: keep out of the fridge. On first use, keep at room temperature for 1–2 hrs before injection. Stable at 2–25 °C. Usually discard any unused after 28 days but check information leaflet for each manufacturer's insulin.
- Have you got the right insulin for that dose and time of day?
- Is it within its expiry date?
- Is the bung clean? If not, clean with alcohol wipe.
- Is the bung damaged? If yes, do not use.
- Does usually clear insulin look clear? If not, do not use.
- If you use a cloudy insulin rotate the pen/vial gently 20 times between your hands.
- Do not shake as it will foam. Clear insulin does not need rotating.
- Expel any air bubbles (if using a syringe do not work the plunger up and down too vigorously or microscopic particles will shear off the syringe into the insulin, causing the plunger to 'stick').
- Use a new syringe and needle each time. Ensure safe disposal.
- If using a pen device, use a new needle each time. Do not resheath. Take it off after the injection and dispose of it safely.

Insulin passport

Every patient on insulin should have 'Safe use of insulin and you' an information leaflet. Print them out from:

    ℘ http://www.leicestershirediabetes.org.uk/uploads/121/documents/Safe%20use%20of%20insulin%20and%20you%20patient%20info%20booklet.pdf.

    People with diabetes on insulin should consider wearing a medical-alert bracelet or pendant.

Preparing insulin for injection

Cloudy insulins—the longer-acting insulins—should be mixed gently by rotating the bottle/pen before drawing up the dose to resuspend the insulin. Without resuspension the amount of insulin complex injected may vary. Over-zealous mixing can introduce bubbles leading to dosage errors.

    Contamination may occur with the introduction of cloudy insulin into the clear bottle by the self-mixer who has forgotten that one should draw up the clear insulin first (➜ p. 170). Another form of contamination is to leave short-acting insulin and zinc suspension insulins in the syringe for more than a few seconds before injection. The short-acting insulin will gradually be converted to slower-acting insulin.

    Obviously, the patient or their carer should give the right insulin for that person for that occasion. Mistakes happen all too easily.

Insulin injection equipment

Ask patients to bring their injection equipment to each appointment so you can check how they use it. The patient should choose the method he/she prefers. Patient preference, vision, and manual dexterity may be a more important factor than which brand of insulin is used. Pen/pump colour or size may be higher on the patient's wish list than the insulin-delivery features.

Syringe and needle

- Basic equipment
- Small and fiddly. Requires very good vision and dexterity, and precision
- Single-use only—throw away safely
- ⚠ The only syringe to use for drawing up insulin is an insulin syringe.
- Needle usually attached—use the 8 mm size or less and a skin fold injection technique in most patients to avoid intramuscular (IM) injection
- 1 ml (100 units), 0.5 ml (50 units), and 0.3 ml (30 units) syringes are available, each marked to allow the right number of units to be drawn up
- May stick with cloudy insulin
- May be supplied with an insulin vial as backup for pen/pump patients
- Used by healthcare professionals

Insulin pens

- Convenient, portable (combine device and insulin), popular.
- Require good vision and dexterity.
- Easy to use by family or carer if patient unable to do so.
- Re-usable—insulin cartridge needs to be inserted; or disposable—preloaded with insulin.
- Need new pen needle each time (length 4 mm, 5 mm, and 8 mm (rarely needed)). Use the shortest that delivers insulin SC.
- Penmate® covers the needle in NovoNordisk pens for needle-phobic patients. ℘ <https://novonordisk.com/diabetes_care/insulin_pens_and_needles/penmate/default.asp>
- Expel insulin from pen ('safety test') before use, following individual manufacturer's instructions. Usually 2 units are expelled, needle-up, before use, more if it is first use of that pen.
- Remove used needle after injection to avoid insulin leaks or air being sucked in as insulin cools. Do not resheath. Dispose of old needle safely.
- Pens available with 0.5, 1, and 2 unit dose adjustment
- Maximum dose varies from 30 to 80 units (Tresiba® FlexTouch 160 units)
- Vary in size, shape, colour, visibility/audibility of dose dialing, memory (or not)—e.g. insulin used/remaining, end-of-cartridge warning, ease of plunger depression
- Use the manufacturer's pen for Lilly, NovoNordisk, and Sanofi-Aventis insulin cartridges (the mechanism is engineered to match that particular insulin, and the cartridge is engineered to fit the pen).

- Autopens® can be used for some insulins. Ensure that the patient has the right Autopen®—they are different:
  - Lilly insulin can be used in their pens or in Autopen®
  - Wockhardt insulin is used in Autopen®
  - Sanofi-Aventis insulins can be used in their pens or in Autopen 24®
- MIMS has the most frequently updated list (➋ p. 152) for insulins and their delivery systems
- DSNs usually have the most expertise in insulin pens and use in real life
- View pens and detailed usage instructions on the manufacturers' websites: Lilly, NovoNordisk, Owen Mumford, and Sanofi-Aventis

Magnifiers are available for people with poor vision. Insulin pen reminders (e.g. Timesulin®) can help reduce forgotten or double doses. All patients on insulin should be considered for insulin pen therapy—it is usually more accurate, convenient, comfortable, and practical.

Insulin jet injectors

These needle-free devices drive insulin spray through the skin. They may help people with needle phobia. The instructions should be followed closely as poor technique may leave lumps, or sore areas at the injection site and insulin may ooze out afterwards. Arms should be avoided. Bruising can occur. Insujet® is an example (European Pharma Group) and uses any insulin cartridge.

Continuous subcutaneous insulin infusion pumps (CSII)

Insulin pumps therapy (CSII) should only be started and managed by trained DSTs (diabetologist, diabetes nurse, and dietitian). The method can be used in adults and children (including babies).

In 2012 there were 183 UK centres delivering CSII with > 13 000 adult patients on pump therapy. Many children also use CSII. Numbers are rising but there are fewer patients in the UK on CSII than in some other countries. Patients may arrive from abroad with pumps and variable knowledge of self-care. Healthcare professionals are likely to encounter pump patients so this section provides some background and safety information. The key point is to contact the DST straightaway if an insulin pump patient comes under your care.

CSII uses continuously infused, short or rapid-acting insulin to provide background (basal) insulin and bolus insulin for meals or high glucose correction. In a 'tethered' pump, insulin is loaded into a special vial within the pump which then pumps it via fine tubing to an indwelling SC cannula. The cannula is left *in situ* for several days. The tubing can be disconnected to allow showers, etc. Many pumps are waterproof. The pump is worn on a belt or in a pocket or clothing (e.g. Animas, Medtronic, Roche), or stuck onto the skin (e.g. Omnipod®). The patient adjusts the infusion rates with buttons (like programming a mobile phone). Mealtime boluses can be started at the press of a button and may be short or long. Some pumps calculate doses based on glucose levels transmitted by CGM devices or entered, along with carbohydrate counts, by the patient. These 'wizards' depend on the insulin sensitivity calculations previously entered by patient or professional, and the insulin doses delivered may not, in fact, be appropriate for the situation.

Pairing of CGM with CSII has allowed the development of computer algorithms to form a closed loop that controls the blood glucose overnight without patient intervention. Work continues on daytime glucose control. This is currently a research project not available for general use.

Who should have an insulin pump?

Patients using CSII (or their carers) should:
- have type 1 diabetes; pumps are rarely used in type 2
- be willing and able to learn and prepared for a lot of 'homework'
- should usually have participated in NICE-compliant type 1 diabetes education
- be persistent, and able and willing to problem-solve
- be emotionally stable (CSII is *not* the solution to psychologically driven 'brittle' diabetes)
- be using basal–bolus insulin regimens already
- be checking SMBG at least four times every day
- be using CHO counting to adjust insulin doses
- be able to calculate insulin doses to correct high blood glucose
- have and use a mobile phone (i.e. be capable of managing the electronic device)
- have good hygiene habits
- be prepared to have a cannula permanently *in situ*

NICE Technology Appraisal TA151 2008 states that CSII is recommended as a possible treatment for type 1 patients > 12 yrs if attempts to reach target HbA_{1c} levels with multiple daily injections result in the person having disabling hypoglycaemia; or HbA_{1c} levels have remained ≥ 8.5 % with multiple daily injections despite the person and/or their carer carefully trying to manage their diabetes. In the UK the diabetologist has to obtain permission from the NHS service commissioners for funding for CSII.

How does the patient manage his/her insulin doses?

See Box 9.1.

Box 9.1 Calculating rapid/short-acting insulin doses

Basal–bolus insulin or CSII

Intensive glucose control is usually started and monitored by DSNs, dietitians, and diabetologists. It is effective but complex and time-consuming.
⚠ There is a risk of misunderstanding and of hypoglycaemia.

These calculations provide an approximation which must be checked by the patient against what actually happens to his/her SMBG. There are other ways of calculating these ratios. Patients starting on insulin pumps or unfamiliar regimens usually reduce the total daily dose (TDD) by 25 % before using it in the calculations below to avoid hypoglycaemia.

Add up TDD of all insulin	= TDD
Insulin-to-carbohydrate (CHO) ratio CHO g covered by 1 unit of insulin	= 500/TDD
Correction dose Glucose fall for 1 unit of insulin	= 100/TDD

Example

John takes:	
10 units analogue insulin with each meal	= 30 units
20 units long-acting insulin at bedtime	= <u>20 units</u>
TDD	= 50 units
John's insulin-to-CHO ratio: 500/TDD = 500/50 = 10g CHO CHO	= 1 unit per 10 g
John's correction dose: 100/TDD = 100/50 = 2 mmol glucose	= 1 unit insulin per 2 mmol glucose
John's meal contains 60 g CHO His pre-meal glucose is 13 mmol/l His target is 7 mmol/l	= 6 units insulin
13 – 7 = 6 mmol/l excess glucose @ 2 mmol fall per unit	= <u>3 units insulin</u>
Total short-acting insulin for that meal	= 9 units insulin

Staff should attend training on using this system before teaching patients e.g. DAFNE (➲ pp. 63–4 and p. 72)

Insulin pump users will:

- have one or more basal insulin rates, e.g. 0.5 units /hr)
- have an insulin-to-carbohydrate ratio, e.g. 1 unit of insulin to 10 g carbohydrate (which may differ for different meals)
- have a correction calculation, e.g. 1 unit of insulin for every 2 mmol glucose above their target glucose (e.g. 7 mmol/l)
- either use the pump's preprogrammed calculator to work out the bolus dose, or do the calculation themselves

Problems with insulin pumps and what to do

Pump patients should have had a thorough education in potential problems and how to manage them. All the pump companies provide 24-hr helplines for equipment problems (common). Back-up for other problems should be provided by the DST managing the patient, ideally via a 24-hr service.

A&E staff and on-call medical teams faced with a pump patient should note the following:

- Essential: Contact the DST immediately.
- ⚠ Hyperglycaemia: these patients have no long-acting insulin depot. If their insulin supply fails (e.g. air in the line, kinked line or cannula) they will develop DKA within hours which may be fatal.
- Glucose ≥ 11 mmol/l, urine, or blood ketones present but otherwise well, normotensive, not shocked: ask patient to give correction dose. Has the patient checked the infusion set and pump? If the correction dose does not lower the glucose or there is a problem with infusion set (common) or pump inject SC insulin, e.g. 6–10 units (or double the patient's usual correction dose), immediately. Use intermittent SC insulin according to finger-prick blood glucose level, adding long-acting insulin if appropriate, until the set or pump problem is resolved.
- ⚠ Glucose ≥ 11 mmol/l, ill, vomiting, hypotensive, ketones present: manage as for DKA. (➔ pp. 216–19) Inject 6–10 units of insulin IM if there is any delay in IV insulin infusion—the patient has minimal insulin depot because he/she is not using long-acting insulin.
- Hypoglycaemia: usual possible reasons (➔ pp. 194–5). In addition, consider dose miscalculation by pump 'wizard' or very rarely, pump runaway. If the pump appears to be malfunctioning, disconnect it, treat the hypoglycaemia and revert to intermittent insulin with syringe or pen. Contact the pump company helpline immediately.
- Glucose < 4 mmol/l, patient able to self-treat: give oral glucose as usual (➔ p. 188). The patient will pause the pump if they usually do so when hypo. Once patient is recovered (i.e. blood glucose ≥ 6 mmol/l and 45 mins after ingesting oral glucose) ascertain why they became hypoglycaemic. Unexplained hypoglycaemia—ask the patient to check pump function. If any doubt, pause or disconnect pump, continue intermittent SC insulin and contact pump company helpline.
- Glucose < 4 mmol/l, patient confused or unable to self-treat: give IV glucose or SC/IM glucagon (➔ p. 190) after disconnecting the pump infusion line from the cannula—it can usually be pulled off the button stuck onto the skin. If profound hypoglycaemia and you cannot disconnect the tubing from the cannula, pull out the abdominal cannula. Insert IV cannula and infuse glucose. Once glucose has risen, ask patients

who are able to do so and compos mentis to reconnect the pump and make any corrections needed. If the patient is not well enough, ensure that the patient has intermittent insulin injection treatment or IV variable rate infusion, depending on their clinical state and according to blood glucose measurements. ⚠ Danger: the patient may go from hypoglycaemia to DKA without his/her pump.

- Infusion site infection. Ask patient to remove cannula (or do so yourself). Send cannula to microbiology if feasible. Give anti-staphylococcal antibiotics. Check patient's personal and pump hygiene, especially site preparation. Treat the infection. Until infection cleared use a completely different site or intermittent subcutaneous insulin injections or IV variable rate depending on clinical condition. Toxic shock syndrome or necrotizing fasciitis are very rare complications.
- Keep the pump with the patient—pumps cost thousands of pounds. If it has to be discontinued, turn it off if you can or simply allow it to continue to pump into a polythene bag (e.g. a blood sample bag). It will produce only a drop of fluid. If malfunction is suspected contact the pump company helpline within 24 hrs. Pumps can be interrogated electronically by the company to detect errors provided that the battery is still working.

Patient help group INPUT: ✍ <http://www.inputdiabetes.org.uk>

Implantable insulin infusion devices

Implantable insulin pumps have an insulin reservoir which can be filled through the skin. The insulin is pumped either directly into a vein or intraperitoneally. They are used in people in whom no other method has succeeded in preventing frequent DKA. They are rarely used. Phone a diabetologist immediately (day or night) if such a patient comes under your care.

Continuous intravenous insulin infusion (III)—inpatients only

An IV insulin bolus works and disappears within 5 mins. It should be used only when SC or IM insulin are inappropriate and there is a delay in establishing an IV insulin infusion (III).

Do you really need to use III at all? III is used too often. It can cause considerable disruption to blood glucose control as well causing severe hypoglycaemia. If the III is stopped without giving SC insulin first patients can develop DKA.

III is not easy to manage. Each hospital should have specific guidance, adopted in liaison with the specialist diabetes team, to which compliance is audited. In the National Diabetes Inpatient Audit (NaDIA) 10.6 % of inpatients were on III of whom 6.5 % were judged to be receiving it inappropriately. Half of all the patients on III had too few blood glucose measurements for safety. Of the inpatients audited, 0.5 % developed new DKA while in hospital.

✍ <http://www.hscic.gov.uk/catalogue/PUB10506>

III is indicated for people with diabetes in the following situations:

- DKA (➲ pp. 216–19)
- Hyperglycaemic Hyperosmolar State (HHS) (➲ pp. 220–2
- Patients undergoing surgery or procedures who will miss >1 meal
- Patients unable to eat and drink normally for other reasons

III key points:
- use fixed rate (FRIII) in DKA and after fluid rehydration in HHS.
- use variable rate (VRIII) when patients cannot eat or drink normally. This used to be called a sliding scale.
- adjust VRIII according to finger-prick blood glucose levels. (➲ p. 436)
- prescribe III on a specific separate chart that includes blood glucose monitoring results and according to NPSA guidance ✍ <http://www. nrls.npsa.nhs.uk/alerts/?entryid45=74287>
- use soluble insulin (Actrapid®, Humulin S®, Insuman Rapid®) 50 units in 49.5 ml 0.9 % sodium chloride in a fully labelled syringe in an appropriate syringe pump (some hospitals produce pre-filled III syringes).
- prescribe appropriate IV fluids to run concurrently with the III e.g. 0.9 % sodium chloride in DKA, or 0.45 % sodium chloride with 5 % glucose, and potassium chloride 0.15 %.

See JBDS guidance ✍ <http://www.diabetologists-abcd.org.uk/JBDS_DKA_ Management.pdf>
- ✍ <http://www.diabetes.org.uk/About_us/What-we-say/ Improving-diabetes-healthcare/Management-of-adults-with-diabetes -undergoing-surgery-and-elective-procedures-improving-standards/>
- continue intermediate or long-acting insulin (usually).
- monitor capillary blood glucose hourly (see guidance) and, if on VRIII, prescribe instructions for insulin adjustment (➲ p. 436), and see JBDS guidance) according to glucose levels.
- specify action to be taken for glucose < 4 mmol/l or persistently > 12 mmol/l, including when to call doctor.
- ⚠ Do not stop III in patients with type 1 diabetes, or those previously managed on insulin without first giving SC insulin—high risk of DKA.
- return to usual insulin regimen (increase dose if still infected or otherwise more insulin resistant) when patient eating and drinking normally.
- stop IIIs at breakfast time.
- give the rapid/short-acting SC insulin at least 30 mins before discontinuing III.
- the person stopping the III must confirm that the SC insulin has actually been injected.
- the intermediate or long-acting insulin should, in most patients, have continued throughout III—if the basal/intermediate dose was reduced it should be returned to normal (depending on patient state).

Disposal of sharps and syringes

All needles, lancets, and syringes are pre-packed and sterilized by the manu-facturers. They are made for single use only.

It is each professional's and patient's personal responsibility to ensure that used sharps and used syringes are disposed of properly.. Pen needles can be removed with a Unigard® pen-needle safety remover. Every patient should use a needle clipper (e.g. B-D Safe-Clip™). Clipped, unusable syringes are put in a sharps box (available on prescription in the UK) to be kept out of reach of children or pets and returned to the chemist, hospital, or surgery for formal disposal. In the UK it is the local council's responsibility to provide safe sharps disposal arrangements. Arrangements can be found on council websites or by telephoning waste management. There is a risk of needle-stick injuries when clipping needles, emptying finger-pricking devices, and handling lancets. Needles and lancets should never be resheathed. Lancets should withdraw the needle out of harm's way.

See Royal College of Nursing guidance including European guidance: http://www.rcn.org.uk/__data/assets/pdf_file/0008/418490/004135.pdf

Administering insulin

Staff administering insulin should follow the prescription. If they have concerns they should query them with the relevant doctor. Inexperienced nurses and doctors have omitted insulin in vomiting type 1 patients precipitating DKA and sometimes death.

- Check the prescription yourself and with the patient.
- Measure all doses of insulin using an insulin syringe or commercial insulin pen device. Never use an ordinary IV syringe for insulin administration.
- Sign that the insulin has been given and when.

Drawing up insulin into an insulin syringe

Drawing insulin into a syringe to the correct dose with no air requires dexterity, concentration, good vision, and a steady hand (Figure 9.1).

- Check insulin is in date.
- Clean bung with alcohol swab. Do not use if bung damaged.
- Attach needle to syringe if necessary.
- Gently rotate bottle 20 times to mix cloudy insulins.
- Hold vial upside down.
- Draw up air and inject into the insulin vial.
- Draw up insulin into syringe.
- Clear air bubbles from syringe.
- Check syringe contains correct insulin dose.
- Inject insulin into fatty layer under skin.
- Count to 10.
- Withdraw needle.
- Press on the hole—do not massage the site.

Insulin pen users should follow the instructions provided by the pen manufacturer and their diabetes nurse. Don't forget to prime the pen first as instructed. After the plunger or slider has been pressed, the pen should be left *in situ* with the plunger or slider held down for a count of 10.

Mixing insulin

Nowadays few people self-mix their insulins. It is difficult and often inaccurate. Isophane (NPH) insulins make stable mixtures with short-acting insulins, but none of the others are stable and should be injected immediately. Other insulins cannot be mixed with Levemir® or Lantus®.

- Gently rotate the bottle to mix insulin
- Draw up air
- Inject air into cloudy insulin bottle
- Put cloudy insulin down
- Draw up air
- Inject air into clear insulin bottle.
- Draw up clear insulin
- Express air bubbles and check you have drawn up correct dose of clear insulin
- Draw up correct dose of cloudy insulin
- Inject

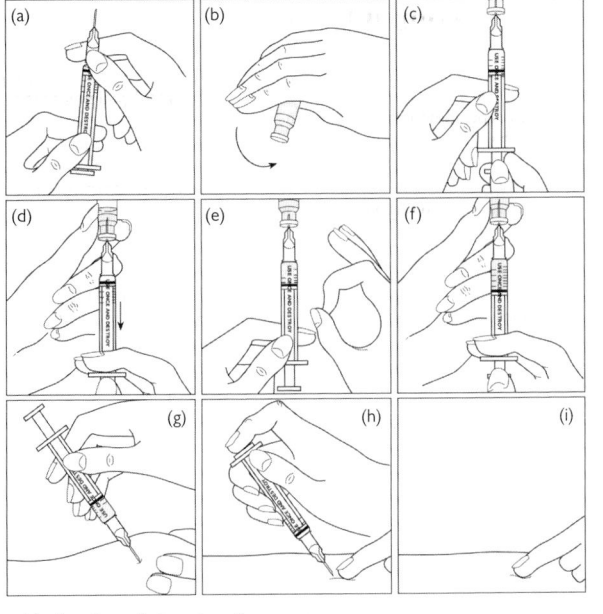

(a) Attach needle to syringe if necessary
(b) Gently rotate bottle to mix insulin
(c) Draw up air and inject into the insulin bottle
(d) Draw up insulin
(e) Clear air bubbles
(f) Check syringe contains correct insulin dose
(g) Inject insulin into fatty layer under skin
(h) Withdraw needle
(i) Press on the hole

Fig. 9.1 Drawing up and injecting insulin.

Injecting insulin

Insulin is injected subcutaneously (SC) into bare skin (Figure 9.2). Injecting through clothes risks infection. A shallow injection may produce a painful intradermal blister with unpredictable insulin absorption. A deep injection which penetrates intramuscularly (IM) will lead to rapid insulin absorption and may cause severe hypoglycaemia. The patient should take a thick pinch of skin and subcutaneous tissue and insert the needle at an angle of 45°. An angle of 90° can be used if there is enough subcutaneous fat. The insulin is then injected, the needle left *in situ* for a count of 10, and then withdrawn.

Some patients press a clean tissue, cotton-wool swab, or finger over the hole for a few moments.

If the skin is dirty it should be washed and dried. Skin cleansing with alcohol or surgical spirit is not usually necessary, and may causing stinging during injection, and skin hardening if used regularly. Bruising occurs occasionally, as does a tiny trickle of blood. Patients need to be reassured that this is most unlikely to mean that the insulin has been injected intravenously. Some doctors advocate withdrawing the plunger before injection to ensure that a vein has not been entered, but many no longer consider this useful.

⚠ Do not inject insulin SC if the patient is shocked, hypotensive, or 'shut down' as it will not be absorbed or work until the patient's circulation improves risking late hypoglycaemia. The IM route can be used if an III cannot be set up promptly.

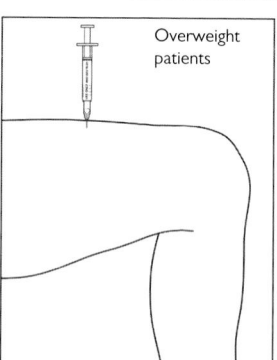
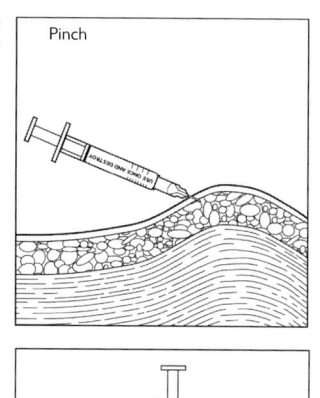

Fig. 9.2 Different methods of injecting insulin.

Insulin injection sites

The most commonly used sites are the thighs, upper buttocks, abdomen, and upper arms. A few patients use their calves and forearms. Rotate sites to avoid over-use and insulin fat hypertrophy. Insulin absorption varies with each injection site. It is most rapid from the abdomen, then the arms, thighs, and buttocks. Therefore a multi-site rotation scheme can cause variability in blood glucose balance, although this may be more of a problem in some people than others. It may be better to use, say, the abdomen during the day and thighs at night, or to use the left and right side of a particular site for a week or two and then change. Patients who are prepared to monitor this closely with blood glucose testing can work out which site is most appropriate for which circumstance.

Patients will all have favourite sites (usually those which are easy to reach) and there will be areas which gradually become numb through repeated use. Occasionally one discovers small black holes in a patient's leg or abdomen into which he/she has been putting insulin for years!

Insulin fat hypertrophy or atrophy

Insulin has a direct effect on fat cells and often causes hypertrophy at over-used injection sites. These unsightly bulges also cause variability in insulin absorption. The commonest area is paraumbilical. Check each visit. Atrophy due to insulin antibodies is rarely seen nowadays. Encourage patients the whole extent of each available injection site.

When should insulin be injected?

Rapid or short-acting insulin should be injected before meals in most patients. Analogue insulins can be injected immediately before or after eating. Other insulins take 10–30 mins to be absorbed. Insulin is given after meals more often than we realize—patients forget, or they have never understood when to give it, or the district nurse is late. If eating is very erratic (e.g. a person with dementia) it may be safer for carers to give rapid-acting insulin once the meal has definitely been eaten, and just give a little longer-acting insulin once a day to prevent decompensation. Basal insulin is often injected at bedtime.

Factors affecting insulin absorption

These are myriad and tend to be forgotten when the patient and diabetes adviser are poring over the blood glucose diary.
- Type of insulin
- Location of injection site
- Amount of subcutaneous fat at injection site
- Depth of injection
- Size of insulin depot
- Temperature of injection site and patient overall
- General state of circulation
- Exercising underlying muscle (e.g. thigh or arms)
- Hypotensive shock (never give subcutaneous insulin in this situation)
- Vasoconstrictor compounds/medication (e.g. nicotine)
- Vasodilator medication (e.g. nitrates)

The amount of insulin cleared from an injection site within 24 hrs can vary from 20 % to 100 % from person to person and within the same person. With such considerable variability in insulin absorption added to the effects of food, exercise, and emotion, the mystery is not why the blood glucose balance is so variable, but why it is possible to control it at all!

Common insulin regimens

See Box 9.2 and Figure 9.3

Starting dose

Varies with the patient! Seek the diabetes specialist team's advice. The approximate rule of thumb for patients new to insulin is 0.5 units/kg (more in infected or otherwise insulin resistant, less if danger from hypoglycaemia or vigorous exercisers) with about half as basal insulin and the rest divided between the meals according to the usual amount of CHO eaten. However, in many cases a smaller amount of insulin can be given at first, especially with patients outside hospital, with gradual increments according to SMBG.

Tailor the treatment to the patient and do not over-treat patients in whom this is neither safe nor desirable (Box 9.1, ⊋ p. 149).

Thrice-daily short-acting insulin and once-daily longer-acting insulin: basal–bolus

This provides sophisticated and flexible insulin treatment which can often allow a very varied lifestyle. Use background (basal) insulin overnight (e.g. isophane (NPH), Lantus®, Levemir®, Tresiba®, or zinc suspension insulin) and give rapid or short-acting insulin before each meal (bolus). Sometimes twice-daily background insulin is needed. Adjust the dose of rapid/short-acting insulin according to blood glucose at that time, food to be eaten, and activity planned. Using CHO counting to adjust the insulin dose more precisely can improve glucose control. Properly used, this regimen can produce normoglycaemia. However, to do so requires a sophisticated use of insulin dose adjustment and careful observation by the patient of their glucose responses to insulin, food, and activity. A basal–bolus insulin regimen does not, in itself, produce better glucose control.

This regimen is popular with patients. Many find that they can move meals and even omit them. However, others still need regular mealtimes and snacks, and all must eat a bedtime snack to guard against nocturnal hypoglycaemia.

Twice-daily injections of a fixed-proportion mixture

This regimen is simple for patients but inflexible and unlikely to produce good glucose control. It is best for patients with little variation in their daily eating and activities. Current options are given on (⊋ p. 153; p. 159). It is probably the easiest regimen to start with and can be converted to a more flexible pattern if required. However, many diabetologists feel patients should start with basal–bolus straight away.

Twice-daily, self-mixed, short-acting, and longer-acting insulin

This has largely been superseded by the basal–bolus regimen. The usual insulins are a short-acting types such as Actrapid® or Humulin® S and an isophane such as Insulatard® g.e. or Humulin® I. This regimen gives four points at which the insulin dose can be adjusted. It is essential that the patient understands this—many do not. It is very prone to dosage error. Full use of this regimen is possible only with knowledgeable SMBG.

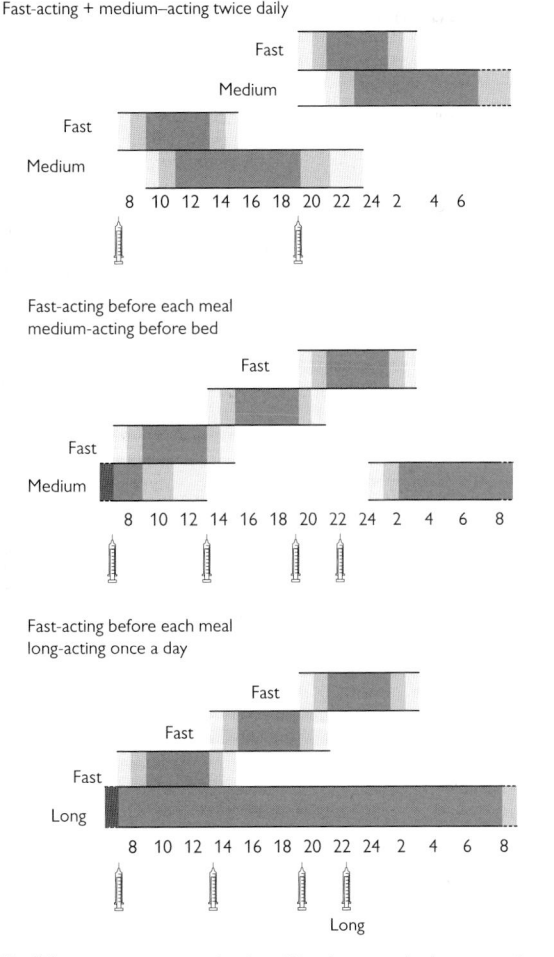

Fast-acting + medium–acting twice daily

Fast-acting before each meal
medium-acting before bed

Fast-acting before each meal
long-acting once a day

Fig. 9.3 Insulin regimens with fast (rapid/short) acting and either intermediate or long-acting insulin. The onset, intensity, and duration of insulin action varies from person to person and from day to day. Insulin action and duration is shorter with rapid-acting insulins than with short-acting. Long-acting insulins usually act throughout 24 hrs but insulin concentrations may rise and fall variably.

Once-daily, long-acting insulin, ± rapid/short-acting insulin

This regimen is used in type 2 patients uncontrolled on oral agents. It may be sufficient to improve glycaemic balance without mealtime insulin. It rarely produces good glucose control unless the patient is making some insulin. Other situations in which it can be useful are when a carer such as a district nurse has to come in to give the insulin to someone who cannot inject his/her own, or for someone in whom the aim of treatment is not normoglycaemia but freedom from symptoms and avoidance of hypoglycaemia or marked hyperglycaemia. The insulin is usually added to the non-insulin agents (→ p. 143).

It is the patient who injects the insulin, not the doctor

The doctor prescribing the insulin is not the person who has to inject it and live with what happens thereafter. The insulin regimen must be tailored to the needs of the each person with diabetes. If the patient cannot control their blood glucose on a particular regimen, finds it hard to use, or loses confidence in it, it should be changed. Clearly, it is worth giving each new regimen a few months' proper trial with full education and continued support. If a patient moves to your clinic from elsewhere on a bizarre insulin regimen which seems totally illogical but appears to satisfy them without obvious safety issues, do not change it until you have had a chance to assess how it works for that person.

Monitoring people on insulin therapy

Honeymoon period

Warn type 1 patients about the possibility of a honeymoon period of diabetes in which the last remaining beta-cells, released from the toxic effects of hyperglycaemia, produce some insulin before succumbing to the continuing autoimmune destructive process. Hypoglycaemia may occur and doses will have to be reduced rapidly. Patients may think that their diabetes has gone away. Warn them about the honeymoon period at the outset to avoid bitter disappointment. Be prepared to reduce insulin doses fast if this occurs, and to increase them again when it ends.

Clinic checks: insulin-treated patients

- Patient knowledge—theory
  - Does the patient know which insulins and how much of each he/she is taking?
  - What is the insulin for?
  - When is each insulin likely to act?
  - Does he/she know how to adjust the dose according to blood glucose levels, diet, and activity?
  - What should he/she do if he/she becomes ill?
  - What precautions should he/she take?
  - Is he/she aware of the risk and symptoms of hypoglycaemia?
- Patient knowledge—practical
  - Does the patient know how to check, store, and draw up his/her insulin? Does he/she know how to inject it?
  - Does he/she know what to do with unused and used sharps and syringes? Have you watched him/her draw up and inject insulin?
  - Does he/she know how to use his/her insulin pen, including changing cartridges? Have you watched him/her do this?
- Insulin passport? (⮕ p. 161)
- Diabetes card/record of insulin used?
- Carrying glucose? Ask to see it.
- Glucagon: Has the patient's partner or relative an up-to-date supply and does he/she know how to use it? (⮕ p. 190)
- Hypoglycaemia: Has the patient experienced this? Does he/she have warning symptoms? Does he/she have nocturnal hypoglycaemia?
- Blood glucose balance (Table 9.1): if the blood glucose is persistently outside your targets for that patient, his/her treatment needs adjusting.
- Type 1 patients: DKA education and ketone testing. Do they need blood ketone testing kit? Do they know how to use it? All patients who have had DKA should have a ketone testing kit at home (⮕ p. 110).
- Clinical state: apart from usual tissue damage monitoring, have any conditions arisen which would alter the insulin regimen? Is there any evidence of side effects of treatment? Have you examined the injection sites?

- Laboratory monitoring: consider checking renal function as this will alter insulin clearance.
- Driving: has the patient told the DVLA he/she is on insulin? Does he/she know how to drive safely on insulin? Has he/she told his/her vehicle insurance company? (➲ pp. 395–400)
- Take-home message: what dose should the patient be taking now? When should it be taken? Write it down.

Remember that patients knows their diabetes far better than you do. Listen to their observations carefully and do not contradict them without due thought. They are usually correct in saying that a particular insulin does not suit them. Even if they do harbour misconceptions, correct them gently with an appropriate explanation.

The whole principle of insulin treatment is that the insulin is adjusted to the patient's lifestyle and not the other way around. People should not have to eat to keep up with their insulin—lower the dose to suit what they want to eat. People should not be prevented from doing particular things because they have to go home and inject their insulin—give them an insulin pen to carry with them. They should not be afraid that hypoglycaemia will ruin their work or a day out. Learn about your patient as a person and fit the diabetes treatment around his/her needs.

Box 9.2 Information for patients on insulin injections

Date started	Date stopped	Insulin brand name(s)	Insulin type*	Injection time(s) with syringe/pen

*Insulin type: analogue / human / porcine / beef

Inject your insulin subcutaneously—this means into the fatty tissue under the skin of the thighs, abdomen, buttocks, or upper arms.

Inject your pre-meal insulin. . . . . minutes before food.

Adjust your insulin dose for food, exercise, and current glucose as shown by your diabetes nurse or doctor.

Eat three meals a day with mid-morning, mid-afternoon, and pre-bed snack unless otherwise advised.

Insulin lowers the blood glucose level and will help to control your blood glucose level.

Sometimes the blood glucose may fall too low (i.e. below 4 mmol/l). This is called hypoglycaemia and may happen if you are taking too big a dose, eat too little, or exercise more than you expect. If you feel muddled, slow-thinking, tingly, unduly emotional or cross, sweaty, or shaky, or notice your heart thumping fast, eat some glucose and then have a big snack. Contact your doctor or diabetes nurse. You may need to reduce your dose of insulin.

Insulin will work only if you inject it regularly as prescribed!

If you are unable to take your insulin for any reason, contact your doctor or diabetic nurse immediately.

Never stop your insulin. If you cannot eat, or are vomiting, contact your doctor immediately or follow the sick day rules he/she has given you.

Always carry a diabetic card and some glucose with you.

Inhaled insulin

Inhaled insulin (Exubera®) was licensed for the treatment of both type 1 and type 2 diabetes but was withdrawn by the manufacturers. In 2014 Afrezza® was licensed by the FDA for use as a rapid-acting inhaled insulin in the USA. At the time of writing Afrezza® is not licensed in Europe. Insulin is well absorbed via the lungs, producing a more rapid glucose-reducing effect than injected insulin. However, there are concerns about adding potential adverse effects on the lungs (including possible lung cancer risk) to the reduction in pulmonary function seen as a complication of diabetes.

Oral insulin

Previously there was no successful method of protecting swallowed insulin from digestive enzymes. Several companies are working on oral insulin products. There are on-going FDA-approved studies of an oral insulin preparation that has been shown to produce a measurable rise in plasma insulin level in type 1 patients.

Islet cell and pancreas transplant

There is a UK islet cell transplant programme for people with type 1 diabetes who have recurrent severe hypoglycaemia with hypoglycaemic unawareness. Diabetic patients with functioning kidney transplants may also have islet cell transplant if they have major problems with glucose control despite optimal care. As in other transplants, immunosuppression treatment is needed. The hypoglycaemia and quality of life improves and some patients become insulin independent. Five yr graft survival 30–50 %; hypoglycaemia free and insulin independent 20–25 %. Many patients need further islet infusions.

℘ <http://guidelines.diabetes.ca/Browse/Chapter20#tbl1> (*Practical Diabetes* 2012; **29**(7): 280–5; doi: 10.1002/pdi.1707).

Pancreas transplants are usually performed at the same time as a kidney transplant in people with type 1 diabetes (simultaneous pancreas kidney transplant (SPK). In the UK, the 5-yr survival rate for pancreas graft (in SPK) is 77 %, patient survival 90 % (⊃ p. 279).

Patients with severe recurrent hypoglycaemia with unawareness may have pancreas-alone transplants. Most patients can stop insulin. Serious perioperative complications are frequent (UK figures: 5-yr graft survival 45 %; patient survival 92 %.) Islet cell transplant would seem a better option in those not needing a kidney transplant.

℘ <http://www.organdonation.nhs.uk/statistics/transplant_activity_report/current_activity_reports/ukt/survival_rates.pdf >

Patients who have had pancreatic or islet-cell transplants should continue to receive annual diabetes review, including retinal screening, whether their glucose is normal or not. Retinopathy usually stabilizes or improves, but may develop or worsen early on. Nephropathy eventually improves over many years. Neuropathy shows little improvement. More research is needed. Patients who become normoglycaemic off all glucose-lowering treatment have 'diabetes in remission' (⊃ p. 21).

Summary

- All staff prescribing or administering insulin must have formal training in safe use of insulin and keep up to date.
- If the patient needs insulin prescribe it—the sooner the better.
- Choose the insulin regimen that suits the patient's needs.
- Only use III if it is really necessary, and follow national and local guidance.
- An insulin regimen will succeed only if the person using it understands how his/her insulin(s) work and can adjust it according to insulin need.
- Remember the factors influencing insulin absorption from the injection site.
- Choose equipment appropriate to the patient's needs and keep up to date with advances in insulin delivery.

Further reading

NICE CG15 ℘ <http://guidance.nice.org.uk/CG15> (N.B. check for updated type 1 guidance)
Scottish Intercollegiate Guidelines Network (SIGN) ℘ <http://www.sign.ac.uk/guidelines/fulltext/116/>

Chapter 10

Low blood glucose: hypoglycaemia

What is hypoglycaemia?

The price of normoglycaemia is often hypoglycaemia. Take care that your zealous quest for a normal glucose to reduce the likelihood of future problems does not create problems now.

For the person who has diabetes, hypoglycaemia can be a terrifying experience to be avoided at all costs. The person may aim for persistent hyperglycaemia, preferring the absence of hypoglycaemia now to the vague and distant threat of long-term tissue damage. Some older patients still cling to old advice to 'keep a little sugar in your urine'. About 1 in 3 people with insulin-treated diabetes will experience hypoglycaemic coma; 2–3 % of insulin-treated patients have frequent severe hypoglycaemia.

Hypoglycaemia occurs in sulfonylurea-treated patients—about a third on glibenclamide experience hypoglycaemia. Patients taking metformin or incretin-effect enhancing drugs are rarely at risk of hypoglycaemia unless the drug is added to other glucose-lowering drugs or taken in overdose.

'When I feel my glucose is low'

Patients often call hypoglycaemic attacks 'hypos'.

For a person with diabetes, hypoglycaemia usually means 'when I feel that my glucose is low and I don't expect it to be'. Some patients discount symptoms before meals, or with exercise, when they expect to feel a little low, and report only episodes which have occurred at other times. Other patients discount episodes which they have successfully treated themselves—for them 'hypoglycaemia' means when someone else had to revive them. Many people with diabetes are unaware of some or all their hypoglycaemic episodes, and many have amnesia for severe hypoglycaemia (➔ p. 186). Some patients deny hypoglycaemia despite recording a value < 2 mmol/l because, to them, the only real hypoglycaemia is that which makes them feel unwell. Symptoms of hypoglycaemia are by definition subjective and vary from person to person and from episode to episode (Table 10.1). Symptomatic hypoglycaemia is not a good way to define hypoglycaemia.

Table 10.1 Common symptoms of hypoglycaemia

Sweating	Weakness
Trembling	Hunger
Inability to concentrate	Blurred vision

Any person with diabetes treated with glucose-lowering medication who behaves oddly in any way whatsoever is hypoglycaemic until proven otherwise.

Source data from *Diabetic Medicine* 1992; **9**:70–5; doi: 10.1111/j.1464-5491.1992.tb01718.x.

When counter-regulatory hormones are released

As the blood glucose falls, it stimulates release of adrenaline, noradrenaline, glucagon, cortisol, and growth hormone. Adrenaline causes tachycardia with palpitations and tremor. Glucagon stimulates glucose release from the liver. In people with diabetes the glucagon response may be blunted or absent, and excess insulin inhibits liver glucose release. This 'emergency' hormonal response is called counter-regulation.

Hypoglycaemia could be defined as the blood glucose level at which the body initiates its emergency response. However, this point varies according to the prevailing blood glucose balance in that person. In people with persistently high blood glucose levels, counter-regulation may occur at blood glucose of ≥ 5 mmol/l. This explains why some patients complain that they feel hypoglycaemic at blood glucose levels not normally regarded as hypoglycaemic. In those whose blood glucose is usually normal, significant counter-regulation may not occur until the glucose is < 2 mmol/l. As patients tend to rely on autonomic symptoms to warn of hypoglycaemia, they may have little time to act before the falling glucose level incapacitates them.

Blood glucose concentration

Hypoglycaemia is usually defined as a laboratory venous plasma glucose < 2.2 mmol/l. However, it is safest to tell patients on glucose-lowering drugs that if their blood glucose is < 4 mmol/l it is too low. 'Make 4 the floor.' They should stop what they are doing and eat or drink glucose. They should check their glucose again soon. In a potentially dangerous situation, or where rapid relief of symptoms of hypoglycaemia is required, they should stop and eat glucose, followed by a snack or meal, and check their blood glucose again soon (⊃ p. 188).

Signs and symptoms of hypoglycaemia

The most frequently reported symptoms are sweating, trembling, inability to concentrate, weakness, hunger, and blurred vision (Table 10.1).

Any patient on glucose-lowering treatment who behaves oddly in any way is hypoglycaemic until proved otherwise.

Changes in thinking and perceiving

Subtle changes in mental function occur before the patient is aware that he/she is hypoglycaemic.

- Altered perception includes blurred vision, *déjà vu,* distancing from the world around, colour changes (e.g. everything turns pink), altered intensity of sound, or other sensation.
- Time slows. Time estimation is involved in assessment of speed and so hypoglycaemia may cause accidents to pedestrians and drivers/riders.
- Poor concentration, short attention span, easily distracted
- Slow decision-making is common.
- Conversation may be slow or hesitant.
- Once a task has been taken on, a hypoglycaemic person may not relinquish it—'I've started so I'll finish'; e.g. continues to drive.
- As the blood glucose level continues to fall the person becomes increasingly confused, although they are often able to articulate this as it happens: 'I'm all anyhow, tee hee!' The confusion may be patchy—e.g. the person may be unable to count but can steer a car (but not safely).

Emotions

- Any out-of-character behaviour may be due to hypoglycaemia: irritation and frustration worsened by attempts to help; fast-rising rage out of all proportion to the problem.
- Depression or tearfulness.
- Everything is wonderful, exciting, or hilariously funny.
- A change in personality may be an early and subtle sign.

Refusal of help

Patients commonly refuse help when hypoglycaemic. They may be convinced that they are coping well (but are not). Patients may also convince relatives that this is so.

Hunger with or without abhorrence of food

- Most symptomatic hypoglycaemic people complain of hunger, and will eat ravenously.
- Food may be rejected. Food refusal is common and shows the split thinking of the hypoglycaemic person. Part of the brain may recognize the hypoglycaemia and the need to eat, while another part is revolted by the food, despite hunger.
- Patients may note a dry mouth.

Panic and hyperactivity

Cerebral irritation may combine with the stirring effects of catecholamines to produce panic, terror, and the desire to flee. Carers may be perceived as pursuers. The lack of glucose for muscle energy does not prevent considerable strength or stamina. Carers or staff may be injured.

Skin colour changes

Adrenaline causes skin pallor, but flushing or blotchy rashes may also occur in hypoglycaemia.

Sweating

- Some patients wait until they experience sweating before diagnosing hypoglycaemia.
- Sweating may be a late phenomenon.
- Sweating has been used in hypoglycaemia alarms which measure changes in skin resistance due to sweating and bleep to awaken a sleeping person (assuming that they are not already unconscious).

Palpitations and tachycardia

- Uncomfortable awareness of the heart's action
- Moderate increase in heart rate
- Systolic blood pressure may rise

Respiratory changes

- Apnoea
- Hyperventilation
- Uncomfortable awareness of breathing
- Cheyne–Stokes breathing, especially in comatose patients

Tingling

Unlike the prolonged paraesthesiae of severe recurrent spontaneous hypoglycaemia, the paraesthesiae of acute hypoglycaemia occur fleetingly, often around the mouth and lips. Paraesthesiae may also occur in the median nerve distribution in the hand, or elsewhere.

Tremor

A falling glucose level can induce a fine tremor of the hands—not always noticeable unless sought.

Dilated pupils

Not always.

Problems speaking or unclear speech

May sound drunk.

Headaches

Both during and afterwards. Patients complain of feeling 'hungover' after nocturnal hypoglycaemia in particular.

Incoordination and unsteadiness

- A lack of coordination may combine with sweating and tremulous hands to cause spillages and breakages.
- Incoordination is seen in most hypoglycaemic people but they may not always realize it themselves.
- Patient feels unsteady and stumbles readily. May appear drunk.
- Bumps into people.
- Occasionally patients exhibit considerable feats of balance, of which they are apparently incapable when not hypoglycaemic.

Weakness

- Generalized muscle weakness—'As if I've run out of petrol'
- Limb weakness
- Hemiplegia

Weariness, sleep, and coma

- Intense exhaustion and a compulsion to fall asleep can overwhelm the hypoglycaemic person.
- Increasing lassitude makes everything too much bother.
- A gradual descent through tiredness and sleep to coma.
- Sudden coma. People prone to the latter should not hold potentially hazardous jobs and should take especial care to avoid hypoglycaemia.

Tonic–clonic seizures or other epileptiform activity

- Fitting is relatively uncommon, usually with nocturnal hypoglycaemia.
- Sleep prevents recognition of early signs of a falling glucose.
- A person who has a fit only when hypoglycaemic is not epileptic and does not usually need anticonvulsants.
- People with epilepsy can fit when hypoglycaemic.

⚠ No symptoms—loss of warning

- Reduced warning is very common occurring in at least 25 % of insulin-treated patients rising to 50 % with > 25-yr duration of diabetes.
- Many patients are unaware of nocturnal hypoglycaemia.
- Symptomless hypoglycaemia is frightening for patients and carers.
- Near-normoglycaemia increases the risk of impaired warning.
- Warning may (but not always) be restored by raising the average blood glucose for a few weeks and eradicating hypoglycaemia.
- Tell patients with poor warning of hypoglycaemia that they must not drive, operate machinery, or perform activities in which confusion or coma could put them or others at risk until warning has been regained.

Diagnosis of hypoglycaemia

A person on glucose-lowering treatment (whether insulin or tablets) who seems unusual or behaves oddly in any way is hypoglycaemic until proved otherwise. Patients and carers should have a high index of suspicion. This can lead to friction: one of my patients pointed out that he can no longer express anger or impatience without being offered sugar.

Clinical suspicion—act in dangerous situations

In a potentially hazardous situation (e.g. swimming or rock-climbing) the person should eat glucose immediately they suspect hypoglycaemia. Delay caused by blood testing allows the glucose to fall further with worsening of symptoms and increased risk of inappropriate behaviour or coma. Rapid recovery proves the diagnosis.

⚠ These people with diabetes may be hypoglycaemic:
- drowsy post-anaesthesia
- smelling of alcohol

Blood glucose < 4 mmol/l

- Finger-prick blood glucose. Wash the finger well with water first. The patient may have been trying to eat glucose.
- If possible take a venous sample for laboratory blood glucose. There may be any diagnostic confusion or medico-legal implications. Do not delay treatment whilst awaiting the results.
- Remember that a finger-prick glucose may be misleading. If in doubt, or the patient is cold or vasoconstricted, take blood for laboratory venous glucose. If you suspect hypoglycaemia give a dose of glucose pending the lab result.

Treatment of hypoglycaemia

In patients capable of swallowing

Start with fast CHO. Follow with slow CHO. Glucose is absorbed most rapidly in liquid form. It is also best absorbed when swallowed alone—fat (e.g. in chocolate) slows absorption of glucose. As an approximate calculation, 10 g of glucose (Box 10.1) raises an adult's blood glucose by 2 mmol/l, and 20 g raises it by 4 mmol/l, but multiple factors influence this. Give adults 15–20 g glucose or equivalent. Try not to over-treat hypoglycaemia but do not hold back if in doubt. Patients on acarbose must use glucose to treat hypoglycaemia as they cannot break down sucrose.

Treat hypoglycaemia as soon as it is suspected. Check finger-prick glucose if possible. If not, give oral glucose immediately. Delay in treating prolongs recovery. If no recovery in 15 mins repeat, completing 3 glucose doses in total if necessary. Check finger-prick glucose at 10–15 mins and repeat this if further glucose doses are needed. If glucose level still not > 4 mmol/l or patient's condition has worsened, dial 999 ambulance (call doctor in hospital setting).

Follow this rapid CHO with slower CHO, e.g. biscuits, sandwich, meal if due. Give more slow CHO if you have used glucagon, to replenish body glycogen stores. Monitor blood glucose regularly for the next 24 hrs. Give the next dose of insulin at the usual time unless the patient has taken an insulin overdose. Review insulin dose—does it need reducing?

Box 10.1 The following contain about 10 g glucose

- three glucose tablets (e.g. Dextrosol®)
- one tube 25 g GlucoGel® or Dextrogel® (glucose gel)
- one-third of an 80 g bottle of GlucoGel® (a whole bottle contains 32 g glucose)
- 50–60 ml or one-sixth of a 380 ml bottle of Original Lucozade® (a whole bottle contains 68 g glucose; other versions contain different quantities of glucose)
- 90ml or one-third of a can of non-diet Coca Cola®
- A third of a carton of original Ribena® (dilute for children)
- 100ml orange juice (without bits)
- two spoonfuls of sugar
- three sugar lumps
- three or four sweets (e.g. fruit pastilles or jelly babies)

Patients who cannot, or will not, swallow safely

Conscious patients who refuse to swallow

Hypoglycaemic patients may irrationally reject food. Patients may spit out glucose or food and/or fight. Persistent firm encouragement usually works. Glucose gel is hard to spit out completely.

If the patient becomes violent, keep back to avoid personal injury. Try to contain the patient in a safe area. Inject glucagon IM. The alternative is to muster sufficient help to achieve robust venous access and give IV glucose.

Unconscious patients, unsafe swallow, uncooperative

Profound hypoglycaemia is uncommon. It is seen most often after insulin overdose, alcohol, excess sulfonylurea or in renal failure.

- ⚠ Dial 999 ambulance out of hospital unless trained to use glucagon. Glucagon must be to hand, and the person using it must be confident in managing such an episode in this particular patient (e.g. family member with similar successfully treated previous episodes).
- In hospital, fast bleep doctor.
- ⚠ Risk of respiratory or cardiac arrest.
- Protect airway. Recovery position.
- If in IV insulin or CSII, stop it (➲ pp. 166–7), but leave IV or SC cannulae *in situ*.
- Give oxygen if convulsing or hypoxic.
- Safeguard patient and staff from injury.
- In non-clinical setting families/carers can inject glucagon.
- Gain IV access via a large vein, tape in cannula securely (care— extravasated glucose can cause ulceration).
- Withdraw blood for laboratory glucose, urea and electrolytes, liver function, and perhaps thyroid function or cortisol.
- Give IV glucose (repeat once if not recovered within 15 min).
- Over 10–15 mins infuse 75–80 ml 20 % glucose IV or 150-160 mls 10 % glucose.
- 50% glucose is not recommended nowadays—it is hypertonic, hard to use, and extravasation is damaging.
- Check finger-prick glucose at 10 mins. If not > 4 mmol/l recheck every 10 mins until it is.
- IV access impossible—inject glucagon IM.
- If patient fails to recover consider steroid lack. Take blood for subsequent cortisol level and inject 100 mg hydrocortisone IV or IM.
- Monitor Glasgow coma scale, heart rate, BP, respirations, oxygen saturations—and, of course, blood glucose.
- Feed patient if safe, or infuse 5 % or 10 % glucose slowly—rate depends on clinical situation.
- Monitor glucose and condition hourly until full consciousness regained and maintained. Keep under medical observation for at least 4 hrs and admit if any of the factors ('after glucose given') apply.
- Do not remove IV cannula until patient ready for discharge.

Glucagon (UK-GlucaGen®)

Use glucagon when IV access cannot be gained, e.g. in the home or if a vein cannot be found safely by a health professional. Glucagon releases glucose from the liver. However, the rise in blood glucose is temporary and there is considerable risk of recurrent hypoglycaemia. Feed the patient before they become hypoglycaemic again. This many be difficult as glucagon can cause nausea.

Contraindications to glucagon use
- Situations in which glucagon may be ineffective:
  - alcohol excess (chronic or acute)
  - fasting or very strict weight-reducing diet
  - anorexia nervosa
  - steroid lack
  - chronic or recurrent hypoglycaemia
  - chronic liver disease
- Sulfonylureas (caution—recurrent hypoglycaemia likely)
- Warfarin (increases plasma level of warfarin)
- Phaeochromocytoma (risk of hypertensive crisis)
- Indometacin (risk of worsening hypoglycaemia)
- Insulinoma or glucagonoma

Use of glucagon
- Teach families and carers how to use glucagon initially, and revise with each new prescription.
- Prescribe for all patients on insulin who have someone who may need to use it.
- Prescribe two kits in case of breakage.
- Hypoglycaemia-prone patients should carry one kit.
- Storage—protect from light and store at 2–8 °C. Can be stored at room temperature.
- Check expiry date regularly. Check fluid is clear and discard if not.
- Place patient in recovery position and protect airway.
- Kit contains a 1 mg glucagon powder vial and 1 ml water for injection in a pre-filled syringe.
- Place kit on clean safe surface so it cannot roll off, e.g. tray on middle of table.
- Inject water into glucagon vial and shake gently until dissolved. Clear air bubbles and inject.
- Adults, and children > 25 kg or > 8 yrs, inject 1 mg SC, IM, or IV.
- Children < 25 kg or < 8 yrs inject 0.5 mg SC, IM, or IV.
- △ Call 999 ambulance if patient not awake in 10 mins.
- Feed patient plenty of slow CHO.
- Beware recurrent hypoglycaemia.

⚠ Insulin overdose

- ⚠ Risk of death (especially if alcohol involved).
- Ice-packs on sites of injection of large insulin overdoses may slow insulin absorption to 'buy time' for treatment.
- What type of insulin was injected? When?
- Treat as discussed previously.
- Call diabetes registrar and consultant immediately.
- Admit to HDU/ICU.
- High risk of cardiac and/or respiratory collapse.
- Monitor potassium very carefully (it will fall as you give glucose). Replace potassium according to potassium levels.
- Get all the previous clinical records urgently.
- Treat concurrent disease with relevant specialist help.
- Obtain psychiatric help once patient able to talk and understand.
- Hypoglycaemic brain damage may take many months to recover and there is a risk of permanent damage.

After glucose or glucagon given

- Check the finger-prick blood glucose in 10–15 min (wash patient's fingers well). It should be ≥ 6 mmol/l.
- Feed patients with carbohydrate (biscuit, sandwich) after recovery from severe hypoglycaemia to sustain the recovery and prevent relapse.
- Wait a further 45 mins to allow brain function to recover from hypoglycaemia before considering leaving the patient alone, or allowing him/her to drive or perform activities potentially hazardous to him/herself or others.
- Elderly people or those with cerebrovascular disease often take longer to 'come to' after hypoglycaemia than younger people.
- ⚠ Keep patients under observation for at least 1 hr from oral glucose or glucagon treatment (4 hrs after IV glucose), and check glucose and mental function before allowing them to leave the clinic or hospital, or before leaving them alone.
- Check for injuries.
- Be particularly careful if the patient wishes to drive immediately or perform dangerous activities, activities which influence other people's safety, or activities which require concentration. If in doubt stop them.
- Hospitalize hypoglycaemic patients (after emergency treatment)
  - on sulfonylurea.
  - elderly patients.
  - those living alone and vulnerable.
  - who have ingested alcohol or drugs of abuse.
  - with renal disease, liver disease, or other significant disease.
  - with psychiatric problems.
  - with suspicion of overdose of insulin or glucose-lowering tablets.
  - if you have concerns about their safety.

- Patients on long-acting insulin should be considered for admission unless they are fully conscious and capable of monitoring themselves and SMBG, and adjusting their food and insulin safely.
- Patients on sulfonylurea treatment or long-acting insulin may have prolonged or recurrent hypoglycaemia until sulfonylurea-stimulated plasma insulin levels fall as the drug is excreted. Monitor finger-prick blood glucose 1–2 hourly for at least 24 hrs and until the glucose is stable. This may take several days with glibenclamide.
- Note that it is difficult to provide advice for all situations as the clinical effect and risk of hypoglycaemia varies considerably. If in doubt, err on the side of caution.
- △ Remember that the patient's ability to judge their own cognitive function is likely to be impaired.
- Inform the diabetes team of the patient's admission.
- The DST should check diabetes self-care, injection, and blood-monitoring technique, and psychological issues. Change diabetes treatment as required.
- Arrange psychological or psychiatric help if required
- Follow up appointment with diabetes nurse or doctor in 1 mth—or sooner if severe hypoglycaemia and vulnerable.

There is an NHS Best Practice Tariff for diabetic adults admitted as an emergency with DKA or hypoglycaemia. It requires:
- referral to the DST on admission.
- patient seen within 24 hrs by a member of the DST.
- education review by a member of the DST before discharge.
- seen by a diabetologist or DSN prior to discharge
- a written care plan (copied to GP).
- patients to be offered access to structured education, with the first appointment scheduled to take place within 3 mths of discharge.

🔊 <http://www.gov.uk/government/uploads/system/uploads/attachment_data/file/214902/PbR-Guidance-2013-14.pdf>

Prevention of further hypoglycaemia

- What glucose level is the patient aiming for (➔ p. 97) Patients aiming for near-normoglycaemia are at risk of hypoglycaemia. Consider adding 2–4 mmol/l or more to the glucose targets, e.g. 4–7 mmol/l becomes 6–9 mmol/l or 8–11 mmol/l (the latter is safer).
- Immediate patient safety comes first.
- Be especially careful to prevent recurrence in patients with jobs or pursuits risking hazard to themselves or others.
- There is a high risk of recurrence in:
  - patients with previous hypoglycaemia.
  - patients who are very frightened of diabetic tissue damage.
  - elderly patients.
  - those with erratic or small meals.
  - renal disease.
  - hepatic disease.
  - those living alone.
  - alcoholics.
  - steroid-dependent patients.
  - dementia.
  - psychiatric or psychological disturbance.
  - 'brittle' diabetes (➔ p. 327).

- At what time of day did the hypoglycaemia originate?
  - Is there a pattern?
  - Beware nocturnal hypoglycaemia.
  - Reduce daily dose by 25–50 %.
  - Reduce the tablet/insulin acting at the risky time of day.
- SMBG before each meal, pre-bed, and during the night for a few weeks.
- Monitor food intake and well-being.

Children—emergency situations only

This book relates to adults only. However, healthcare professionals may encounter hypoglycaemia requiring immediate action in children. ⚠ Do not use hypertonic 50 % IV glucose which can be fatal in children. Read the BNF for Children ℛ <http://www.bnfc.org> which advises the following:

- By mouth: child 2–18 yrs, 10–20 g glucose (➋ p. 188) repeated after 10–15 min if necessary.
- If still hypoglycaemic or oral route cannot be used:glucagon injection 1 mg/ml SC, IM, IV, according to weight:
  - Child 1 mth to 2 yrs, 500 mcg (0.5 ml)
  - child 2–18 yrs, body weight < 25 kg, 500 mcg (0.5 ml)
  - child 2–18 yrs, body weight > 25 kg, 1 mg (1 ml).
- If prolonged hypoglycaemia or unresponsive to glucagon after 10 min:
  - 10% glucose IV infusion by IV injection into large vein
  - child 1 mth–18 yrs, 2–5 ml/kg (glucose 200–500 mg/kg).
⚠ Get expert paediatric help immediately.

Recurrent hypoglycaemia in insulin-treated patients

Hypoglycaemia due to excess rapid-acting insulin usually responds rapidly to glucose treatment. However, if hypoglycaemia is due to longer-acting insulin it may recur after the initial dose of oral or IV glucose.

Recurrent hypoglycaemia may be seen in patients trying to normalize their blood glucose, in people whose lifestyle or eating patterns have changed, in those who have misunderstood (or never had) diabetes education, and in various other circumstances (Box 10.2). Recurrent severe hypoglycaemia may be due to manipulation by psychologically disturbed patients and can be hard to detect. General measures are as follows.

- First, safeguard the patient.
- Stop them driving or doing dangerous jobs or pursuits (➋ p. 395–400).
- Refer to DST urgently for assessment and education.
- Remove all risk of hypoglycaemia by raising the blood glucose to a constant level of > 10 mmol/l.
- Reduce all insulin doses by 25–50 %. Warn of the need to increase insulin during infection (phone DSN).
- Check insulin administration technique (from drawing up to injection, including timing—human insulin may need to be given closer to meals, even at the table).
- Ensure that food intake is evenly spaced throughout the day—three meals and three snacks (a pre-bed snack is vital).
- Test blood glucose before each meal and before bed (check technique), and during the night (about weekly or more often if severe nocturnal hypoglycaemia).
- Once the hypoglycaemia stops, the blood glucose will gradually be returned towards normal by gentle insulin adjustment.
- Sometimes such patients require hospital admission.

Box 10.2 Causes or risk situations for hypoglycaemia

Hypoglycaemia unawareness
Recent hypoglycaemia or incompletely treated hypoglycaemia
Recurrent hypoglycaemia—'hypos beget hypos'
Nocturnal hypoglycaemia

Too much insulin/non-insulin drug (one-off or over-strict glucose control)
Tightening control at new diagnosis of complication (e.g. retinopathy)
Extra insulin/sulfonylurea/hypoglycaemic drug dose by mistake
Deliberate insulin/sulfonylurea/hypoglycaemic drug overdose

Inappropriate insulin type for person or circumstance
Prescribing error (especially in hospital)
Insulin prescribed or given at the wrong time
Insulin not matching time of meal (oral or enteral) (especially in hospital)
Drawing up or injection errors (patient or staff)
Use of emergency fast-acting insulin ('as needed' or 'prn')
IV insulin infusions (III) including lack of accompanying IV glucose
Injection site problems (lipohypertrophy or atrophy)
Moving away from lipohypertrophy to inject
Rotating injection sites, e.g. leg to abdomen
Staff/family giving regular medication to previously non-concordant patients
Warming injection site, e.g. bath or hot weather
Exercise of muscle under injection site

Lack of diabetes education (patient or staff)
Poor vision or hearing limiting understanding of information
Language problems
Insufficient AMBG or SMBG
Inappropriate response to high AMBG or SMBG

Too little CHO (e.g. mistaken idea that 'diabetics can't eat starch')
Usual snacks omitted (e.g. in hospital or out and about)
Unaccustomed fibre
Change in diet content or timing (holiday, hospital)
'Nil by mouth' pre-operatively
Cancellation of procedure or surgery, and rebooking next day
Lack of appetite
Slimming
Fasting (including Ramadan, and intermittent fasting diets)

Increased exercise (one-off, e.g. running for a bus)
Mobilizing the previously chair-bound or bed-bound, or after illness or injury
Increased regular exercise and training effect

Change of circumstance (e.g. new job/redundancy, marriage/separation)
Erratic lifestyle
Hospital admission
Care home admission
Changing country of residence

Alcohol
Street drugs
Medication interacting with non-insulin drugs
β-blockers (reduce warning symptoms of hypoglycaemia)
Herbal or complementary remedies (e.g. karela)

Very young
Adolescent
Very old

Intensive glucose control pre-conception or during pregnancy
Early pregnancy
Late placental insufficiency
Breast feeding

Kidney disease
Renal dialysis

Severe liver impairment
Recovery from infection
Very severe infection

Gastroenteritis
Coeliac disease and other causes of malabsorption
Vomiting
Delayed gastric emptying or diabetic diarrhoea (autonomic neuropathy)
Dental problems

Bariatric surgery (immediately after)

Major loss of body tissue (e.g. amputation, large tumour removal)

Steroid lack
Cessation of therapeutic steroids
Thyroid lack
Pituitary failure
Malignancy

Emotional problems
Mental illness
Dementia

Terminal illness (end-of-life care)

Hospital or care facility staffing lack or excessive workload

Criminal act (very rare)

Causes of hypoglycaemia

Once the person is thinking clearly, review the sequence of events which led to the hypoglycaemic episode and derive lessons for future prevention. Often, the cause is obvious—late for work, no breakfast, running for the train, late business meeting, missed lunch, miscalculated insulin dose, unexpected activity e.g. missed bus, walked home.

Patients may forget the incident entirely, and so it is important to inform diabetes carers what happened.

Too much insulin

- Deliberate overdose.
- Insulin dose excessive for patient's current needs.
- Inappropriate increase in insulin dose by the patient or their carers.
- Check that the patient understands the time of maximum insulin action and its usual duration (Table 9.2 (➲ p. 152); Figure 9.5 (➲ p. 175)).

Unexpectedly rapid absorption of insulin

The insulin may arrive in the circulation earlier than expected—as from an IM injection, or if the circulation to a subcutaneous site is increased (e.g. by warmth, baths or showers may do this), or by exercising the muscle underneath. Absorption from an abdominal injection is faster than from the arm, which is faster than from the leg.

Too much sulfonylurea or meglitinides

Hypoglycaemia may arise early in treatment if a new patient is started on a weight-reducing diet and oral hypoglycaemics at the same time. There is considerable variation in response to oral hypoglycaemics—2.5 mg glibenclamide may render one patient severely hypoglycaemic and have no obvious effect on blood glucose in another. Always start cautiously. The medication should be given with meals. Pay attention to the recommended dosage intervals and avoid large doses in the evening. Occasionally, sulfonylureas are taken in deliberate overdose by the patient, or by a depressed family member or friend. Meglitinides may also cause hypoglycaemia. Addition of pioglitazone or incretin-effect enhancers may trigger hypoglycaemia because of their additional hypoglycaemic effect although on their own hypoglycaemia is uncommon.

Too little food

Probably the most common cause of hypoglycaemia. An accidentally missed meal, deliberate dieting (especially in young women), avoidance of disliked foods, missed snacks, and spoiled cooking can all contribute. The introduction of large amounts of fibre into the diet of someone usually on a low-fibre diet may also cause hypoglycaemia. This can occur in hospital, on a new diet, or on diabetic group holidays.

Exercise

Hypoglycaemia may be caused if the person has failed to eat enough to fuel the exertion, or has too much insulin in their system, preventing glucose release by the liver. Planned exercise is best coped with by reducing insulin or hypoglycaemic tablets beforehand and, if the exercise is vigorous, by eating more. Unexpected exertion (e.g. ran out of petrol so walked to garage) commonly causes hypoglycaemia. The hypoglycaemia can occur at the time of the exertion and for up to 48 hrs afterwards, e.g. at night. This can be explained to patients as 'the body reorganizing its glucose stores after exercise'. Eat carbohydrate to cover unplanned exertion (➲ pp. 239–40).

Alcohol

Alcoholics with insulin-treated diabetes run a high risk of severe, perhaps fatal, hypoglycaemia. Although 1–2 units of alcohol are unlikely to cause hypoglycaemia, one large drink on an empty stomach may be enough to precipitate or aggravate hypoglycaemia. Every year patients find themselves guests of the constabulary who assume, at least initially, that a person who smells of alcohol, and is behaving oddly, is drunk. This is one reason why every person with diabetes who is on glucose-lowering treatment should carry a diabetic card and glucose.

Drugs

β-blockers, especially non-selective ones, may reduce the warning of hypoglycaemia. β-blockers and other hypotensive drugs, such as guanethidine and clonidine, may reduce the response to hypoglycaemia. Some drugs potentiate the hypoglycaemic action of sulfonylureas and repaglinide (aspirin and NSAIDs, warfarin, sulfonamides, clofibrate). ACE inhibitors may cause hypoglycaemia (Table 8.2, ➔ p. 127).

Renal impairment

This can cause severe hypoglycaemia in both insulin-treated and sulfonylurea-treated patients. If a patient has falling insulin or tablet requirements, check their renal function.

Autonomic neuropathy

This may lead to delayed gastric emptying. Pyloric obstruction can delay food digestion and absorption. Patients with severe autonomic neuropathy may not recognize hypoglycaemia.

Malabsorption

Coeliac disease is commoner in people with diabetes than those without.

Liver impairment

Can cause hypoglycaemia in a patient without diabetes. Its presence requires very careful insulin dose adjustment and frequent food intake (say, every 2 hrs). As most sulfonylureas and repaglinide are metabolized in the liver, they should be used with great caution in hepatic impairment or profound hypoglycaemia will ensue. Avoid pioglitazone.

Steroid insufficiency

Check for steroid lack (adrenal or pituitary) in patients with inexplicable recurrent hypoglycaemia whether or not they have diabetes. Addison's disease is more frequent in patients with type 1 diabetes than in the general population. Cessation of therapeutic steroids can also cause hypoglycaemia.

Hypothyroidism

Check for thyroid hormone lack in patients with inexplicable recurrent hypoglycaemia.

Malignancy

This is another cause of spontaneous hypoglycaemia in non-diabetics, but it may precipitate puzzling recurrent hypoglycaemia in people with diabetes.

Severe infection

This is a rare cause of unexplained hypoglycaemia.

Hypoglycaemia and hypothermia

Hypoglycaemia and cold are a potentially lethal combination. Glucose is essential for normal thermoregulation—hypoglycaemic people cannot shiver (*Clin Sci* 1981; **61**:463–9). Check venous glucose in everyone with hypothermia. If this is difficult, give glucose anyway. This particularly applies to people suffering from exposure in the mountains, at sea, or in other cold/wet/windy situations.

Never do a finger-prick blood glucose on someone with cold, vasoconstricted fingers, as the result, if obtained at all, will be hard to interpret. Use venous blood on a strip and send the sample to the laboratory as well (some glucose strips are not calibrated for venous blood).

Responsibility

Major efforts must be made to prevent hypoglycaemia. These include repeated patient and professional education. People with diabetes clearly have a choice about whether or not to accept medical advice. However, doctors and other health care professionals must ensure that patients understand that hypoglycaemia may not only cause them to injure themselves, but may also cause injury to others, e.g. while driving a car or operating machinery, or require the rescue services, perhaps risking the lives of rescuers. Record your advice. (Driving, see ➔ p. 400)

Carry glucose and a diabetic card

People with diabetes on glucose-lowering treatment, whether insulin or non-insulin medications, should carry glucose on their person. They must be taught when to take it and replenish it once eaten. A diabetic card or medical alert bracelet or pendant may help others to help them.

Summary

- Hypoglycaemia frightens patients and others and may cause harm. Prevent it.
- Hypoglycaemia is common in people taking insulin or sulfonylureas.
- Hypoglycaemia is a laboratory venous blood glucose < 2.2 mmol/l. Patients on insulin or glucose-lowering tablets with a blood glucose < 4 mmol/l should stop and eat glucose or bring forward a snack or meal. ('Make 4 the floor')
- Hypoglycaemia produces many symptoms, but patients can learn to recognize their early symptoms to allow prompt treatment.
- For practical purposes, anyone with diabetes on insulin or glucose-lowering tablets who behaves oddly in any way should be assumed to be hypoglycaemic. Staff and carers should have a high index of suspicion.
- The treatment of hypoglycaemia is glucose taken either by mouth or intravenously. Glucagon should be used only if glucose cannot be injected IV.
- After treatment the cause should be sought and preventive measures instituted. Re-educate the patient (and staff if appropriate).

⚠ Essential further reading

All healthcare professionals caring for people with diabetes should be trained in the management of hypoglycaemia. Relevant detailed advice can be found here:

The Hospital Management of Hypoglycaemia in adults with diabetes mellitus (2010)
🖰 <http://www.diabetes.org.uk/About_us/What-we-say/Improving-diabetes-healthcare/The-hospital-management-of-Hypoglycaemia-in-adults-with-Diabetes-Mellitus/>

Recognition, treatment, and prevention of hypoglycaemia in the community (2011)
🖰 <http://www.trend-uk.org/documents/Trend_report_to_print.pdf>

Safe use of insulin e-learning suite, including 'The safe management of hypoglycaemia' 🖰 <http://www.healthcareea.co.uk/theinsulinsafetysuite >

High blood glucose: hyperglycaemia

What is hyperglycaemia?

One aim of diabetes care is to restore the blood glucose towards normal. This is not the only aim; resolution of symptoms, prevention and treatment of tissue damage, control of other metabolic imbalance, and, above all, a good quality of life are equally or more important.

Hyperglycaemia would usually be regarded as a fasting glucose of > 7.0 mmol/l or a random glucose level > 11.0 mmol/l; i.e. within the diabetic range. Before defining hyperglycaemia for a particular patient, set the patient's blood glucose target zone. (➜ pp. 40–1). Table 7.1 (➜ p. 97). The aims must be tailored to each individual's situation.

For practical purposes, hyperglycaemia is the blood glucose level above the target zone for an individual patient. However, most patients have 'one-off' levels above their target zone from time to time. The occasional random value > 11.0 mmol/l is no worry. Action is required only if hyperglycaemia persists. This may mean immediately in a patient in whom you are aiming for strict normoglycaemia (e.g. a pregnant woman with diabetes), or after observing the glucose levels for a few days in others. It is important not to cause hypoglycaemia by overzealous normalization of the blood glucose. It is also vital to identify dangerous hyperglycaemia promptly.

Causes of hyperglycaemia

There are a number of causes of hyperglycaemia (Box 11.1).

Box 11.1 Causes of hyperglycaemia

Lack of insulin
Lack of non-insulin medication
Failure to respond to non-insulin medication
Too much food
Too little exercise
Infection
Injury—accidental or surgical
Acute coronary syndrome or other acute illness
Menstruation
Pregnancy
Emotional stress
Drugs
Hormonal (e.g. Cushing's syndrome/steroid therapy)

Lack of insulin

- Insulin dose forgotten, omitted, too small, leaked out of the injection site, poorly absorbed from the injection site.
- Insulin dose insufficient for everyday needs.
- Insulin dose insufficient because of increasing insulin demands, as in any situation when the stress hormone response is triggered (e.g. in infection).
- Young girls may omit or reduce insulin to cause hyperglycaemia and hence weight loss (➔ p. 414).
- Insulin omitted because of vomiting or hypoglycaemia (usually wrongly, ➔ pp. 170–3).
- IV insulin (III) not set up, run out, or not going into patient.

Lack of non-insulin medication or failure to respond to it

- Failure to adjust non-insulin hypoglycaemic drugs despite hyperglycaemia.
- Dose of medication insufficient for everyday needs.
- Forgotten or omitted medication.
- Increasing insulin demands due to illness.
- Medication may be vomited or pass through rapidly with diarrhoea.
- Inadequate pancreatic insulin production—insulin treatment needed.

Too much food

- One-off high due to large or unusual meal, e.g. Christmas (teach patients to increase glucose-lowering treatment relating to that meal).
- Hidden CHO (e.g. unfamiliar food, ready meal, or eating out).
- Slim or underweight patients may need both more food and more insulin.
- Overweight patients should be encouraged to return to their diet.

Too much IV glucose
Unmonitored glucose infusions in hospital are a frequent cause of hyperglycaemia in diabetic inpatients.

Too little exercise
Reduces energy expenditure, e.g. a previously active person changes to a sedentary job.

Infection
This is a common cause which should always be sought assiduously in a patient with unexplained hyperglycaemia. Insulin requirement rises rapidly with a developing infection, and then falls equally fast as it resolves.

Injury
May cause stress hormone release and increased insulin demands. Thus people with diabetes who have accidents or who undergo surgery require careful glucose monitoring.

Acute coronary syndrome (ACS) or other acute illness
ACS may be the presenting feature of diabetes, especially in Asian patients. As the myocardial infarct can be silent or produce atypical symptoms, do an ECG in any older patient with unexplained hyperglycaemia.

Menstruation
May be preceded by hyperglycaemia (⟳ p. 334) due to sex hormone fluctuations. Patients may not always volunteer this explanation of repeated hyperglycaemia.

Pregnancy
Can cause unexpected hyperglycaemia in young women, whether or not they are using contraception.

Emotional stress
This has unpredictable effects on the blood glucose. In theory, any stress which stimulates catecholamine release would be expected to raise the blood glucose. While hyperglycaemia is the usual response, some patients become hypoglycaemic under severe stress (e.g. fear) because of increased clearance of insulin from the injection site. Another effect of stress may be to influence the patient's management of his or her treatment. Anxieties about hypoglycaemia can lead to persistent hyperglycaemia. Severe psychological disturbance can be manifested by insulin omission or overdose.

Drugs
Hyperglycaemia may be caused by medication, including steroids (e.g. asthma treatment), thiazide diuretics, tricyclic antidepressants.

When to take action

There are a number of danger signs to look out for—see Box 11.2.

The blood glucose is only one factor to be considered. Review the duration of hyperglycaemia and its cause. A one-off high glucose following a birthday party is rarely a cause for concern, although the lesson learned is to increase the amount of insulin injected before another similar party. Persistent hyperglycaemia or hyperglycaemia in an ill person needs action immediately. Note that the level of the blood glucose may not match the patient's degree of illness. Patients can have life-threatening acidosis and a blood glucose of 12 mmol/l. Other patients walk into clinic, apparently well, with a blood glucose of 30 mmol/l.

Never consider the blood glucose without assessing the patient as a whole. This will also help you to identify patients whose general condition is such that they must be managed in hospital, those who need frequent assessments as their condition might deteriorate, and those in whom there is time to adjust the blood glucose balance gradually.

Is the patient ill?

First, decide if the patient appears unwell or not. Then consider the degree of hyperglycaemia. Your priority is to identify patients who should be managed in hospital. Then act to control the blood glucose concentration.

Check ketones (➔ p. 110)

Check finger-prick blood ketones (best option) or urinary ketones:
- patient ill or vomiting, or emergency attender and glucose > 11 mmol/l
- patient appears well and glucose > 15 mmol/l.

If blood ketone ≥ 3 mmol/l or urinary ketones > 2+ treat for DKA (➔ pp. 216–19).

Box 11.2 Danger signs

⚠ Admit patients with these signs to hospital 999

- Altered consciousness
- Confusion
- Vomiting
- Abdominal or chest pain
- Altered respiration
- Infection
- Dehydration
- Hypotension
- Blood ketones ≥ 3 mmol/l—DKA

⚠ Suspicion of diabetic ketoacidosis? HOSPITAL 999

DKA is still a major cause of death in people with insulin-treated diabetes < 50 yrs old. A Danish review (1996–2000) found a mortality rate of 4 % (*Diab Res & Clin Prac* 2007; **76**:51–6; doi:10.1016/j.diabres.2006.07.024). In Birmingham (2000–09) the mortality rate was 1.8 % (*Br J Diab & Vasc Dis* 2009; **9**:278–82; doi: 10.1177/1474651409353248).

The most prominent symptom is vomiting, a feature which always signals possible danger in diabetes. Treat DKA promptly and effectively. It should always be managed in hospital (➋ p. 217–8).

If the patient can swallow and is not vomiting, encourage oral water. If available, infuse 0.9 % sodium chloride, 500 ml/hr IV during transfer (unless risk of fluid overload, e.g. heart disease). If there is considerable delay to transfer to hospital consider giving one dose of rapid or short-acting insulin (e.g. Apidra®, Humalog®, Insuman® Rapid, NovoRapid®, or Actrapid®, Humulin® S) 0.1 unit/kg body weight IM. Initiation of fluid replacement should come first. Send a written record of your treatment to hospital with the patient.

Ill hyperglycaemic patients without ketones

These patients may also require hospital assessment. If very unwell it may be appropriate to treat them for DKA with IV fluid and IM insulin.

⚠ These suggestions must be adapted to each patient's clinical state.

Infection

Evidence of infection anywhere is a danger sign. Infections in people with diabetes require prompt treatment which usually needs to be more intensive and longer lasting than in those without diabetes. As metabolic chaos can rapidly ensue during an infection, any patient with more than a minor infection should be assessed in hospital. Remember that blood glucose rises rapidly in the presence of infection. A patient's insulin dose may double, and people usually controlled on non-insulin drugs often need insulin.

⚠ *All* patients with *any* evidence of foot infection should be assessed promptly by the diabetes specialist foot team (DSFT) (➋ p. 308–9). Check your local arrangements.

Pregnancy

Pregnant women should be managed by a DST. Any problems with diabetes management should be referred on the same day to the diabetes team linked to obstetrics. High glucose can harm the foetus acutely or chronically (➋ p. 342–4).

Elderly patients and children

It may be difficult to assess elderly patients clinically; they may have severe hyperglycaemia with little clinical evidence. Have a low threshold for seeking hospital assessment of a hyperglycaemic elderly person. The same applies to young children.

Non-diabetic illness

Diabetes can make the treatment of any other illness more difficult, and most other illnesses can cause hyperglycaemia. The presence of diabetes may determine the outcome of a coexisting illness. Such patients who become hyperglycaemic should be assessed in hospital. It is often better to refer the patient via the DST who can then coordinate care with other disciplines. Alternatively, notify the DST when referring a patient so that they can help to supervise care.

Does the patient have symptoms of hyperglycaemia?

The symptoms of hyperglycaemia are mainly thirst, polyuria, and nocturia. The patient may also have general malaise and lethargy. These symptoms are unpleasant, so treat the hyperglycaemia quickly. The blood glucose level at which they occur varies from person to person, and some people appear to adapt to persistently high blood glucose concentrations. If the patient's only problem is symptomatic hyperglycaemia and they are not unwell in other ways, they can usually be managed at home by the GP and/or the diabetes team.

Start or adjust treatment on the day the patient is seen. Review the patient within a week. Provide a contact number for immediate help if their condition deteriorates. If there is no response despite further treatment adjustment, help seek help from the DST.

Management of hyperglycaemia

It is assumed that other urgent treatment has been initiated and that other problems (see Box 11.1) have been addressed. This section is very difficult to write because management which seems appropriate in theory is not always practical. Assess each patient fully and adjust treatment to his/her particular situation. Remember that there are huge variations in the effect of blood glucose upon symptoms and clinical condition, and in the response of blood glucose to treatment.

Preventive vs reactive care

- *React* to a one-off high glucose with a one-off correction dose of insulin if required, and learn why it happened.
- *Prevent* persistent hyperglycaemia at a particular time of day by reviewing the SMBG diary and adjusting glucose-lowering treatment to reduce the glucose at that time.

The same approach can be used to correct hypoglycaemia—react to a one-off low glucose with immediate treatment. Prevent repetition by reviewing the timing and circumstances of the hypoglycaemia and adjusting treatment.

General measures

Check SMBG technique

Check that the patient is using strips and meter correctly and that the results in the diary are at the times stated. Timing errors are common—is the meter clock right? Review or download the glucose meter.

Check medication

Is the patient taking what you think they are—right amount, right time? Has other medication been started or stopped?

Check total calorie and CHO intake

Is the patient eating too much for his/her needs? If so, advise reduction. Refer to the dietitian.

Increase exercise

Regular exercise within the training zone (➔ p. 238) which will help to reduce the blood glucose long term. Many people feel unable to make this commitment but it can be explored. Making an effort to walk regularly; using stairs will help. Patients unable to manage a full exercise programme can still increase their exercise level (➔ p. 237).

Correct causes

Review the list of causes (Box 11.1) and treat any applying to your patient.

Insulin-treated patients

Check medication and technique

Check that you and the patient are both talking about the same insulin and the same doses. Observe insulin pen use or drawing up, injection sites, injection process. Is it too shallow? Does insulin leak out?

If these are all satisfactory, consider whether it is appropriate to increase insulin (Table 11.1), decrease food, or increase regular exercise, or all three.

Table 11.1 Insulin increase to reduce blood glucose

Time of high blood glucose	Insulin dose to increase
Before breakfast	Pre-dinner or pre-bed intermediate-/long*-acting
Before lunch	Pre-breakfast rapid or short-acting
Before main evening meal (dinner)	Pre-breakfast intermediate-/long*-acting
	Pre-lunch rapid or short-acting
Before bed	Pre-dinner rapid or short-acting
	Pre-breakfast long*-acting

*It is assumed that the patient is injecting a long-acting insulin (e.g. Lantus®) once daily.

Correction dose

Every person with diabetes has one-off highs. Some patient learn to use correction doses (Box 9.1, ➲ p. 165–6). Others should consider missing the next snack, reducing the meal, or take some exercise.

Adjust usual insulin

If the blood glucose is > 11 mmol/l for ≥ 3 days and any underlying condition (e.g. premenstrual state) has not resolved, action should be taken.

Acute hyperglycaemia in sick people—increase insulin

Rapidly rising emergency hormones (e.g. bacterial or viral infection) can require rapid insulin increase. High-dose steroids for acute asthma require immediate insulin increase (or often insulin injections in those on other forms of hypoglycaemic treatment). This usually occurs in the context of illness, e.g. an infection. Don't forget to reduce the insulin dose as the patient recovers and the glucose falls.

An example of sick-day rules for a person with diabetes is shown in Table 11.2. Agree sick-day rules for each patient on insulin before they need them.

Chronic hyperglycaemia in 'well' people—increase insulin

Consider the time of peak action and length of action of the insulin acting at the time of hyperglycaemia. Increase one type of insulin at one injection time, wait 2 days for rapid or short-acting insulin, 3 days for intermediate-acting insulin, and 5 days for long-acting insulin, and then review. Make further changes as appropriate. It is usual to increase the insulin by 2 units at a time (1 unit in patients on < 20 units/day or in patients especially sensitive to insulin) (see Table 11.1).

Reduce or redistribute carbohydrate food

Reduce CHO eaten at main meals or redistribute it to other times of day. Balance the calorie intake to the patient's dietary needs. It is unwise to stop snacks, and the pre-bed snack should never be stopped. People who have to get home from work (especially if driving or cycling) should always have a mid-afternoon snack. See Table 11.3.

Table 11.2 Sick-day rules for a person with insulin-treated diabetes

If you are unwell your blood glucose will usually rise as your body releases emergency hormones. This means that you will nearly always need more insulin than usual, even if you are not eating. You also need fluid to prevent dehydration, and carbohydrate at meal times.

1. Measure your blood glucose 6-hourly; that is, before the times you would normally eat and before bed. Test your blood or urine for ketones.

2. DO NOT STOP YOUR USUAL INSULIN

   Be prepared add extra insulin to each dose

Blood glucose	Insulin (adapt dose to the patient)*
≤ 11 mmol/l	No extra units
11.1–16.9 mmol/l	2 extra units
17–21.0 mmol/l	4 extra units
≥ 22 mmol/l	6 extra units
	*If total daily dose > 50 units double the extra units
	Reduce the extra doses as you get better and glucose falls

3. Drink plenty of sugar-free fluid (100 mls/hr). Try to eat carbohydrate foods at meal times; if you cannot eat try drinking milk with added sugar, original Lucozade®, non-diet Coca Cola®, or Pepsi Cola®, or other sugary drinks or juice.

4. CALL FOR HELP SOONER RATHER THAN LATER

   Give the extra insulin and get help:

   If your blood glucose is > 22 mmol/l on two occasions

   If your blood glucose is > 11 and your blood or urine shows ketones

   If you are vomiting and unable to keep fluids down

   If you feel too ill to measure your blood glucose

   If you do not know what to do

YOUR HELP TELEPHONE NUMBER IS

More detailed instructions for people with type 1 diabetes who have been taught how to use them can be found at: ✆ <http://www.leicestershirediabetes.org.uk/438.html>

Patients on non-insulin hypoglycaemic medication

Increase hypoglycaemic drugs

First, check that the patient is actually taking the medication as advised. The dose should be increased gradually and with care not to induce hypoglycaemia. Do not exceed the recommended dose. It is often better to look at the food pattern if there is isolated hyperglycaemia during the day. Most drugs should be given two or three times daily at meal times. Modified release drugs are usually given once daily. Add a second or third agent if on the maximum dose of existing treatment (➜ p. 143).

Stop medicines that are not working despite being taken as advised.

If the patient is persistently hyperglycaemic on maximum doses of non-insulin agents, they need insulin. This should be started without delay (➜ pp. 149–50).

Reduce carbohydrate food

Dietary changes are similar to those for insulin-treated patients, although people on non-insulin drugs rarely need snacks. For people who are overweight, reduction in food intake combined with increased exercise is the best way of improving glycaemic balance. See Table 11.3.

Sick-day rules on non-insulin medication

Unwell patients should continue their glucose-lowering tablets or injections. They should perform SMBG 4–6 hrly (hence the benefit of teaching everyone with type 2 diabetes on glucose-lowering medication how to check finger-prick glucose).

Individual patients on glucose-lowering medication that can be increased (e.g. meglitinides) should be given specific instructions about this, for hyperglycaemia when well and unwell. However, many non-insulin medications cannot be adjusted so patients who feel unwell and whose glucose is > 13 mmol/l should phone their GP or DSN for advice.

All unwell patients should drink at least 100 ml/hr non-sugary fluids, and eat (or drink) carbohydrate at meal times (see Table 11.2).

People too unwell to drink should phone the GP or emergency services straightaway.

Vomiting with abdominal pain may be a danger sign in patients on metformin (lactic acidosis) or on incretin-effect enhancers (pancreatitis) and such patients should stop these drugs and phone their GP or 999 straightaway.

Table 11.3 Carbohydrate reduction to reduce blood glucose

Time of high glucose level	Carbohydrate food to reduce
Mid-morning	Breakfast
Before lunch	Mid-morning snack/breakfast
Mid-afternoon	Lunch
Before main evening meal	Mid-afternoon snack/lunch
Before bed	Main evening meal

Summary

- Hyperglycaemia means a blood glucose concentration in the range for the diagnosis of diabetes.
- Define hyperglycaemia for each patient.
- In an acute situation, assess the patient's condition, then the level of blood glucose.
- Ill patients should be transferred to hospital regardless of their blood glucose. Hyperglycaemia in pregnant women, elderly patients, and children should be managed by the DST, usually in hospital.
- Patients with severe symptoms need prompt treatment.
- DKA is a medical emergency requiring urgent treatment in hospital. It is preventable. It can be fatal.
- Causes of hyperglycaemia are insufficient insulin or hypoglycaemic drugs, excess food, too little exercise, infection, injury (accidental or surgical), myocardial infarction or other acute illness, menstruation, pregnancy, emotional stress, and drugs.
- Treatment of hyperglycaemia includes treating the cause, if possible, and controlling the glucose by increasing hypoglycaemic therapy, reducing food, or increasing exercise.
- React to a one-off high glucose by adjusting hypoglycaemic treatment, food, or exercise that day. Prevent persistent high glucose levels by studying the pattern and adjusting hypoglycaemic treatment, food, and exercise.
- Provide sick day rules tailored to each patient's situation before they are needed.
- If the glucose cannot be controlled, seek the diabetes team's help early.

Chapter 12

Diabetic ketoacidosis (DKA) and hyperosmolar hyperglycaemic state (HHS)

DKA or HHS?

Diabetic high glucose emergencies are usually divided into acidotic and non-acidotic states, but some patients have components of both and the division is not rigid. It depends on the patient's body habitus (internal and external), the way in which fat and other body tissues respond to actual or relative insulin deficiency and dehydration, and the influence of coexisting conditions or medications (Table 12.1). The division is useful to help plan fluid replacement, thrombosis risk, and prognosis. However, it is important to adjust treatment to each patient and to fine-tune it according to clinical response. Rigid attempts to label the high glucose problem are not always helpful. If in doubt, treat as hyperosmolar hyperglycaemic state (HHS).

DKA is, by definition, a state in which high levels of ketones make the blood acid. HHS used to be called hyperosmolar non-ketotic hyperglycaemic state (HONK) and hyperosmolar hyperglycaemia non-ketotic state, and it is a situation in which the main problem is gross dehydration and high glucose levels producing hyperosmolar blood. The glucose levels may be extreme (311 mmol/l has been recorded: *Diabetes Care* 1990; **13**:1812; doi: 10.2337/diacare.13.2.181). It usually occurs in older patients with multiple health problems with a history of several days of worsening health. These patients may show ketones, but not at the levels found in DKA.

Table 12.1 DKA or HHS?

Test	DKA	HHS	Severely illcontact HDU/ICU
Consider contacting ICU for all patients with DKA or HHS.			
Blood glucose	> 11 mmol/l or known diabetes	> 11 mmol/l Usually > 30 mmol/l	> 40 mmol/l
Blood ketone	≥ 3 mmol/l	< 3 mmol/l	> 6 mmol/l
Venous/arterial pH or	< 7.3	Normal	< 7.1
Venous bicarbonate	< 15 mmol/l	> 15 mmol/l	< 5mmol/l
Calculated osmolality * (2 × sodium) + glucose + urea		> 320 mosmol	All patients with HHS
			Clinically very ill
			Confused or unconscious
			Heart rate < 60 or > 100 bpm
			BP < 90 systolic
			Oxygen saturation < 92 % on air
			Potassium < 3.5 mmol/l
			Anion gap > 16**
			Child or elderly
			Pregnant
			Heart disease or Comorbidity

*There are many calculations. This follows JBDS guidance.

**Anion gap = (sodium + potassium) − (chloride + bicarbonate)

DKA

- ⚠ Any suspicion of DKA requires immediate 999 transfer to hospital.
- Caused by absolute or relative insulin lack.
- A major diabetic emergency—preventable, predictable, treatable.
- Mortality 1–4 %—the most common cause of death in diabetic patients < 50 yrs of age.
- One in 200 diabetic inpatients developed new DKA in English hospitals after admission in 2012–13 (NaDIA). If the patient dies, prosecution may follow; see ℘ <http://www.bbc.co.uk/news/uk-england-st oke-staffordshire-26279657> DKA may recur if Ill is stopped after successful treatment without SC insulin being restarted.
- ℘ <http://www.hscic.gov.uk/catalogue/PUB10506>

This chapter relates to adults ≥18 yrs (DKA in children and young people should be managed by paediatric diabetologists, (➲ p. 230)). Doses of fluid and insulin are given for guidance but treatment must be tailored to the individual patient. Seek senior advice and DST advice in all patients.

Symptoms

- Vomiting (most common symptom)
- Tiredness, malaise, weakness
- Thirst, polyuria
- Weight loss
- Deep and rapid respiration—'air hunger'
- Anorexia, abdominal pain, diarrhoea, or constipation
- Symptoms of diabetic complications
- Symptoms of precipitating condition
- May be few symptoms

Signs

- Ketotic breath—'rotten apples, pear drops'
- Hyperventilation—over breathing
- Tired, unwell
- Dehydration, weight loss
- Tachycardia, hypotension
- Hypothermia
- Vomiting ± coffee grounds—due to haemorrhagic gastritis
- Abdominal tenderness
- Gastric retention
- Full bladder or polyuria—if not, very dry
- Evidence of diabetic complications
- Evidence of precipitating condition
- Coma; rare—either very ill or other cause
- N.B. should not be hypoxic—this means there is a lung problem

Causes

- Infection—most common cause
- Too little or no SC insulin
- IV insulin not started as prescribed, not running, or stopped without giving SC insulin
- Psychological factors
- Too much food, especially sugars
- Lack of education (patient or staff)— insulin omission by patient or staff in vomiting patients
- New diabetes mellitus
- Alcohol abuse
- Exercise with insulin lack
- Acute coronary syndrome
- Stroke
- Gangrene
- Surgery
- Trauma
- Any illness
- Gynaecological problems
- Pregnancy
- Manipulation
- Stress—exclude other causes

Diagnosis

See Table 12.1.
- History—exclude DKA in any vomiting insulin-treated diabetic patient
- Examination—may find little, may be dehydrated and hypotensive
- Capillary glucose > 11 mmol/l—if shut down use venous blood on strip strip—or known type 1 diabetes with lower glucose level
- Urine ketones positive. Blood ketones ≥ 3 mmol/l
- Venous pH < 7.3 (arterial blood testing is not required for pH testing as the venous/arterial difference is minimal. Arterial blood may be needed for checking oxygen saturation)
- Bicarbonate < 15 mmol/l
⚠ DO NOT DELAY TREATMENT AWAITING LABORATORY RESULTS

Management

Initial management
- Resuscitation: airway, breathing, circulation
- Aim door to needle time < 15 min
- Good IV access
- Take venous bloods
- 1000 ml 0.9 % sodium chloride IV over 1 hr
- After IV fluids flowing, start FRIII 0.1 units/kg/hr soluble insulin (e.g. Actrapid®, Humulin S®)
- Protect pressure areas, especially feet
- Inform diabetes registrar or consultant diabetologist

Tests
- Finger-prick capillary blood glucose + ketone (beware cold fingers, always send blood for laboratory venous glucose as meters have an upper limit to readings)
- Venous blood pH unless hypoxic on pulse oximetry
- Urgent laboratory venous glucose, U&E, creatinine, FBC
- Use point-of-care (POCT) biochemistry system (e.g. blood gas analyser) quality-controlled by laboratory to monitor progress
- Later LFT, TFT, lipids, blood cultures, CRP
- Dipstick urine
- MSU, throat swab, microbiology swab any lesion
- Pregnancy test
- 12-lead ECG with continuous cardiac monitor thereafter
- Chest X-ray
- Consider abdominal X-ray

Aims of treatment
Start initial resuscitation within 15 mins. Then:
- Gradual return to normal
- Rehydrate over 24 hrs; use IV fluid and insulin to correct DKA
- Aim for:
  - a glucose fall of 3 mmol/l/hr
  - a blood ketone fall of ≥0.5 mmol/l/hr
  - a venous bicarbonate rise of 3 mmol/l/hr
  - a gradual venous/arterial pH rise over 24 hrs

Actions
- Consider ICU/HDU for each patient (see Table 12.1)
- Good IV access
- Oxygen if hypoxic (unless respiratory disease risking CO_2 retention)
- Nasogastric tube if severe vomiting, gastric retention (occurs in severe DKA and may cause aspiration), coma. Take care with NG tube insertion—this may trigger cardiac arrest in severe DKA, presumably from vagal stimulation
- Consider urinary catheter if incontinent or not passed urine within 1 hr, immobile, coma
- IV fluids and electrolytes
- Insulin
- Treat precipitating condition (e.g. antibiotics for infection)
- Prophylactic low molecular weight heparin
- Contact seniors and DST

Treatment

Fluids (depends on patient—beware fluid imbalance)
- Fluid deficit averages 6 litres, but may be as much as 10 litres. Rate of infusion must be tailored to each patient's clinical condition, age, and comorbidities.
- Reduce rate in elderly, cardiac disease, if bicarbonate > 10 mmol/l (mild acidosis).

- Use 0.9 % sodium chloride to correct fluid deficit. Infuse:
  - 1000 ml in 1 hr
  - 1000 ml in 2 hrs twice
  - 1000 ml in 4 hrs twice
  - 1000 ml in 6–8 hrs, continued as needed
  - Maintain ongoing review of fluid balance, and at 12 and 24 hrs

Insulin
- Continue the patient's usual dose and timing of long-acting insulin (e.g. Lantus® or Levemir®). Wait until SC tissues are normally perfused in shocked patients.
- Fixed rate insulin infusion (FRIII) 0.1 units/kg/hr soluble insulin (e.g. Actrapid®, Humulin S®).
- If there is a delay in setting up insulin infusion inject rapid or short-acting insulin 0.1 units/kg IM once (unless already given pre-admission).
- Continue FRIII until pH > 7.3 mmol/l and finger-prick blood ketones < 0.5 mmol/l.
- Glucose and insulin are needed to clear ketones and acidosis. If these are not improving check all infusions, pumps, lines, and cannulae.
- If blood glucose < 14 mmol/l but pH < 7.3 or blood ketones > 0.3 mmol/l or bicarbonate < 18 mmol/l, infuse 10 % glucose at 125 mls/hr in parallel with the 0.9 % sodium chloride to keep the blood glucose 8–14 mmol/l.
- Urine ketones are not helpful in monitoring recovery from DKA and will still be found after blood ketones have normalized.
- Measuring bicarbonate is not helpful after 12 hrs.
- Continue FRIII until patient eating properly.
- Restart usual SC insulin at breakfast time and discontinue the FRIII at least 30 mins later (➲ pp. 167–8).

Potassium
- Patients are potassium-depleted.
- Potassium < 3.5 mmol/l on admission means gross potassium depletion (e.g. laxative abuse). ⚠ Risk of cardiac arrest. Seek immediate senior advice as these patients need a lot of potassium replacement. Admit to HDU/ICU.
- Potassium 3.5–5.5 mmol/l use 0.9 % sodium chloride infusion with 40 mmol/l potassium.
- Do not give potassium if K > 5.5 mmol/l or patient anuric.
- Beware known renal failure—care with potassium replacement.

Bicarbonate
- Sodium bicarbonate is not indicated and may impede recovery.

Phosphate
- While phosphate is depleted in DKA there is no evidence of benefit from replacing it. Consider replacement if there is evidence of muscle weakness.

HHS

- ⚠ A dangerous condition with a mortality of > 10 %. It is difficult to manage successfully. Get diabetologist help immediately and refer patients to HDU/ICU.

Symptoms and signs

- Patients are often elderly but HHS can occur in young people. It is commoner in African–Caribbean patients in the UK. Many of the clinical features are the same as DKA. Patients with HHS often present with symptoms of a urinary tract infection and confusion. They may have had profound thirst (quenched with sugary drinks in younger patients), polyuria, and polydipsia. Vomiting is not common and the patients will not be hyperventilating. They may arrive moribund after many days preceding decline. Some patients have features of both DKA and HHS.

Causes

- The patients are likely to have type 2 diabetes. Causes are as for DKA. The most common cause is infection (especially urinary or chest) and the patient is often on diuretics and may have cardiac disease and/or renal impairment.

Diagnosis

See Table 12.1.

There are no formal diagnostic criteria for HHS but the cardinal feature is gross dehydration, usually with hypovolaemia, with an osmolality > 320 mosmol, and very high glucose without sufficient ketoacidosis to satisfy diagnostic criteria for DKA. Patients may be misdiagnosed as having a stroke (or HHS may have been precipitated by a cerebrovascular event).

Management

There may be initial failure to recognize the danger – staff may believe 'she's just a bit confused'. It may take 72 hrs or more for the patient with HHS to recover. Gradual improvement is safest.

Initial management

- Resuscitation: airway, breathing, circulation.
- Aim door to needle time < 15 mins.
- Good IV access.
- Take venous bloods.
- 1000 ml 0.9 % sodium chloride IV over 1 hr.
- Do not start insulin unless blood ketones > 1 mmol/l or ketonuria > 2+ and do not give starting dose of insulin (Joint British Diabetes Societies (JBDS) guidance (➔ pp. 221–2)).
- Patients are often confused or aggressive—get help early if needed.
- Urinary catheter to measure fluid output accurately.
- Protect pressure areas, especially feet.
- Treat cause of HHS, e.g. infection.
- Give prophylactic low molecular weight heparin if there are no contraindications (some diabetologists would fully anticoagulate).

- Review all treatment for comorbidities.
- Inform diabetes registrar or consultant diabetologist.

Tests
- As for DKA, but you will need to use near-patient analyser or laboratory to measure glucose at first in most patients. Calculate osmolality (unless your laboratory can measure it hourly) using ((2 × sodium) + glucose + urea).

Fluids (depends on patient—beware overload)
- The key issue in HHS is severe dehydration. Fluid replacement will bring the glucose concentration down. Fluid deficit may be > 10 litres. Rate of infusion must be tailored to each patient's clinical condition, age, and comorbidities. Care in elderly, cardiac, or renal disease. This guidance is taken from JBDS in patient group recommendations which should be consulted for their detailed advice (➜ p. 231).
- Stop diuretics.
- Aim for a fall of 3–8 mosmol/kg/hr.
- Use 0.9 % sodium chloride to correct fluid deficit.
- If systolic BP < 90 infuse 500 mls 0.9 % sodium chloride over 15 mins and get senior advice (ideally diabetologist). Repeat this if BP still < 90 while awaiting senior input. If BP still < 90 consider additional cause, e.g. myocardial infarct. Call ICU.
- If systolic BP > 90 infuse 0.9 % sodium chloride:
  - 1000 ml in first hr.
  - Then 500–1000 ml per hr aiming for a positive fluid balance of 2–3 litres by 6 hrs.
  - Further fluid according to response aiming for a positive fluid balance of 3–6 litres by 12 hrs.
- If the patient or the blood tests are not improving, check all infusions, pumps, lines, and cannulae. Confused patients may dislodge them.
- The plasma sodium level will rise. Providing the osmolality is falling at ≥ 3 mosmol/kg/hr continue 0.9 % sodium chloride.
- If osmolality is not falling and positive fluid balance inadequate, increase rate of 0.9 % sodium chloride infusion.
- If plasma sodium is rising and osmolality is not falling and fluid balance is adequate, change to 0.45 % sodium chloride.
- If plasma osmolality falling too fast (≥ 8 mosmol/kg/hr) slow down IV fluids.
- If blood glucose not falling each hour and positive fluid balance inadequate, increase rate of IV sodium chloride infusion.
- If blood glucose not falling each hour and positive fluid balance adequate start insulin as stated below.

Insulin
- HHS patients are often more insulin-sensitive than those with DKA. Hypoglycaemia is very dangerous in these patients and great care must be taken with insulin use.
- Aim for a glucose fall of < 5 mmol/l/hr to a level of 10–15 mmol/l.

- If usually on insulin continue the patient's long-acting insulin (e.g. Lantus® or Levemir®) in most cases (but wait until SC tissues are normally perfused in shocked patients).
- Do not continue non-insulin medications.
- Start insulin if blood ketones > 1 mmol/l or ketonuria >2+; or if blood glucose is no longer falling despite appropriately positive fluid balance.
- Use a fixed rate insulin infusion (FRIII) 0.05 units/kg/hr soluble insulin (e.g. Actrapid®, Humulin S®).
- FRIII may need to change to VRIII according to response. Take diabetologist advice.
- Take diabetologist advice about when to stop III and what treatment the patient should continue for glucose lowering.

Potassium
- Patients are potassium-depleted but less so than in DKA.
- Many of these patients have renal impairment so take care to avoid hyperkalaemia.
- Potassium < 3.5 mmol/l on admission means gross potassium depletion.
  ⚠ Risk of cardiac arrest. Seek immediate senior advice as these patients need a lot of potassium replacement. Admit to HDU/ICU.
- Potassium 3.5–5.5 mmol/l use 0.9 % sodium chloride infusion with 40 mmol/l potassium.
- Do not give potassium if K > 5.5 mmol/l or patient anuric.

Phosphate and magnesium
- Neither is normally given in HHS. Consult the diabetologist.

Monitoring DKA and HHS

Bedside monitoring
- LOOK AT THE PATIENT (hourly at first).
- Can the patient talk normally?
- Pulse, BP, respirations, pulse oximetry (hourly).
- Fluid input/output—hourly.
- Neurological observations if impaired conscious level (e.g. Glasgow coma scale chart).
- CVP hourly if used.
- ECG monitor—look at T waves (peaked if high potassium) and rhythm.

Laboratory/POCT monitoring
- Venous pH every 2–4 hrs until pH > 7.3 if acidotic on admission.
- U&E every 2–4 hrs.
- Venous glucose every 2 hrs until < 30 mmol/l (or below maximum meter limit).
- If glucose within meter range, finger-prick glucose hourly unless BP low/cold; if so, use laboratory venous reading.
- Finger-prick ketone every 2–4 hrs until < 0.5 mmol/l (use venous blood if patient shut down).
- In HHS calculated osmolality hourly for first 6 hrs.
- Reduce frequency of monitoring thereafter according to patient state and response (see JBDS guidance, ➲ p. 231).

Lessons learnt the hard way
Take it seriously
- Take DKA/HHS seriously. Don't delay!
- Make diagnosis and start treatment within 15 mins.
- Put all patients with suspected DKA/HHS into the resuscitation area.
- One-to-one nursing until stable, or longer if very ill.
- Call medical registrar and/or diabetes registrar, then diabetologist.
- Consider referral to HDU or ICU for all these patients.

Get the previous records
Previous clinical records must be available within an hour of patient's arrival in hospital. Many patients admitted with DKA/HHS will be under your local diabetes service. Many will have had previous admissions with DKA. Old clinical records may indicate risk (e.g. known cardiac or renal disease), and speed diagnosis and management.

Admit the patient to the diabetes ward or ICU/HDU
Patients should be cared for by staff expert and experienced in their management. They are more likely to spot problems, or unusual clinical responses. Patients usually go home sooner.

Review the patient yourself

Patients with DKA/HHS should improve gradually from your first intervention. A doctor/senior nurse should talk to the patient once an hour for at least the first 6 hrs, and 4 hourly thereafter. If the patient cannot talk there is a serious problem. The most common reason for failure to improve is treatment not happening, e.g. cannula fallen out. Medical wards are busy places and nurses are stretched to the limit.

Patients who do not look ill—but are!

Patients who usually run high glucose levels tolerate them well. They may have problems with self-care or manipulate their management. Although you often see them in clinic with glucose > 20 mmol/l, always check their ketone levels—you may be able to pre-empt an admission in DKA. Some patients tolerate DKA remarkably well. They may be vomiting and a little dry but with no other signs. However, they may still be significantly acidotic and dehydrated. Always take a vomiting or sugary diabetic patient seriously.

Use blood ketone strips to assess ketosis (➲ p. 110)

- Use blood ketone strips to diagnose DKA and monitor progress.
- The predominant ketone in DKA is β-hydroxybutyrate. This is what the blood ketone strips measure.
- Blood ketones 1.5–2.9 mmol/l and not acidotic may progress to DKA. Give insulin *immediately* to prevent DKA. Consider admission, fluids, and insulin infusion (➲ pp. 205–7).

Urine ketone strips measure acetone, which is a less helpful indicator of ketosis. Also, the urine will have been in the bladder for varying lengths of time and indicates past, but not necessarily present, ketosis (➲ p. 91).

Missed infection

- Infection is the most common cause of DKA/HHS and patients may not have a fever.
- People with diabetes may behave as if they are immunocompromised.
- Most patients with DKA will have a slightly raised WBCC—this cannot be used as a marker for infection. Marked elevations usually indicate infection. Measure CRP but this may not be raised in infection.
- Viral infections can trigger DKA/HHS.
- Bacterial infections may be due to multiple organisms.
- If in doubt give broad-spectrum antibiotics—the patient is too ill to await microbiological results.
- Fungal infections may be hard to diagnose, and may be systemic and not just superficial. Candida is the most common (albicans or glabrata).

Hypothermia

- The temperature in DKA/HHS may be normal or low.
- Hypothermia is common in DKA/HHS and has a high mortality.
- Measure temperature with a low-reading thermometer.
- Lack of fever does not rule out infection.

Glucose 'not high enough'

Patients who have eaten little for some time, or who have liver disease, can have severe DKA with a glucose < 11 mmol/l. Look at the whole picture, not just the glucose level. N.B. Alcohol excess can cause ketoacidosis.

Normal or low potassium on admission

The potassium should be raised in insulin lack. Normal or low potassium usually means severe, often chronic, potassium lack (do not forget laxative abuse). Give potassium in the first bag of saline. Such patients may need large doses of potassium IV and therefore may need HDU nurses to administer this. Watch the T waves on the ECG to monitor the effect of the potassium on the heart.

Normal or high sodium concentration on admission

- The sodium should be low if the glucose is high due to insulin lack.
- If the sodium level appears normal or high the patient may be severely dehydrated.
- The calculation to correct the sodium for glucose concentration is about 0.4 mmol/l sodium per mmol of glucose (*Am J Med* 1999; **106**: 399–403; doi: ℘ http://dx.doi.org/10.1016/S0002-9343(99)00055-8). But the relationship between sodium and glucose is non-linear as the glucose rises so the correction should be regarded as approximate only. Example: plasma glucose 30 mmol/l and sodium 135 mmol/l corrects to sodium ~ 147 mmol/l (0.4 × 30 = 12, 135 + 12 = 147).
- Infuse IV 0.9 % sodium chloride initially in all patients (➲ pp. 217, 220–1).

Raised urea and creatinine

Dehydration can cause marked rises, e.g. creatinine > 500 micromol/l. Some of these patients will have acute-on-chronic renal disease. Proteinuria suggests the latter (in the absence of a UTI). Also, low urine output despite plentiful fluid replacement may indicate poor renal function. Check previous laboratory results and past records.

Bizarre or dramatic changes in glucose levels

- Check cannula and lines. Has there been a delay in refilling an empty insulin pump or replacing a bag of fluid?
- Check that insulin has been given—and at the right dose.
- Suspect manipulation, especially if the patient is psychologically disturbed. Rarely, patients substitute water for insulin in the pump.

Abnormal oxygen or carbon dioxide concentrations

- The arterial oxygen level should be normal. If the patient is hypoxic, he/she has cardiac or respiratory disease or fluid overload, aspiration of gastric contents, or are developing very severe complications of DKA such as pulmonary oedema or adult respiratory distress syndrome (ARDS). Urgently seek and treat the cause of hypoxia. Start with repeat CXR.
- In DKA the arterial CO_2 should be low because of hyperventilation. If is it not, the patient may have respiratory disease causing CO_2 retention, or they may be so ill that they have respiratory depression.

Complications of DKA and HHS

⚠ Cardiac and/or respiratory arrest

- Institute all usual cardiac arrest procedures.
- Call diabetes registrar or consultant diabetologist.
- Patients may arrest because the severity of their condition has not been appreciated.
- Check for hypoglycaemia immediately.
- Ensure treatment (fluids, insulin) has been given.
- DKA causes major potassium shifts—check it.
- Ensure infection and other precipitants have been treated.
- Even young patients with DKA may have had a myocardial infarct.
- Consider aspiration of gastric contents.
- Even if the situation appears hopeless carry on full resuscitation for at least twice the usual time to allow some correction of the metabolic issues—remarkable recoveries can occur.
- Transfer to ICU if resuscitation successful.

Patient not recovering

- The patient should have improved clinically every time you see him/her. If not:
- Check treatment: is IV cannula still in and working? Are infusion lines patent? Have all drugs/fluids all been given according to prescription?
- Check diagnoses: consider other causes of acidosis. Other cause(s) of DKA/HHS. Missed infection?
- Further events (e.g. silent myocardial infarct or stroke).
- Additional new or existing diagnoses.

Hypoglycaemia

- Common and dangerous
- Caused by over-enthusiastic insulin infusion
- Aim for glucose fall of 3 mmol/hr in DKA, < 5 mmol/hr in HHS
- Use IV glucose to control rate of fall (➲ p. 219) (➲ pp. 167–8)

Cerebral oedema

- Needs ICU/HDU. Can be fatal
- Has been linked to use of concentrated bicarbonate solutions, over-rapid fall of glucose, excessive use of hypotonic electrolyte infusions
- Signs/symptoms:
  - headache
  - drowsiness
  - irritability
  - bradycardia
  - hypertension
  - slowing of respiratory rate
  - reduced Glasgow coma scale
  - neurological signs (e.g. cranial nerve abnormalities, papilloedema, seizures)
  - hypoxia
  - respiratory arrest

- Management:
  - slow insulin infusion rate.
  - give mannitol
  - get consultant diabetologist help
  - transfer to ICU

Central pontine myelinolysis
Has occurred in HHS and is thought to be due to over-rapid shifts in osmolality.

Persistent hypotension
- Consider ICU/HDU
- Too little fluid—or not enough to overcome glycosuric effect
- May be due to cardiac dysfunction, including silent myocardial infarct
- Is it solely DKA? Consider lactic or renal acidosis
- Consider septic shock
- Consider excessive/persistent hypotensive medication or overdose of any drug

Pulmonary aspiration
- Needs ICU/HDU
- Why did you not insert a nasogastric tube earlier?
- Has patient's risk of aspiration changed since your initial assessment because of vomiting with impaired gag reflex (stroke, reduced conscious level), or gastric retention and massive vomiting
- Management:
  - oxygen
  - empty stomach via nasogastric tube
  - vigorous chest physiotherapy and suction as appropriate
  - antibiotics (e.g. cephalosporin and metronidazole)

Pulmonary oedema
- Needs ICU/HDU
- Too much fluid, too fast
- Cardiac disease—new or existing
- Early ARDS (see ARDS)
- Low albumin (patient very ill or prolonged illness)
- Management:
  - slow or stop IV infusion
  - consider diuretics or cardiac support medication
  - may need non-invasive or invasive ventilation

Adult respiratory distress syndrome (ARDS)
- Needs ICU/HDU
- Hypoxia and crackles in very sick patient
- Usually patient obviously very ill on admission and already on ICU
- Requires ventilation
- High mortality

Thromboembolism

- Dehydrated sugary patients have hypercoaguable blood and don't move much.
- Are you giving enough fluid?
- Patient should have been on prophylactic low molecular weight heparin.
- Increase this to treatment dose in patients with proven thromboembolism and in those with HHS at high risk of this.

Pressure sores or foot ulcers

Failure to protect the feet and pressure sores is unforgivable. Every person admitted to hospital must have a foot risk assessment on admission and full foot protection (p. 305).

Rhabdomyolysis

Can occur after HHS and cause renal failure.

Muscle weakness

Consider phosphate replacement.

Fetal distress/death

In pregnant women with DKA obtain obstetric opinion as soon as initial resuscitation is done. There is a risk of fetal death in maternal DKA.

A fetus of viable age should be monitored as it may need to be delivered if the fetal heart slows unduly. However, the risk of *any* surgery in an acidotic patient is considerable (she may die), and the mother must be resuscitated and her pH improved before any surgery can be contemplated.

The next stage

- To be managed by DST.
- Review usual diabetes treatment. Is it the right treatment for this patient? Did the treatment contribute to the DKA/HHS?
- Change glucose-lowering treatment if it has been inappropriate.
- Start SC insulin 30 mins before stopping III at breakfast time (➲ pp. 167–8). An episode of DKA demands long-term insulin treatment in most patients. Some patients with HHS may return to oral hypoglycaemics.
- Elucidate cause (gather evidence from patient, relatives, health professionals inside and outside hospital, social services).
- Once the patient is recovering, the problem (DKA) and its cause must be fully explained and steps taken to prevent recurrence.
- Teach patients and carers to use blood ketone testing and ensure that the relevant meter and strips are provided.
- Note that the DKA may have been precipitated by inappropriate insulin reduction by a health care professional who should be identified and constructively educated.
- There is an NHS Best Practice Tariff for diabetic adults admitted as an emergency with DKA (➲ pp. 191–2).

Follow-up

- Every patient admitted with DKA must be followed by the specialist diabetes service.
- All such patients should be seen by a DSN.
- Follow-up appointment intervals vary according to the patient and local arrangements, but a month is reasonable.
- African–Caribbean patients may have ketosis-prone type 2 diabetes (➲ pp. 18–19), and about half will subsequently be able to manage on diet and oral hypoglycaemic agents for some years.

Prevention of DKA/HHS

- Education of patients and staff in primary, community, and secondary care.
- Monitor glucose and adjust treatment.
- If ill—never stop insulin, monitor glucose, monitor ketones, ask for help.
- Address psychological problems.
- Plan surgery.
- Plan pregnancy.
- Treat infection promptly and fully.
- Identify high-risk patients—previous DKA, 'brittle' diabetes, youthful non-attenders. The DSN should keep in touch with them.
- Always admit vomiting type 1 diabetics unless you or the patient are very experienced.
- Ensure that patients and carers seek advice if they feel increasingly unwell or have an infection.
- Ensure regular checks on older patients with diabetes who take diuretics or have renal impairment.
- N.B. Patients with previous DKA or HHS are at risk of another episode—increase contact and professional review.

DKA/HHS in children <18 yrs of age

- Diagnostic features are similar in adults and children.
- HHS is rare but may occur in African–Caribbean teenagers.
- Treatment of DKA in children demands specialist paediatric expertise.
- Contact on-call paediatric registrar or consultant paediatrician immediately.
- Guidelines for the management of DKA in children are on the BSPED website: <http://www.bsped.org.uk/clinical/clinical_endorsedguidelines.html>

Summary

- DKA and HHS are potentially fatal.
- DKA and HHS are usually preventable.
- The most common cause is infection.
- DKA and HHS are medical emergencies requiring immediate treatment—door to needle time < 15 mins.
- DKA and HHS are the product of insulin deficiency and tissue (especially fat) response to this.
- Vomiting in insulin-treated patients is a key symptom of DKA.
- Blood ketones ≥ 3 mmol/l = DKA.
- DKA and HHS. Infuse 0.9 % sodium chloride first. Include potassium as indicated.
- DKA fixed rate insulin infusion then infuse glucose as needed in parallel to 0.9 % sodium chloride to clear ketones and avoid hypoglycaemia.
- HHS—patients are severely dehydrated. Start treatment with fluids first, then consider low-dose insulin. Sodium usually rises but this is not necessarily an indication to change from 0.9 % sodium chloride.
- Treat precipitating cause.
- Monitor the patient very closely, both clinically and with bedside or laboratory tests.
- The most common cause of failure to respond to treatment is failure of treatment to be given.
- Complications of DKA/HHS include cardiac arrest, hypoglycaemia, cerebral oedema, central pontine myelinolysis, hypotension, aspiration, pulmonary oedema, ARDS, thromboembolism, rhabdomyolysis, fetal distress/death. Many of these complications are preventable.
- Start or restart insulin therapy carefully and reliably to avoid a return of DKA/HHS.
- Educate patient and staff to prevent recurrence.
- Ensure diabetologist follow-up.

Further reading

All doctors in roles in which they may need to treat DKA or HHS should read the Joint British Diabetes Societies Inpatient Care group (JBDS) guidance:

The management of Diabetic Ketoacidosis in adults (2010)
☏ <http://www.diabetologists-abcd.org.uk/JBDS_DKA_Management.pdf>
The management of the hyperosmolar hyperglycaemic state (HHS) in adults with diabetes (2012)
☏ <http://www.diabetologists-abcd.org.uk/JBDS/JBDS_IP_HHS_Adults.pdf>

Chapter 13

Exercise

Prevention of type 2 diabetes

Regularly supervised exercise programmes ± dietary advice has been shown in international studies to reduce the risk of developing type 2 diabetes in people with impaired glucose tolerance: NICE Public Health Guidance 38; Lancet 2006: **368**:1673–9; doi:10.1016/S0140-6736(06)69701-8. *Lancet* 2009; **374**:1677–86; doi:10.1016/S0140-6736(09)61457-4. This effect is as good as, or better than, giving metformin. Successful participants required frequent (e.g. every 1–2 ths) individualized advice and encouragement from physical trainers ± dietitians and other healthcare professionals.

Exercise is good for people with diabetes

Regular exercise:
• improves blood glucose balance in both type 1 and type 2 diabetes although the benefit appears greater in the latter.
• increases insulin sensitivity.
• improves glucose tolerance.
• aids weight reduction.
• reduces the risk of coronary heart disease.
• makes many people feel good.

Exercise, insulin, and glucose

In a non-diabetic, exercising muscles first use their stored glycogen. Muscle cells contain a glucose transporter called GLUT4. Insulin and/or muscle contraction stimulates the movement of GLUT4 to the cell surface. GLUT4 then 'opens the door' into the cell and glucose is taken up passively from the bloodstream as needed, e.g. during exercise for energy and after exercise to replenish glycogen stores. As the blood glucose concentration falls, pancreatic insulin release is reduced, glucagon rises, and glucose is released from the liver glycogen stores to 'top up' the blood glucose concentration. If CHO has been eaten, this will be absorbed into the bloodstream and insulin will be released, if necessary, to store it in the liver and/or facilitate its use by the exercising muscles. Liver glycogenolysis will cease while the glucose derived from the meal is distributed. However, if exercise continues and the blood glucose level falls, insulin release will fall and liver glycogenolysis will again release glucose into the circulation. With prolonged exercise, adrenaline and glucagon levels rise, glucose and insulin levels fall, and fatty acids are released as fuel.

This process can still occur in a person with diabetes treated by diet alone, and to a large extent in patients being treated with metformin. However, as soon as sulfonylureas or, particularly, insulin injections are introduced, the fine-tuning of glucose balance in exercise is disturbed.

The effects on blood glucose and other biochemistry, such as lipids, in a person with insulin-treated diabetes who exercises depend on the amount of circulating insulin and how much food has been eaten (Figure 13.1). The crucial difference between the diabetic and non-diabetic athlete is that there is no fine on–off control of insulin release.

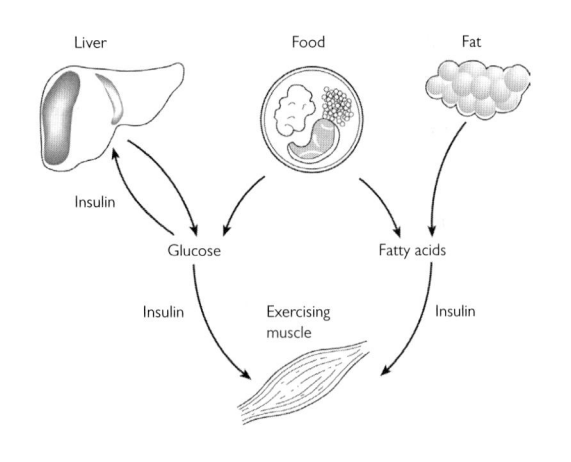

	At rest	**Brief excercise**	**Longer excercise**
Food	Glucose and fat absorbed into the blood	Glucose and fat absorbed into the blood	Less glucose and fat absorbed as some blood diverted to muscle
Insulin normal	Released from the pancreas according to blood glucose	Less insulin released from pancreas as glucose falls	
diabetic	Released from the injection site	More released from injection site as circlulation to muscles and skin increases	
Liver	Stores glucose as glycogen*	Starts to release glucose^	Releases a lot of glucose^
Fat	Stores fatty acids*	Starts to release fatty acids^	Releases a lot of fatty acids^
Muscle	Stores glucose as glycogen*	Converts glycogen to glucose for energy^	Takes up glucose and fatty acids and uses them for energy*

* Needs insulin
^ Blocked by insulin

Fig. 13.1 Exercise, food, and insulin.

Someone who is insulin-deficient is likely to have a high blood glucose. Exercise will further increase the blood glucose as the stress hormone response releases glucose from the liver. As exercise continues, the muscles take up glucose from the bloodstream (much of this uptake is insulin-independent although insulin will move more GLUT4 transporters to the muscle cell surfaces). However, this effect is unlikely to outweigh that of hepatic glucose release. Fat breakdown, lipolysis, which occurs in prolonged exercise to provide free fatty acids as an additional fuel, may be followed by ketone formation in insulin deficiency. Any food eaten will merely serve to exacerbate the hyperglycaemia, thus exercise may worsen hyperglycaemia and promote ketosis in an insulin-deficient person.

Hypoglycaemia may ensue in someone who has a large subcutaneous reservoir of injected insulin, especially if they increase the circulation to the injection site by the exercise. As before, the exercising muscles will use their stored glycogen. The presence of insulin ensures good glucose uptake by the exercising muscles. However, high plasma insulin concentrations inhibit glucose release from the liver, further reducing the blood glucose concentration. Hypoglycaemia rapidly ensues. This situation can be prevented by eating CHO which will be absorbed and top up the blood glucose level as exercise proceeds. Glucose absorption from the gut is not dependent on insulin.

In patients taking sulfonylureas, the drugs enhance pancreatic insulin release, as well as improving tissue glucose uptake. Thus they may produce hyperinsulinaemia and can cause exercise-induced hypoglycaemia.

Which form of exercise and how much?

To derive full benefit from exercise it should be regular—at least 20–30 min on at least 5 days each week. The aim should be to keep the heart rate within the training zone, i.e. between 60 % and 85 % of the maximum heart rate (Table 13.1). (ADA advises at least 50–70 %.) The heart rate should not exceed the maximum, which is calculated by subtracting the age from 220. Two or three 10-minute episodes are nearly as good as one longer one. Obese patients who are not reducing calorie intake may have to do double this exercise requirement to lose weight.

All exercise programmes should start gradually, building on existing exercise capacity and capability. Long-term success is improved by continued contact or support after the initial programme.

Exercise does not have to be weight-lifting or marathon running. A brisk walk will maintain the pulse rate within the training zone. Furthermore, exercise which does not reach the training zone, such as gardening or gentle swimming, can be helpful in improving well-being and maintaining a full range of joint movement.

Exercise may be anaerobic (e.g. sprint), aerobic (e.g. running, swimming, dancing), or resistance (e.g. weight-training) or a combination of these. All forms of exercise have been shown to improve glucose levels, but aerobic physical exercise is likely to reduce the HbA_{1c} more. Exercise is often added to a weight-reducing diet. Note that exercise has beneficial effects on its own (e.g. improved glucose control).

Table 13.1 The training zone

Age (yrs)	Heart rate (beats/min)		
	Training zone		Maximum
	60 %	85 %	
15	123	174	205
20	120	170	200
25	117	166	195
30	114	162	190
35	111	157	185
40	108	153	180
45	105	149	175
50	102	145	170
55	99	140	165
60	96	136	160
65	93	132	155
70	90	119	150
75	87	123	145
80	84	119	140

To derive greatest benefit from exercise the heart rate should be within the training zone for at least 20 mins on most days. First aim for the lower end of the training zone (60 %), or lower in someone who has not exercised recently. Do not use this calculation for people with autonomic neuropathy.

Helping people with diabetes to exercise safely

Use common sense. Always start gradually. The exercise activity(ies) chosen must be practical and fit in with everyday life in all seasons. Patients should seek expert advice (e.g. a trainer or join a club/gym) for activities that are out of the ordinary for them. If it hurts, stop.

Controlling the blood glucose

Diet-treated diabetes

No special measures need to be taken regarding blood glucose balance if the glucose is well controlled on diet alone.

Non-insulin-treated diabetes

Metformin alone usually presents no problem, although if insulin sensitivity increases and weight is lost, the metformin dose may be reduced.

Unexpected or vigorous exercise in patients taking sulfonylureas occasionally causes hypoglycaemia, which may be prolonged. In this case, the person should check his/her blood glucose during or after exertion and eat some CHO if necessary. If hypoglycaemia ensues, the person should eat a series of small snacks until he/she is sure that the blood glucose has stabilized. The blood glucose must be checked regularly for at least 24 hrs.

If the exercise is planned, it is better to reduce the dose of sulfonylurea or meglitinide before the exertion so that hypoglycaemia is prevented. If too much CHO is eaten to cover the exertion, excess insulin will be released and this may compound any late exercise-induced hypoglycaemia. If the exercise is regular, a long-term reduction in sulfonylurea dosage may be possible.

Incretin-effect enhancing drugs are relatively new agents and experience of vigorous exercise when on them is limited. These drugs suppress glucagon which is needed for glucose release from the liver. However, a study in non-diabetics given exenatide found that glucose levels rose during exercise and fell later. Many patients will also be taking other drugs that could cause hypoglycaemia so the combination needs to be looked at. The other drugs may need to be reduced before exercise.

Insulin-treated diabetes

Exercise is a common cause of hypoglycaemia. It is preferable to reduce the insulin acting during the exertion (and afterwards if exercise is vigorous or prolonged exercise). Eating extra can result in an increase in weight, especially in type 2 diabetes.

In general, advise 15–30 g glucose before exercise. If the exercise is very vigorous, unusual, or hazardous, take about 15–45 g every 30–60 mins and afterwards. Tailor advice to the individual patient and situation. Encourage blood glucose testing as the symptoms of hypoglycaemia can be hidden by the sweating, tachycardia, and breathlessness of exercise. For prolonged exertion it is theoretically helpful to eat some high-fibre CHO as well.

For planned exercise, the insulin acting during the time of exertion should be reduced beforehand. If the extent of the exertion is unknown (as in learning a new sport) it is better to reduce the insulin by about 20–40 %

for the first few occasions. Inject the insulin away from any exercising muscle. Take care to avoid the risk of hypoglycaemia while swimming or driving home. The next meal should contain extra high-fibre CHO to prevent subsequent hypoglycaemia. The next dose of insulin may also need to be reduced after vigorous or endurance exercise. Hypoglycaemia may occur up to 24 hrs after exercise as the body replenishes its glycogen stores.

There is no simple calculation for the amount of insulin dose reduction and the amount of extra CHO. Each person has to work it out for him/herself. The key is SMBG. This should be done four times a day (before each meal and before bed) and also immediately before and after the exercise until it has become familiar. As people train regularly, they will need less extra food for exercise and less insulin reduction.

Glucose control in dangerous activities

This applies mainly to people on insulin injections. In some sports (e.g. suba-qua diving, hang-gliding) a person could die if he/she becomes confused or comatose. Other sports involve taking responsibility for others, as either coach or leader, or in sharing safety (e.g. belaying a climber). There is little or no margin for error and the individual must ensure that hypoglycaemia will not occur. It is safer to have a buddy who knows about the diabetes and what to do if hypoglycaemia occurs.

Reduce the insulin dose which acts during the activity by 20 % (50 % if hypoglycaemia prone or no warning of hypoglycaemia). The last meal before the activity should contain more CHO than usual. Eat an appropriate double snack if there has been a long preparation time for the activity, especially if this has involved exercise (e.g. rowing out to a diving point, walking to the base of a climbing route). Check SMBG before starting the hazardous activity. If it is < 6 mmol/l eat an additional snack and recheck SMBG after 15–30 mins. Immediately before starting the activity (e.g. just before putting foot to rock) eat 15 g glucose. The aim is for the activity to take place on rising glucose from gut absorption which is independent of insulin concentration.

The same principles can be applied for situations in which hypoglycaemia could let the person down (e.g. in competition) or let others down (e.g. team sports). The difficulty lies in balancing freedom from hypoglycaemia and safety vs impairment of performance by hyperglycaemia. Each sportsperson has to spend some time experimenting for themselves. Start sugary and then refine.

There are few activities which are unsuitable for people with diabetes. Only patients who are competent and confident in glucose self-management and who have informed support from a diabetologist should undertake high-risk activities such as scuba diving or ice climbing. Unplanned 'one-off' holiday activities are particularly dangerous as equipment and supervision vary, food may be unfamiliar, and communication may be difficult (➲ p. 401–2).

Both patients and professionals may find helpful advice on RunSweet, a site about diabetes and sport: 🖰 <http://www.runsweet.com/index.html>

Fit to exercise?

Doctors and nurses are frequently asked to confirm fitness to exercise. In general, if the patient can walk briskly without problems he/she is usually fit to start an exercise programme. Areas to consider are:
- hypoglycaemia awareness or not (see advice about glucose)
- heart
- feet
- eyes
- autonomic neuropathy

Heart

- No symptoms. Diabetes may modify cardiac symptoms so their lack cannot guide the degree of exercise that can be undertaken. At the time of writing routine cardiac screening before exercise is not recommended. In patients with macro- or microvasculopathy, seek symptoms of cardiac disease and consider cardiology assessment before they start an exercise programme.
- Known cardiac disease. Ask a cardiologist's advice. Appropriate exercise is good for people with coronary heart disease, but only with the advice of a cardiologist after any treatment required has been instituted.

Foot

- Look at the feet—are they at risk? (⊃ p. 305)
- All patients should have appropriate footwear for their chosen activity. Ask the podiatrist if advice is needed.
- Neuropaths must be careful to avoid injuries, rubs, and blisters, and increased callus formation on pressure areas.
- Charcot feet—avoid weight-bearing exercise. Risk of multiple fractures.
- Foot ulcers—avoid weight-bearing exercise.
- Patients with peripheral arterial disease should keep their feet warm in cold weather, and always protect them.
- Seek and treat athletes' foot.

Eyes

Unstable proliferative retinopathy is a contraindication to exercise (especially resistance) as it could cause blindness from vitreous haemorrhage. Seek ophthalmologist's advice after treatment.

Autonomic neuropathy

⚠ Cardiac autonomic neuropathy can cause sudden death. ADA 2014 states 'individuals with diabetic autonomic neuropathy should undergo cardiac investigation before beginning physical activity more intense than that to which they are accustomed.' <http://care.diabetesjournals.org/content/37/Supplement_1/S14.full.pdf>

Autonomic neuropathy can also cause postural hypotension and hypoglycaemic unawareness (⊃ p. 282).

What to tell a trainer or exercise supervisor

Patients should tell anyone supervising their exercise that they have diabetes. If they are on most non-insulin treatments there are unlikely to be any significant issues. Insulin-, sulfonylurea-, or meglitinide-treated patients should explain that they have adjusted their diet and treatment for the exercise and that problems are unlikely. However, they should ensure that the supervisor knows the symptoms of hypoglycaemia and where the patient's glucose is kept.

Most national sporting bodies are aware of diabetes and will have guidance. Diabetes UK can also help. Also see RunSweet (➡ p. 240).

Summary

- Regular exercise can prevent diabetes in people with impaired glucose tolerance.
- Regular exercise is good for people with diabetes.
- Patients on insulin (and sometimes sulfonylureas/meglitinides) should reduce their medication for planned exercise. They need to eat extra CHO to fuel exercise.
- Take care to avoid hypoglycaemia, especially in high-risk sports and in those with poor warning.
- Check fitness to exercise—cardiovascular disease, foot problems, neuropathy, autonomic neuropathy, and retinopathy.
- Give appropriate advice to patients with diabetic tissue damage.
- Consult Diabetes UK for further advice about individual sports.

Chapter 14

Diabetic tissue damage

Diabetic tissue damage

In most people's minds diabetes is sugar trouble, yet most of the problems of diabetes arise not from fluctuating glucose levels, but from its many tissue complications (Table 14.1). Diabetes is a chronic multisystem disorder of which one manifestation is hyperglycaemia. Damage occurs over months and years, often silently.

Many of the tissue complications of diabetes are preventable and although we still have much to learn about the causes of diabetic tissue damage, we can at least work on reducing the damage due to factors we have identified. Diabetes is for life. The quality of that life and its extent will be largely determined by the development of tissue damage and its extent.

Diabetic tissue damage is usually divided into that which occurs only (or predominantly) in diabetes, and that which is more common in people with diabetes but does occur in others.

Microvascular disease—thickening of the basement membrane of capillaries causing leakage or blockage to the transfer of nutrients and waste substances—is virtually specific to diabetes. This is associated with retinopathy, nephropathy, and neuropathy. These and other changes, such as cheiroarthropathy and dermopathy, may be linked to glycosylation of proteins (➔ p. 107–8).

Macrovascular disease—atherosclerosis—is common in the non-diabetic population, but is much more frequent in people with diabetes.

As most medical and nursing training relates to body systems, the following discussion of tissue damage is conducted by system rather than by aetiology. In most instances symptoms are a late feature of diabetic complications. By the time the patient is aware of a problem it may be too late to treat it, therefore a major part of diabetes care is screening patients for evidence of tissue damage and for risk factors of tissue damage (Box 14.1).

Box 14.1 Prevention of diabetic tissue damage

- Treatment must be safe and practical for each patient
- Help people with diabetes to learn how to work with the diabetes team:
  - to feel as well as possible
  - to reduce the risk of developing diabetic tissue damage
  - to recognize tissue damage early, if present
  - to slow deterioration of existing tissue damage
- Reduce risk factors
- Stop smoking
- Exercise regularly
- BP (without postural hypotension)
  - 130/80 in most patients
  - 120–129/75–80 in kidney, eye or cerebrovascular disease
- Fasting and premeal plasma glucose 4–7 mmol/l without hypoglycaemia, i.e. if safe
- HbA$_{1c}$ 48–58 mmol/mol (6.5–7.5 %) without hypoglycaemia, i.e. if safe (➲ pp. 108–9)
- *Keep BMI between 18.5 and 25 kg/m^2
- Assess all patients for the need for statin therapy (Box 3.2, ➲ pp. 38–40)
- Detect and treat microalbuminuria
- Avoid added salt

* BMI unhelpful in very muscular people. BMI upper limit in Asian/African–Caribbean or Chinese people = 23 kg/m^2. See Chapter 3 for detailed discussion of rise factors and targets.

Mortality

Having diabetes shortens your life. The National Diabetes Audit (NDA) Mortality Analysis followed 2 160 516 million people with diabetes known to be alive for the year 2010/11 and recorded all deaths using formal death notifications.

In England, there were 75 669 deaths among those with diabetes, 23 300 more than expected in an age- and sex-matched general population. Overall, the risk of death for patients with type 1 diabetes was 2.3 times higher than the general population, whilst that for type 2 patients was 1.3 times higher. Among people with diabetes aged 15–34 yrs women were seven times more likely to die, and men four times more likely to die than their non-diabetic compatriots. Mortality varied considerably by geographical region and primary care trust. There appears to be a trend towards reducing excess mortality, but it is too early to be sure. ⅏ <http://www.hqip.org.uk/assets/NCAPOP-Library/NCAPOP-2013-14/NDA2011-2012Report2ComplicationsMortalityINTERACTIVEPDF26-11-13.pdf>

A previous similar analysis for 2007/8 noted that only 6.7 % of the death certificates in people with diabetes mentioned diabetes. Just 4934 (1.1 %) gave diabetes as the cause of death, yet many are highly likely to have died from complications of diabetes that would not have occurred at all, or occurred sooner than expected than in non-diabetics.

The Emerging Risk Factors Collaboration analysed 97 prospective studies: 715 061 adults with no history of vascular disease and at least one year of follow-up were studied, including 40 116 with diabetes.

A 50 yr old with diabetes was likely to die six years sooner than a counterpart without diabetes. This excess mortality in people with diabetes was attributable to vascular causes (58 %), cancer (9 %), and other causes, e.g. kidney or liver disease, infection (30 %).

After adjusting for age, sex, smoking status, and BMI, the hazard ratios for people with diabetes vs those without (hazard ratio = 1.0) for death were:
* any cause 1.80 (95 % confidence intervals 1.71–1.90)
* cancer 1.25 (1.19–1.31)
* vascular 2.32 (2.11–2.56)
* other causes 1.73 (1.62–1.85)

Further adjustment for systolic blood pressure and cholesterol did not significantly alter these ratios, but adjusting for fasting glucose or HbA_{1c} did, reducing the hazard ratios towards the non-diabetic group. Thus being sugary appears to have a substantial influence on mortality.

Cancer deaths associated with diabetes were liver, pancreas, ovary, colorectum, lung, bladder, and breast. Non-cancer, non-vascular causes of death associated with diabetes were renal disease, liver disease, pneumonia and other infectious diseases, mental disorders, nonhepatic digestive disorders, external causes, intentional self harm, nervous-system disorders and chronic obstructive pulmonary disease (COPD) (*N Engl J Med* 2011; **364**:829-41; doi: 10.1056/NEJMoa1008862).

This excess mortality can be reduced by intensive risk factor improvement. UKPDS showed reduced mortality at 20 yrs with an initial 10 yrs intensified glucose control (➲ pp. 40–1). The Steno study showed that intensive multi-factorial risk factor control in people with type 2 diabetes and microalbuminuria reduced cardiovascular mortality (*N Engl J Med* 2008; **358**:580–59; doi: 10.1056/NEJMoa0706245).

There is evidence that life expectancy is improving. The Pittsburgh Epidemiology of Diabetes Complications study found that, for people with type 1 diabetes diagnosed at < 17 yrs old, those diagnosed between 1965 and 1980 had 15 yrs greater life expectancy than those diagnosed between 1950 and 1964 (*Diabetes* 2012; **61**:2987–92; doi:10.2337/db11-1625). A Danish study also found a decline in mortality (*Diabetologia* 2013; **56**:2401–4; doi: 10.1007/s00125-013-3025-7).

Table 14.1 Tissue complications of diabetes

Eyes	Retinopathy, maculopathy, cataract, squint, dry eyes, retinal/vitreous detachment, corneal damage, glaucoma
Ears	Deafness
Smell and taste	Reduced
Kidneys	Nephropathy, renal failure, chronic pyelonephritis
Nervous system	Neuropathy—sensory, motor, autonomic; involving many nerves or one
Heart	Ischaemic heart disease, cardiomyopathy, cardiac failure
Lungs	Impaired function
GI tract	Oral and dental problems; dysmotility of oesophagus, stomach, intestine, gall bladder; anorectal problems
Liver	Non-alcoholic fatty liver
Peripheral arterial disease	Anywhere, especially legs
Feet	Ulcer, infection, gangrene, amputation
Brain	Stroke, transient ischaemic attack, dementia
Sexual function	Erectile dysfunction, reduced female arousal, vaginal dryness
Skin and soft tissue	Dermopathy, necrobiosis lipoidica, bullosis diabeticorum, scleroderma, 'diabetic hand', periungual telangiectasia, mastopathy, carpal tunnel syndrome
Muscles	Sarcopenia, reduced uterine contractility
Ligaments	Dupuytren's contracture, cheiroarthropathy, frozen shoulder
Skeletal system	Charcot joint, osteopenia, osteosclerosis, diabetic osteoarthropathy
Cancer	Increased risk of some cancers
Infection	Increased risk and diminished response to treatment

Cardiovascular disease (CVD)

- Heart
- Hypertension
- Peripheral arterial disease (PAD)
- Cerebrovascular disease

CVD is two to five times as common in people with diabetes as in the general population. Premenopausal diabetic women are about as likely to have a myocardial infarct as diabetic men. The NDA 2011/12 for England and Wales showed that people with diabetes were more likely than non-diabetics to have a hospital admission for angina (↑76 %), for myocardial infarction (↑55 %), and for heart failure (↑73 %). Patients with these conditions had significantly greater short-term mortality than non-diabetics: 1.5 times for angina, 2.4 times for myocardial infarct, and 5.2 times for heart failure.

Advanced glycosylation end-products (AGE) are implicated in atherogenesis in diabetes. Raised insulin levels are associated with increased cardiovascular risk. Diabetes is a procoagulant state. Additionally, diabetic patients have dyslipidaemia and hypertension, and may be obese.

Prevention and reduction of cardiovascular risk

People with diabetes should pay attention to the same risk factors as those without diabetes. It seems likely that all these risk factors have a more detrimental effect on people with diabetes. The main risk factors are smoking, hypertension, obesity, and hyperlipidaemia.

Glucose

It used to be thought that glucose concentrations were not directly linked with large vessel disease. However, the DCCT (➋ pp. 40–1) showed a reduction in plasma cholesterol concentrations in the intensively treated patients and a trend towards less cardiovascular disease in those with near-normoglycaemia. In UKPDS (➋ pp. 40–1) patients with intensive glucose control on metformin had a lower risk of fatal myocardial infarct than these on conventional glucose control. The sulfonylurea and insulin groups did not, however, show a significant reduction in cardiovascular events with intensive glucose lowering. More detailed studies in patients with CVD have shown that outcome is worse with hyperglycaemia, e.g. sugary patients have larger myocardial infarcts.

A meta-analysis including > 27 000 people with diabetes showed an overall reduction in cardiovascular events with intensive glucose control. but no significant reduction in mortality. There was an increase in hypoglycaemia (*Diabetologia* 2009; **52**:2288–98; doi: 10.1007/s00125-009-1470-0).

Smoking

Smoking shortens the life of a person with diabetes by about 6 yrs. Diabetic smokers have a similarly increased risk of CVD to non-diabetics. Overweight, hypertensive, diabetic women who are taking oral contraceptives are at especially high risk of cardiovascular complications. Some studies have also shown that smokers were more likely to have nephropathy and retinopathy than non-smokers.

Obesity

Obesity is common in people with type 2 diabetes and can occur in insulin-treated patients, especially if they are eating to keep up with their insulin. To help patients lose weight safely, reduce their glucose-lowering treatment as they start their reduced-calorie diabetes diet. Tell patients about the risk of hypoglycaemia. Some patients on insulin or oral hypogly-caemic drugs may be able to stop them if they lose weight. Patients treated by diet alone may need medication if they gain weight. Beware of the weight loss of uncontrolled diabetes. Record the patient's height and update this in new records (pp. 78–80).

Hypertension (pp. 257–8)

Over 10 yrs, each 10 mm Hg reduction in systolic BP reduces CVD death by 15 % (*Br Med J* 2000; **321**:412–19; doi: http://dx.doi.org/10.1136/bmj.321.7258.412).

Lipids

Both cholesterol and triglyceride may be raised in diabetes. In addition, lipo-proteins are glycosylated and this process may be involved in atherogenesis.

A study of 209 180 people found that mean levels of total cholesterol and HDL differed little with various fasting times. Calculated LDL varied up to 10 %. Triglyceride varied by up to 20 % (*Arch Intern Med* 2012 Dec 10; **172**(22) 1707–10; doi:10.1001/archinternmed.2012.3708). Patients on insulin may become hypoglycaemic on fasting and random lipid levels are safer. Request fasting levels (give advice on hypoglycaemia avoidance) only if triglycerides are raised.

JBS3 recommends non-fasting samples to measure total cholesterol and HDL cholesterol. These values are used in the JBS3 cardiovascular risk cal-culator to derive non-HDL cholesterol (total cholesterol–HDL cholesterol, likely to become the key measure in the future) to calculate heart age and expected survival without heart attack or stroke. The calculator includes risks for people with diabetes. The excellent graphics can be used to help patients understand their risks. <http://www.jbs3risk.com/pages/risk_calculator.htm>

Most people with diabetes > 40 yrs old have sufficient risk factors for CVD for lipid-lowering treatment with statin to be prescribed regardless of their lipid levels (NICE CG 66) and JBS3 (Box 3.2, pp. 38–40). Reducing LDL by 1 mmol/l reduces CVD risk by 21 % and mortality from all causes by 10 % (pp. 38–40). Intensify statin therapy if CVD is present.

Triglyceride

The main lipid abnormality in diabetes is hypertriglyceridaemia. Plasma triglyceride is elevated in about a third of patients with type 2 diabetes. Patients with type 1 diabetes who are insulin deficient also have high triglyc-erides. A few patients have extremely high plasma triglyceride levels and their serum is milky with chylomicrons. These patients may have eruptive xanthomata, abdominal pain, and pancreatitis, with malaise, tingling, and impaired cerebral function.

Cholesterol

Total cholesterol is more likely to be raised in type 2 than in type 1 patients. HDL cholesterol has the same inverse relationship to coronary heart disease and other conditions due to atheroma as in non-diabetic people. HDL cholesterol is more often reduced in women with type 2 diabetes than in men. The abnormalities related to HDL cholesterol are more closely linked with triglyceride than with total cholesterol.

Seek and treat secondary causes of hyperlipidaemia

- Factors affecting triglyceride levels:
  - glucose control
  - alcohol
  - obesity
  - liver disease
  - chronic kidney disease
  - nephrotic syndrome
  - thiazides
  - β-blockers
  - myeloma
- Factors affecting cholesterol levels:
  - hypothyroidism
  - cholestasis
  - nephrotic syndrome
  - eating disorders
  - diuretics

Raised triglyceride and reduced HDL cholesterol (< 1 mmol/l) increase the risk of CVD. For triglyceride levels > 1.7 mmol/l, institute rigorous blood glucose control and reduction of alcohol intake. If the triglyceride is between 2.3 mmol/l and 4.5 mmol/l use atorvastatin or higher doses of simvastatin. Triglyceride levels > 4.5 mmol/l are unlikely to respond to a statin so use a fibrate (e.g. fenofibrate). Monitor liver function (guidance for statins is LFTs before treatment, at 3 mths and 12 mths, or if symptoms, NICE CG 67). Stop statin if transaminase 3× ULN). Guidance for LFT monitoring in patients on fibrates is less clear; it would seem reasonable to follow the statin guidance.

CVD screening

There is less consensus about the timing and frequency of some screening for cardiovascular disease and its risk factors in diabetes than there is for microvascular disease. It seems sensible to check for evidence of CVD annually in people with diabetes. The Cardiovascular Outcome Strategy (2013) suggested that a standardized CVD assessment to seek the other six conditions be undertaken on any patient in primary or secondary care presenting with any of:

- hypertension
- hypercholesterolemia
- coronary heart disease
- stroke
- type 2 diabetes
- kidney disease
- peripheral arterial disease (PAD)

⌘ <www.gov.uk/government/uploads/system/uploads/attachment_data/file/217118/9387-2900853-CVD-Outcomes_web1.pdf>

Heart

People with diabetes are more likely to have coronary atheroma than the general population. A third of newly diagnosed type 2 diabetic patients will have an abnormal ECG at diagnosis. Diabetes also causes cardiac small vessel disease with basement membrane thickening as in the retina. This probably contributes to the higher frequency of cardiomyopathy and heart failure in people with diabetes, with or without coronary artery disease.

On diagnosis of diabetes check:

- Symptoms of CVD (e.g. angina, intermittent claudication)
- Smoking history
- Family history of CVD
- Height and weight
- BP
- Pulse (atrial fibrillation?)
- Heart size, sounds, and evidence of failure
- Peripheral pulses
- ECG (give patient a copy)
- Chest X-ray if smoker, hypertensive, evidence of respiratory or cardiac disease, tuberculosis-prone
- Cholesterol and triglyceride

Screen patients annually (or as stated) thereafter

- Cardiovascular symptoms
- Smoking
- Family history—new events?
- Weight (assess in relation to height)
- BP
- Peripheral pulses
- Cardiac examination if symptoms, otherwise every 5 yrs
- ECG if symptoms and every 5 yrs routinely
- Cholesterol and triglyceride (2–3 mthly if elevated, every year if normal)

Angina

- Some patients will present with classic symptoms of angina pectoris
- Silent ischaemia is common
- In autonomic neuropathy the symptoms may be different or less pronounced, and there is a greater likelihood of silent ischaemia
- Have a low threshold for requesting cardiological investigations
- Patients may be difficult to diagnose and treat, so seek cardiology advice early
- If the exercise ECG or other dynamic testing is positive it should be followed by coronary angiography
- Diabetic patients usually have diffuse and extensive coronary atheroma

Acute coronary syndrome (ACS)

This includes acute myocardial infarction (AMI), both ST elevation (STEMI) and non-ST elevation (NSTEMI).

General
- ⚠ Have a very low threshold for urgent hospital referral with any symptom which might indicate AMI or acute coronary syndrome.
- Presenting symptoms may be atypical, including painless breathlessness or acute malaise or tiredness, pain anywhere in the chest, right arm pain, and chest tenderness as well as traditional presentations.
- About one in four patients with ACS have diabetes (*Arch Intern Med 2004*; **164**:1457–63; doi:10.1001/archinte.164.13.1457). As many as half of all South Asian ACS patients may have diabetes.
- One in three deaths of diabetic patients are due to AMI.
- The risk is twice to four times greater than that of the general population.
- Patients under 30 yrs old may have AMI.
- Women with diabetes of any age are at risk of AMI, which is less likely to be diagnosed and treated adequately.
- Diabetic patients have a higher mortality from ACS than other patients. In one study, those with NSTEMI had about an 80 % increased risk of death within 30 days, and those with STEMI a 40 % increased risk (*JAMA* 2007; **298**:765–75; doi:10.1001/jama.298.7.765).
- Acute hyperglycaemia or DKA may be due to "silent" AMI.
- Perform a troponin test in all diabetic inpatients whose condition deteriorates without good cause.

Care in hospital
The European Societies for Cardiology (ESC) recommendations on revascularization for people with diabetes (2013) are:
- '[o]ptimal medical treatment should be considered as preferred treatment in patients with stable coronary artery disease (CAD) and diabetes mellitus (DM) unless there are large areas of ischaemia or significant left main or proximal left anterior descending lesions.
- Coronary artery bypass grafting (CABG) is recommended in patients with DM and multivessel or complex (SYNTAX Score > 22) CAD to improve survival free from major cardiovascular events.
- Percutaneous coronary intervention (PCI) for symptom control may be considered as an alternative to CABG in patients with DM and less complex multivessel CAD (SYNTAX score ≤ 22) in need of revascularization.
- Primary PCI is recommended over fibrinolysis in DM patients presenting with STEMI if performed within recommended time limits.
- In DM patients subjected to PCI, drug-eluting stents rather than bare metal stents are recommended to reduce risk of target vessel revascularization.
- Renal function should be carefully monitored after coronary angiography/PCI in all patients on metformin.
- If renal function deteriorates in patients on metformin undergoing coronary angiography/PCI it is recommended to withhold treatment for 48 hrs or until renal function has returned to its initial level.' (*Eur Heart J* 2013; **34**:3035–87. doi:10.1093/eurheartj/eht108)
- Give diabetic patients standard medical treatment for ACS. They may gain even greater benefit than those without diabetes.

- Do not give thrombolytic therapy to patients with unresolved proliferative retinopathy or current vitreous haemorrhage (rare).
- Patients with any glucose reading > 11 mmol/l should have careful glucose control using VRIII for at least 24 hrs with an appropriate concentration of IV glucose, depending on fluid needs and eating ability. Monitor and replace potassium as necessary. Stop VRIII once glucose controlled and eating normally and transfer safely to other glucose-lowering therapy (NICE CG 130) (➔ pp. 167–8).
- Avoid hypoglycaemia which can cause dysrhythmias or cardiac arrest. This means meticulous blood glucose monitoring, including at 2 a.m. and especially at weekends.
- The DIGAMI study (*Br Med J* 1997; **314**:1512–15; doi: http://dx.doi.org/ 10.1136/bmj.314.7093.1512) initially suggested that a year of intensive insulin therapy reduced mortality after AMI. Later studies were not convincing, and patients often suffered hypoglycaemia when this was attempted under non-study conditions. Intensive glucose lowering with insulin regardless of glucose levels is not advised (NICE CG130). Insulin should be used only if clinically indicated. Hyperglycaemia may require different treatment in new/transient vs in known diabetes, and in STEMI vs NSTEMI. More research is needed.
- Control blood glucose with usual medication appropriate to the patient once the acute phase of ACS is over.
- Provide standard medication post ACS (e.g. long term aspirin, clopidogrel if NSTEMI, β-blocker, ACE inhibitor, intensive statin).
- Every patient without known diabetes admitted with ACS should have a blood glucose test and HbA$_{1c}$ on admission.

Cardiac failure

- Two to five times more common in people with diabetes than in those without, with or without symptoms of myocardial ischaemia.
- Of all hospital admissions with heart failure, 28 % involve a person with diabetes (NDA 2011–12).
- Mortality within one year of admission for heart failure five times that of people without diabetes (➔ pp. 250–2).
- Diabetic cardiomyopathy is due to both microvascular disease and ischaemia. There may be interstitial and perivascular fibrosis.
- Hypertension causes left ventricular hypertrophy.
- Silent AMI can cause both impairment of ventricular function and increased risk of dysrhythmia.
- May be preceded by a reduction in left ventricular function which can be found in asymptomatic young people and children with diabetes.
- May have both diastolic and systolic impairment.
- Failure of diastolic relaxation of the left ventricle. Reduced ejection fraction on exercise causes exertional dyspnoea.
- Note that people with diabetes may have a higher serum B-type natriuretic peptide (BNP) than non-diabetics with the same heart failure score (*Exp Ther Med* 2013; **5**: 229–32; doi: 10.3892/etm.2012.760). In type 1 diabetes BNP is higher in those with complications than those

without (*Diabetes Care* 2012; **35**:1931–6; doi:10.2337/dc12-0089). It is also an independent predictor of mortality in diabetic nephropathy (*Diabetologia* 2005; **48**:149–55; doi: 10.1007/s00125-004-1595-0).

- Autonomic neuropathy may be associated with inability to raise a tachycardia when appropriate, and dysrhythmia. Postural hypotension may be severe with low cardiac output and diuretic treatment.
- Cardiac failure can cause hyperglycaemia and rising insulin requirements.
- Diuretic treatment of cardiac failure may worsen renal function, especially if there is pre-existing diabetic nephropathy.
- Hepatic congestion may worsen the effects of non-alcoholic steatohepatitis (NASH (➜ pp. 290–1)), hopefully temporarily.

Atrial fibrillation (AF)

Diabetes is a strong independent risk factor for AF and flutter. (*Int J Cardiol* 2005; **105**:315–18; doi:10.1016/j.ijcard.2005.02.050). A 10-yr US study found an AF prevalence of 3.6 % vs 2.5 % in age- and sex-matched non-diabetic patients. After full adjustment for other risk factors, diabetes was associated with a 26 % increased risk of AF among women (HR 1.26) but not men (HR 1.09) (*Diabetes Care* 2009; **32**:1851–6; doi:10.2337/dc09-0939).

Treatment of cardiac disease

- Drugs as for non-diabetic patients (see warnings (➜ pp. 259–63)).
- Pay careful attention to heart failure management (see NICE CG 108).
- Cardiac disease is more severe and more likely to prove fatal in people with diabetes so it should be managed with greater therapeutic 'aggression' than in non-diabetic people, with earlier intervention including coronary artery bypass grafting if indicated. Implantable cardioverter-defibrillators are effective in people with diabetes. The devices are likely to act more often, and diabetic patients have a higher mortality than those without diabetes (*Circulation* 2013; **128**:694–701; doi: 10.1161/CIRCULATIONAHA.113.002472).
- Stop smoking.
- Healthy eating with low salt intake.
- Alcohol < 21 units/wk men, < 14 units/wk women.
- Resume appropriate weight for height.
- Exercise safely (➜ pp. 239–41).
- Vigorous statin therapy for all (unless contraindicated) to reduce non-HDL cholesterol to < 2.5 mmol/l and LDL cholesterol to < 1.8 mmol/l.
- Control hypertension.
- Control hyperglycaemia as this may improve cardiac function.
- Monitor renal function.

Hypertension

Hypertension is found in at least a third of people with diabetes (Box 14.2). As with other tissue damage, hypertension is uncommon in people with newly diagnosed type 1 diabetes but is frequent in those with type 2 diabetes. Hypertension is three times more common in type 2 diabetes than in the non-diabetic population. Rare causes of hypertension (e.g. Cushing's syndrome, phaeochromocytoma, acromegaly) will be found more often in people with diabetes than in the general population. Non-diabetic renal causes should be considered.

Follow NICE CG 127 guidance for measuring blood pressure (BP). Use the right cuff size. Note that a clinic BP > 140/90 requires ambulatory BP measurements for confirmation unless severe hypertension is present. Goals for people with diabetes are around 130/80 in uncomplicated diabetic patients and 120–129/75–80, in those with kidney, eye or cerebrovascular damage. This more rigorous level is harder to achieve and carries greater risk of postural hypotension, falls, and side effects of medication. Set a realistic and safe target for each patient (➲ pp. 37–8).

Patients can self-measure BP, although this has not been proven to improve outcome in diabetic patients. They should check the BHS website ⌨ <http://www.bhsoc.org//index.php?cID=246> for a list of approved devices and follow the device instructions meticulously. Self-measurement is not suitable for patients in AF.

Box 14.2 Tests in people with hypertension

Electrolytes
Urate
Creatinine + eGFR
Cholesterol and triglyceride
Full blood count
Urine microalbumin:creatinine ratio, microscopy, culture if indicated
ECG (seeking left ventricular hypertrophy; consider echocardiogram)
Chest X-ray if clinically indicated
Consider renal ultrasound
(Urinary catecholamines and free cortisol, other endocrine tests if indicated)

Treatment of hypertension

Follow NICE CG 66 guidelines. Vigorously encourage lifestyle measures as required. Most patients will require medication:

- Use ACE inhibitor. Use ARB if patient intolerant of ACE inhibitor. Do not combine ACE inhibitors and ARBs.
- African–Caribbean: use ACE inhibitor and calcium-channel blocker.
- Any age or ethnicity:
  - BP not controlled—add calcium-channel blocker or thiazide diuretic.
  - BP not controlled—use ACE inhibitor/ARB with calcium-channel blocker and thiazide diuretic.
  - BP not controlled—more diuretic or α- or β-blocker.
- Woman of childbearing potential—advise contraception before treating hypertension. If the patient is planning conception refer to specialist diabetic preconception service. Discussion of therapeutic options (➲ pp. 259–63).
- Statin for all unless contraindication. Aim for total cholesterol < 4 mmol/l, LDL cholesterol < 2 mmol/l.
- Stop smoking.
- Healthy eating.
- ↓Salt intake.
- ↓Alcohol (1–2 units a day or less).
- Regular exercise.
- Resume appropriate weight for height.
- Stress reduction and relaxation.
- Check lying and standing BP and seek symptoms of postural hypotension, especially in neuropathic patients (➲ p. 282).
- Warn patients on β–blockers that they may have reduced warning of hypoglycaemia.
- Check concordance. The most common cause of failure to reach the desired target is failure to take the tablets.

Drugs in management and prevention of diabetic cardiovascular disease and hypertension

For all these drugs please read the current BNF and SPCs for full information. They all have extensive lists of interactions and side effects. This section notes issues important in diabetic patients but is not exhaustive.

Angiotensin-converting enzyme (ACE) inhibitors (ARBs if ACE-inhibitor intolerant) are the first-line treatment, followed by calcium-channel antagonists, thiazides, and β-blockers.

- Avoid these drugs in pregnancy, and in women of childbearing potential not using contraception unless essential (see ➋ pp. 340–1). Avoid these drugs in breastfeeding women.
- Once-daily preparations are more likely to be remembered than multiple-dosage regimens.
- Beware hypotension, particularly postural hypotension, which may be worse in patients with autonomic neuropathy. Ask about postural dizziness or light-headedness, and measure lying and standing BPs.
- ACE inhibitors, ARBs, β-blockers, and diuretics can all cause fluid or electrolyte imbalance.
- Drug interactions are common. Check them before prescribing.
- Most of these drugs can cause erectile dysfunction.

ACE inhibitors

Captopril, enalapril, fosinopril, lisinopril, perindopril, and ramipril have all been shown to be effective in reducing adverse measures in people with diabetes. The benefits shown with different drugs in different trials in diabetic patients in reducing BP, improving the outcome of AMI, preventing cardiovascular events, and reducing microalbuminuria are likely to be a class effect. However, their licensed indications vary, and at the time of writing the only ACE inhibitors which specifically mention diabetes in their SPCs are captopril, ramipril, and lisinopril. This does not mean that other ACE inhibitors cannot be used for hypertension and treatment of cardiac disease in diabetic patients; however, it seems sensible to use those which have been studied in diabetic patients. Captopril is less commonly used nowadays than other ACE inhibitors. Ramipril has been studied extensively.

Cautions
- Check U&E pre-treatment and regularly on treatment.
- Renal impairment: seek specialist advice before prescribing. Dosage reductions shown on SPCs.
- Beware renal artery stenosis: most likely in hypertensive patients with severe PAD. If BP uncontrolled on three agents, consider renal artery stenosis. Danger of renal failure.
- Avoid in aortic stenosis, mitral stenosis, and hypertrophic cardiomyopathy.

- First-dose hypotension varies with different agents but is more likely in fluid-depleted patients (e.g. those on diuretics) or in autonomic neuropathy.
- ACE inhibitors can occasionally induce hypoglycaemia in patients on glucose-lowering treatment. Warn patients.

Angiotensin II receptor antagonists (ARBs)

Have also been shown to be of benefit in diabetes (losartan and irbesartan are licensed for nephropathy). They appear to have a better side-effect profile with less likelihood of cough than ACE inhibitors but require the same cautions. Do not combine ARBs and ACE inhibitors.

Calcium-channel antagonists

Amlodipine, felodipine, nifedipine (long-acting), and others. Calcium-channel antagonists do not cause fluid, electrolyte, or glucose changes. They do cause vasodilatation, and this may result in headache, flushing, or ankle swelling. Class II agents (such as those described) are less likely to depress cardiac contraction than Class I agents such as verapamil.

Diuretics

Bendroflumethiazide and hydrochlorothiazide have both been shown to be safe and effective in diabetes. Thiazides were used in UKPDS (➜ pp. 37–8). Although they may increase blood glucose, this was not a problem and neither was electrolyte disturbance. Measure U&E pre-treatment and regularly thereafter. Diuretics combined with β-blockers seem particularly likely to cause hypokalaemia in clinical practice. Bendroflumethiazide 2.5 mg is usually sufficient to achieve a hypotensive effect. Thiazides should be used with care in pregnancy (and only in a specialist centre).

β-blockers

Not first line. Atenolol was shown to be safe and effective in UKPDS, but has since been shown to be inferior to losartan in reducing cardiovascular mortality and morbidity in diabetic hypertensive patients (LIFE, RENAAL, ➜ pp. 37–8). NICE CG 108 (chronic heart failure) supports the use of β-blockers licensed for the treatment of heart failure due to left ventricular dysfunction in people with diabetes.

Cautions

- Warn patients (especially if on insulin) that β-blockers reduce warning of hypoglycaemia.
- Avoid in patients with asthma or COPD.
- Avoid if bradycardia or heart block.
- Avoid in uncompensated heart failure.
- Avoid in severe peripheral arterial disease.
- May cause exertional tiredness, cold extremities, sleep disturbance, and bradycardia.

Anti-platelet drugs

Aspirin

- The benefit of low-dose aspirin in primary prevention of CVD in people with diabetes is unproven so it should not be used (*Br Med J* 2009; **339**:b4531; doi: http://dx.doi.org/10.1136/bmj.b4531).
- Aspirin (75–100 mg) should be used long-term for secondary prevention in people with diabetes who have established CVD as in non-diabetic patients.
- Control BP to < 145/90 first.
- Exclude contraindications.

Clopidogrel, prasugrel, ticagrelor

All these drugs have been used in people with diabetes. Prasugrel or ticagrelor are more potent than clopidogrel. JBS3 recommends combining either prasugrel or ticagrelor with low-dose aspirin in patients with acute coronary syndrome. Use combined treatment for up to a year after the acute event after which low dose aspirin should be continued indefinitely.

Glycoprotein IIb/IIIa inhibitors

Use as for non-diabetic patients. Early studies suggested that these drugs were particularly effective in people with diabetes but this was not confirmed by more recent research. (ECS 2013).

Lipid-lowering drugs

The Heart Protection Study (HPS) (*Lancet* 2003; **361**:2005–16; doi:10.1016/S0140-6736(03)13636-7) demonstrated convincingly that simvastatin reduced major coronary and vascular events, strokes, and revascularization requirement in people with diabetes regardless of initial lipid values. Similar results were obtained for atorvastatin and pravastatin. Advice at the time of writing is to use the most cost-effective statin initially, moving to atorvastatin if maximum doses are ineffective or not tolerated.

Statins

Atorvastatin, fluvastatin, pravastatin, rosuvastatin, and simvastatin have all been studied in people with diabetes. Simvastatin, pravastatin, and atorvastatin have been used in large lengthy studies which included people with diabetes (➲ p. 38–40). Statins can lower LDL cholesterol by up to 40 % with a slight increase in HDL and reduction in triglyceride. Atorvastatin is the most potent triglyceride-reducing statin. Simvastatin at a dose of 80 mg daily can also lower triglyceride, but this dose may increase adverse effects. Pravastatin is less likely to interact with warfarin than other statins. Rosuvastatin may achieve greater reduction in LDL. Different statins have different side-effect profiles in individual patients. These drugs work best if taken before bed.

NICE recommends simvastatin to 40 mg daily or the statin with the lowest acquisition cost, taking into account required daily dose and product price per dose. JBS3 advocates atorvastatin as first-line therapy now that it is off patent. SIGN advocates atorvastatin 10 mg as starting dose.

Prescribe statins for most people with diabetes aged over 40 yrs and younger patients with complications (for details see Box 3.2, (➲ pp. 38–40)):

Add ezetimibe if cholesterol still above target despite full-dose statin, or unable to tolerate statin or increased dosage.

Precautions for statins and fibrates
- Stop/do not give statins if creatine kinase (CK) > 5 times ULN.
- Check liver function before starting statins and at 1 mth, 6 mths, and 1 yr. Stop/do not give statins if any liver function test > 3× ULN.
- Do not give statins to women of childbearing potential unless they are using reliable contraception. Colestyramine has been used in severe hypercholesterolaemia in pregnancy—risk of vitamin deficiency.
- Hyperlipidaemia in transplant patients should be managed by specialist centres, as should familial hypercholesterolaemia.
- Note the extensive list of drug interactions with statins including hypotensive or CVD drugs and antibiotics—see BNF.

Side effects of statins
Statins are for life. Long-term studies show that statins are generally well tolerated although there has been recent debate about the frequency of adverse effects. The MHRA reviewed the issue (2014) and states: '[t]he benefits of using any statin in its licensed indication outweigh the risks in most patients.' Genetic factors have been implicated in the risk of myopathy.
   ℘ <http://www.mhra.gov.uk/Safetyinformation/DrugSafetyUpdate/CON418521>

   A review (*Am J Cardiol 2006;* April 17; **97**(8A):52–60C; doi:10.1016/j.amjcard.2005.12.010) estimated the following incidence per 100000 person-yrs:
- statin alone—rhabdomyolysis 3.4 (×10 with fibrate)
- myopathy—11
- peripheral neuropathy—12
- liver failure—0.5 (as for general population)

Studies in non-diabetic patients showed an increased prevalence of diabetes in long-term statin users. This has led to a modification of the class effect warning about these drugs by the Heads of Medicines Agencies in Europe: '[s]ome evidence suggests that statins as a class raise blood glucose and in some patients, at high risk of future diabetes, may produce a level of hyperglycaemia where formal diabetes care is appropriate. This risk, however, is outweighed by the reduction in vascular risk with statins and therefore should not be a reason for stopping statin treatment. Patients at risk (fasting glucose 5.6 to 6.9 mmol/L, BMI> 30 kg/m2, raised triglycerides, hypertension) should be monitored both clinically and biochemically according to national guidelines.' ℘ <http://www.hma.eu/fileadmin/dateien/Human_Medicines/CMD_h_/Product_Information/PhVWP_Recommendations/CMDhPhVWP0422012.pdf>

   In the CORALL study of people with diabetes, HbA_{1c} increased slightly but significantly after either atorvastatin or rosuvastatin use (*Diabet Med* 2012; **29**:628-31; doi: 10.1111/j.1464-5491.2011.03553.x).

Fibrates
Second-line agents—bezafibrate, ciprofibrate, fenofibrate, and gemfibrozil. These drugs reduce both cholesterol and triglyceride. Control glucose first. Use as first-line agents in patients whose genuinely fasting triglyceride is > 4.5 mmol/l with or without elevated cholesterol. Care should be taken to improve glucose control and reduce alcohol intake in these patients. Also use fibrates in patients with isolated hypercholesterolaemia who cannot tolerate statins.

Under specialist supervision fibrates may also be added to statin in patients with raised cholesterol and a triglyceride > 2.3 mmol/l. This increases the risk of rhabdomyolysis so the dose of statin should be reduced.

The 5-year FIELD study in people with type 2 diabetes found that fenofibrate was associated with less need for retinal laser treatment than placebo but more pancreatitis (*Lancet* 2005; **366**:1849–61; doi:10.1016/S0140-6736(05)67667-2).

Ezetimibe

This inhibits intestinal absorption of cholesterol. Ezetimibe is used on its own in patients unable to take statins. It can be added to a statin if further lipid lowering is needed but this increases the risk of rhabdomyolysis. It may cause gastrointestinal side effects, headache, fatigue, and myalgia. Pancreatitis is one of the rare side effects. Do not use in women who could become pregnant.

Bile-acid sequestrants

Colesevalam, colestyramine, or colestipol. Rarely used nowadays. Use if patients cannot tolerate other agents, or in combination for severe hypercholesterolaemia. Bile-acid sequestrants often cause gastrointestinal side effects and are poorly tolerated. Use in patients with high cholesterol but avoid if triglycerides are raised. Start with half a sachet before a meal and increase gradually. Other medication should be taken 1 hr before or 4 hrs after the bile-acid sequestrant. This medication may cause reduction in absorption of fat-soluble vitamins. Bile acid sequestrants are sometimes used in pregnancy.

Nicotinic acid or acipimox, omega-3-fatty acid compounds

Nicotinic acid and acipimox are not well tolerated because they cause flushing, acipimox less so.

Omega-3-fatty acid compounds are sometimes used to lower triglyceride. Some experts do not recommend them.

All these drugs are usually managed in specialist clinics and are used in patients who cannot tolerate other agents, or in combination for severe hypercholesterolaemia. Do not use in women who could become pregnant.

Soluble fibre

Ispaghula husk increases soluble fibre in the gut and can reduce cholesterol. It may cause gastrointestinal side effects but can be used as a 'natural' lipid-lowering agent for patients who prefer this or who cannot tolerate other drugs. Ispaghula should be introduced gradually. It may slow glucose absorption and cause hypoglycaemia.

Diabetic women of childbearing age

- Women aged 12–50 yrs may become pregnant.
- Most CVD drugs are contraindicated in pregnancy.
- Not planning pregnancy—advise reliable contraception while taking CVD medication drugs.
- Planning pregnancy (pp. 338–1)—refer immediately to specialist peri-pregnancy diabetes clinic. The risks of the cardiovascular condition should be weighed against the risks of pregnancy, and the risks of CVD drugs on the foetus. The DST will liaise with the relevant specialist clinics, e.g. cardiology.

Peripheral arterial disease (PAD)

After 20 yrs of diabetes, half of all men and two-thirds of women over 60 yrs old have no foot pulses. People with diabetes are four times as likely to have PAD as non-diabetics, and 23 times more likely to have a major amputation. Half the people requiring major amputation have diabetes. There are geographic variations in the frequency of amputation to which organization and delivery of clinical care may contribute (*Diabetologia* 2012; 55(7):1919–25; doi: 10.1007/s00125-012-2468-6). Prevention of amputation is discussed in Chapter 15 (➲ pp. 302, 313). The presence of PAD in diabetes increases the increased risk of dying from CVD by 70–80 %.

Screening

- Screen all patients on diagnosis and annually thereafter.
- Seek PAD in patients with other CVD.
- Check smoking history. Ask about intermittent claudication.
- Look at the feet for evidence of ischaemia and feel the anterior and posterior tibial pulses.
- Measure cholesterol and triglyceride.

Assessment

- Patients may have calf or buttock pain.
- Palpate femoral, popliteal, ankle, and foot pulses.
- Listen for femoral bruits.
- If the patient has symptoms or absent pulses, check with a Doppler probe.
- Measure ankle:brachial pressure index (ABPI). Because diabetes can produce widespread peripheral arterial calcification, non-compressible arteries can produce a falsely elevated reading. ABPI ≤ 0.9 or ≥ 1.40 indicates a high risk of occlusive PAD (*J Vasc Surg* 2008; **48**:1197–203; doi:10.1016/j.jvs.2008.06.005).
- Duplex ultrasound is usually the first test in patients being considered for revascularization. This is usually followed by contrast-enhanced magnetic resonance angiography (monitor renal function, stop metformin). Local diabetes and vascular teams should agree protocols.

Warning signs

- Gradually worsening symptoms. Refer the patient to a vascular surgeon.
- Rest pain. Telephone the diabetologist or vascular surgeon to arrange for admission under their joint care.
- ⚠ Critical ischaemia—red, painful. Poor capillary refilling. Same-day review—diabetologist and vascular surgeon.
- ⚠ Acute ischaemia—white/blue, cold, pulseless, painful foot/limb. Transfer to hospital immediately, to be seen same day by the vascular and diabetes teams.
- ⚠ Gangrene—transfer to hospital same day, to be seen by the vascular and diabetes team that day.
- Any foot problem in addition to PAD (➲ pp. 303–4).

Treatment

- See NICE CG 147.
- Stop smoking forever (➲ p. 36).
- Supervised exercise programme (check first for risk of worsening diabetic foot problems).
- Low-fat diet.
- Vigorous statin therapy for all (unless contraindicated) to reduce non-HDL cholesterol to < 2.5 mmol/l and LDL cholesterol to < 1.8 mmol/l.
- Antiplatelet drugs (➲ p. 261).
- Stop β-blockers.
- Control blood glucose.
- If the treatments do not relieve symptoms, or if there is limb-threatening ischaemia, refer for revascularization.
- Naftidrofuryl oxalate may relieve symptoms in patients in whom exercise has not done so or where revascularization is unsuitable or not desired.
- Intermittent claudication can improve spontaneously as collaterals open up.

The consequences of PAD are disastrous and all patients should be assessed jointly by a vascular surgeon and diabetologist. Angiography is performed in patients with worsening symptoms or whose limb is at risk and who would be suitable for surgery. It usually reveals multiple stenoses with diffuse distal disease. Angioplasty is sometimes possible and both proximal and distal arterial bypass are being used increasingly. Amputation is discussed on (➲ pp. 311–12).

Stroke and transient ischaemic attacks

Both transient ischaemic attack (TIA) and stroke are common in people with diabetes. Stroke is four times more likely in women with type 1 diabetes and twice as likely in type 2 diabetes than in non-diabetic women (*Diabetes Care* 2007; 30:1730–6; doi: 10.2337/dc06-2363). The relative risk of stroke in diabetics compared with non-diabetics was 3.70 for men and 4.35 for women (*Stroke* 1997; 28:1142–6; doi: 10.1161/01.STR.28.6.1142). From 2010–12 over 35 000 people with diabetes in England and Wales were admitted at least once with a stroke; a prevalence of 1.79 %, and an additional risk (vs the general population) of 34.1 %. NDA: ⌘ <http://www.hqip.org.uk/assets/NCAPOP-Library/NCAPOP-2013-14/NDA2011-2012Report2ComplicationsMortalityINTERACTIVEPDF26-11-13.pdf>

Diabetic patients are more likely to die or be disabled after a stroke than those without diabetes (*Diabetes Res Clin Pract* 2005; 69:293–8; doi:10.1016/j.diabres.2005.02.001). In England and Wales they were four times more likely to die within a year (NDA). In a European study '[d]iabetic patients, compared with those without diabetes, were more likely to have limb weakness ($P < 0.02$), dysarthria ($P < 0.001$), ischemic stroke ($P < 0.001$), and lacunar cerebral infarction ($P = 0.03$)'. They were also more likely to be disabled (*Stroke* 2003; 34:688–94; doi: 10.1161/01.STR.0000057975.15221.40). A US study found that 31 % of patients with ischaemic stroke had diabetes and that they were less likely to receive thrombolytic therapy than non-diabetic patients. They were less likely to be discharged home, and had a higher rate of in-hospital death (*Stroke* 2010; 41:e409-17; doi: 10.1161/STROKEAHA.109.572693). They concluded that better treatment was required.

Several studies of people with or without known diabetes have shown that a high admission glucose predicts poor clinical outcome. 'Admitting hyperglycemia was common among patients with acute ischemic stroke and was associated with increased short- and long-term mortality and with increased inpatient charges' (*Neurology* 2002; 59:67–71; doi: 10.1212/WNL.59.1.67). Patients with fatal stroke had higher HbA$_{1c}$ than those with non-fatal stroke (UKPDS 66 *Diabetes Care* 2004; 27:201–7; doi:10.2337/diacare.27.1.201). There are current trials on intensive glucose control in stroke; early results show increased risk of hypoglycaemia with insulin infusion.

'Type 2 diabetic patients found to have incidental carotid bruits have > 6 times the risk of first stroke in the first 2 yrs than patients without a bruit and should receive intensified management of vascular risk factors'. (*Stroke* 2003; 34:2145–51; doi:10.1161/01.STR.0000087360.91794.11).

Management of TIA and stroke in diabetic patients

- Check finger-prick and laboratory glucose to exclude hypoglycaemia which can mimic stroke.
- If patient is on glucose-lowering medication and glucose < 4 mmol/l give 150–160 mls 10 % glucose IV (➜ p. 189) and reassess patient.

- Manage as for non-diabetic patients with prompt referral to the specialist stroke team and transfer to the stroke unit. See NICE CG 68 (2008): ℘ <http://www.nice.org.uk/nicemedia/pdf/CG68fullGuideline.pdf>
- Assess for other cardiovascular disease—patients may have had ACS as well.
- Assess for other diabetic tissue damage—visual problems and neuropathy make rehabilitation more complex.
- Contact diabetes team promptly.
- Control blood glucose with usual tablets if, patient can swallow, glucose < 11 mmol/l, and dose can be adjusted to control glucose.
- If unable to swallow or glucose ≥ 11 mmol/l set up careful VRIII (➔ pp. 167–8) with sodium/glucose/potassium solution in parallel (e.g. 0.45 % sodium chloride with 5 % glucose, and potassium chloride 0.15 %; or 0.45 % sodium chloride with 5 % glucose, and potassium chloride 0.3 %).
- There is no clear guidance on optimal management of hyperglycaemia after acute stroke. A UK observational study of glycaemic control and outcomes suggested keeping the glucose ≤ 10 mmol/l. (*Br J Diab & Vascular Dis* 2010; **10**;287–91; doi:10.1177/1474651410390310). Glucose should remain > 4.0 mmol/l.
- Monitor finger-prick glucose hourly aiming to keep the glucose between 6 mmol/l and 10 mmol/l (seek local DST guidance) (➔ pp. 434–6).
- ⚠ Do not allow patient to become hypoglycaemic. Treat all glucose levels < 4 mmol/l unless on diet with or without metformin.
- Glucose control is difficult with enteral (nasogastric) feeding. Read JBDS guidance 'Glycaemic management during the inpatient enteral feeding of stroke inpatients with diabetes'. Tailor treatment to patient. ℘ <http://www.diabetologists-abcd.org.uk/JBDS/JBDS_IP_Enteral_Feeding_Stroke.pdf>
- Aim for a glucose level of 5–8 mmol/l pre-feed and 6–12 mmol/l while feeding. Many patients can be managed on SC insulin or non-insulin medication with DST advice. For type 1 diabetic patients start with VRIII on admission. Prescribe 10 % glucose IV when no feed running and nil by mouth—high risk of hypoglycaemia. Convert to SC insulin after DST advice and stop VRIII safely(➔ pp. 167–8).
- ⚠ Pressure sores are more likely in diabetic patients, especially if they have PAD or neuropathy. Be very careful to protect pressure areas.
- Institute intensive statin therapy as for ACS and PAD.
- Prescribe antiplatelet therapy as for non-diabetic patients with cerebrovascular disease.

Eyes

Diabetic eye disease is a common cause of blindness among people of working age in the Western world (Table 14.2). People with diabetes should be enrolled in a national screening programme (e.g. the NHS Diabetic Eye screening programme: ℘ <http://diabeticeye.screening.nhs.uk/>). Vigorously encourage them to attend. Identify patients who are unable to attend screening and ensure they get it. If there is no local system for ensuring screening, liaise with your local eye clinic. Only if you are fully trained in diabetic ophthalmoscopy should you screen the patient's eyes yourself. However, it is important to examine the eyes in symptomatic patients.

'Diabetic retinopathy is a chronic progressive, potentially sight-threatening disease of the retinal microvasculature associated with the prolonged hyperglycaemia and other conditions linked to diabetes mellitus such as hypertension.' Royal College of Ophthalmologists (RCOphth) ℘ <http://www.rcophth.ac.uk/page.asp?section=451>

Diabetic eye disease is common. After 25 yrs of diabetes most patients will have retinopathy (97 % in a Danish study; *Diabetologia* 2009; **52**:1829–35; doi: 10.1007/s00125-009-1450-4). Before this, the incidence depends largely on the age of onset of diabetes and the type of diabetes. In Liverpool 45.7 % of type 1 patients and 25.3 % of type 2 patients had diabetic retinopathy. Sight-threatening eye disease was associated with increasing duration of diabetes (Odds Ratio 1.09 per yr; double that in men) (*Diabet Med* 2002; **19**:1014–21; doi: 10.1046/j.1464-5491.2002.00854.x). Children with duration > 5 yrs can develop retinopathy. Type 1 patients diagnosed under the age of 30 yrs are unlikely to have retinopathy on diagnosis but develop it steadily after ~ 3 yrs. About 1 in 5 patients with maturity-onset type 2 diabetes will have retinopathy at diagnosis.

Digital retinal photography, fluoroscein angiography, and optical coherence tomography (OCT) have all provided more detailed information about diabetic eye disease which is often much more extensive than ophthalmoscopy would suggest.

Comorbid conditions (including CVD and depression) are common in people with diabetic retinopathy which is also associated with increased mortality.

Sight-threatening diabetic retinopathy seems to be lessening. A meta-analysis found that in patients without baseline retinopathy, proliferative diabetic retinopathy (PDR) developed in 6.3 % of people in studies published in 1975–85 vs 2.0 % in 1985–2008. Severe visual loss was 2.0 % vs none. In patients with baseline retinopathy, PDR developed in 39.7 % vs none, with severe visual loss 17.5 % vs 5.4 % (*Diabetes Care* 2009; **32**:2307–13; doi:10.2337/dc09-0615). This suggests both reduction in risk factors and better care of retinopathy.

Preventing diabetic eye disease

Factors which have been implicated are high blood glucose, hypertension, the contraceptive pill, and alcohol. High blood glucose and hypertension have definite links; the others are less clear. A link with smoking has been suggested but is unclear. Diabetic retinopathy may progress rapidly during pregnancy.

Hyperglycaemia

Patients with persistent hyperglycaemia are much more likely to develop diabetic retinopathy than those with near-normal blood glucose levels. Normalization of the blood glucose slows the rate of development of retinopathy. However, it seems sensible to reduce the blood glucose gradually, over ~ 4–8 wks, as a sudden return to normal may worsen retinopathy in the short term.

Hypertension

This can cause retinopathy in its own right, but uncontrolled hypertension may be associated with severe diabetic retinopathy. Control BP to < 120–129/75–80 taking care to avoid postural hypotension.

Other factors

Retinopathy may worsen in pregnancy. Pregnant women must have their eyes screened as soon as pregnancy is diagnosed and again later in pregnancy. It is probably sensible to avoid oral contraceptives in women with a marked background of proliferative retinopathy.

Smoking should be stopped anyway, and excess alcohol intake is inadvisable.

Screening

Every patient with diabetes, including those with diabetes in remission (➌ p. 21), should attend their free annual digital retinal photographic eye check (e.g. NHS Diabetic Eye screening programme). Check that they have actually attended. The NHS provides free sight tests for people with diabetes which they should also attend. Mobile services are available for those who cannot travel.

Screen all patients on diagnosis of diabetes and annually thereafter. (Recent evidence suggests that some patients do not need annual screening but the interval has not been changed at the time of writing).

Warning symptoms

- Deterioration in vision. Check the patient's visual acuity with a Snellen chart. Use pin-hole correction if acuity is worse than 6/6 in either eye.
- If the visual acuity is worse than 6/9 despite pin-hole correction, refer the patient to an ophthalmologist. (N.B. If the patient is hyperglycaemic, it is advisable to retest the eyes after the blood glucose has returned to normal—hyperglycaemia may cause temporarily blurred vision.) If the pin-hole resolves the impairment of visual acuity, advise the patient to visit an ophthalmic optician or optometrist. Patients should not buy expensive spectacles until their blood glucose level is stable, preferably near normal.
- 'Floaters', blobs, or wisps across the vision. The patient may have had a vitreous haemorrhage (Figure 14.1). Examine the eye and refer to an ophthalmologist for urgent assessment.
- None—that is why retinal screening is essential.

Table 14.2 Eye problems in diabetes

Orbits	Fungal infections via sinus (rare)
Lids	Ptosis, inflammation
Eye muscles*	Mononeuropathy causing squint
Refraction	Changes or blurring—often fluctuate with glucose level
Tears	Dry eyes
Cornea	Reduced sensitivity, scratches, ulcers
Iris	Rubeosis iridis, neovascular glaucoma
Ciliary body	Premature presbyopia (long-sightedness)
Lens	Cataract, refraction problems
Vitreous	Posterior detachment
Retina	Diabetic retinopathy (haemorrhages, exudates, new vessels), lipaemia retinalis, arterial occlusion, central retinal vein occlusion, detachment
Macula	Maculopathy (exudates, ischaemia, oedema)
Intraocular pressure	Glaucoma
Optic nerve*	Swelling (papilloedema), optic atrophy, new vessels on disc

*Consider other causes.

Source data from *J Am Optom Assoc* 1990; **61**:533–43, and Ariffin A, Hill RD, Leigh O, *Diabetes and primary eye care*. Oxford: Blackwell Scientific, 2002.

Squint or ptosis

Squint may occur acutely, often with associated pain, as a sign of diabetic mononeuropathy. The 3rd, 4th, or 6th nerve may be affected. In 3rd-nerve palsy due to diabetes, pupillary function is often intact. The squint may gradually resolve. Beware the coincidental brain tumour. Refer patients with a new squint to the medical on-call team or a neurologist same day.

Ptosis may occur with Bell's palsy (7th nerve).

Lens

Age-related cataract occurs earlier in people with diabetes than in others. If the patient has a cataract in either eye and they have impaired visual acuity, or you cannot see the retina, refer them to an ophthalmologist.

Patients under 30 yrs old with cataracts should be seen by an ophthalmologist that week; acutely developing juvenile cataract can cause blindness within days. These are sometimes described as 'snow-flake' cataracts. Osmotic shifts may also cause reversible cataracts.

The optic nerve

Rarely, diabetes can cause optic neuritis visible as papilloedema. Refer to an ophthalmologist but also consider other causes of papilloedema, e.g. raised intracranial pressure. New vessels can occur here.

The retina

Diabetic retinopathy is divided into proliferative (new vessels present), and non-proliferative (or background) or preproliferative. Macular involvement is termed maculopathy.

Non-proliferative retinopathy

Microaneurysms and/or dot haemorrhages are seen (Figure 14.1). They will not impede vision, are potentially reversible, but may progress. There may also be hard exudates—shiny, clearly defined, yellowish fatty exudates. A prompt referral is needed if these exudates are at the macula.

Preproliferative retinopathy

A sign of diabetic ophthalmopathy. Larger blot haemorrhages with tortuous dilated capillary remnants (intra-retinal microvascular anomalies or IRMA) may be present. Veins also have bulges (beads) and extra loops on them. Cotton-wool spots are pale and poorly defined. The retina may be pale. There are likely to be more changes on fluoroscein angiography. Refer to an ophthalmologist.

Proliferative retinopathy

Neovascularization indicates proliferative retinopathy. Fine tangles of tiny vessels are most often seen near the optic disc but can occur anywhere, including at the periphery of an otherwise normal-looking fundus. Disc vessels are particularly likely to bleed. Contact the ophthalmologist—the patient should be seen within 2 wks.

Vitreous haemorrhage

Vitreous haemorrhage (Figure 14.1) should not happen—it is largely preventable. Bleeding occurs when the fragile new vessels are damaged. Red or black blobs ('tadpoles', 'floaters') or wisps float across the patient's vision. A big bleed may be like a curtain. The haemorrhage may clear, but some people may develop severe permanent visual impairment. Telephone the ophthalmologist for a same-day appointment. The more bleeding, the harder it may be to visualize the bleeding vessels and attempt to photocoagulate them.

Maculopathy

Because the patient's problem is at the fovea, using a pin-hole to correct visual acuity may make it worse. This is the area of best vision so problems here require urgent treatment. If there is a ring of hard yellow exudates around or near the macula this may impair the best vision. If the little pink dot which marks the fovea is blurred or if the whole macula appears swollen, the patient should be seen by an ophthalmologist straightaway—they may need urgent anti-vascular endothelial growth factor (VEGF) treatment. OCT may reveal previously undetected intra-retinal fluid and is now used routinely in most eye clinics.

Advanced eye disease

Even if the interior of the eye appears completely disorganized with fibrous bands pulling on the retina and detaching it, vitreous surgery and other specialist techniques may be helpful. Rubeosis (i.e. new vessels on the iris causing glaucoma) may occur, but it may be treatable. Such patients should be seen by an ophthalmologist within a week.

Other retinal problems

Thrombosis of retinal arteries and veins, and glaucoma are more common in people with diabetes than in the general population. They all require prompt ophthalmological advice.

Retinopathy grading

There are several different grading systems. The English Diabetic Eye Screening programme uses:

R0—no retinopathy
R1—mild background retinopathy
R2—preproliferative retinopathy
R3A—active proliferative retinopathy
R3S—stable treated proliferative retinopathy

Further information can be found at:
🖱 <http://diabeticeye.screening.nhs.uk/gradingcriteria>
RCOphth Diabetic Retinopathy screening guidelines 2012 (minor update July 2013) 🖱 <http://www.rcophth.ac.uk/page.asp?section=451>

(a) CATARACT

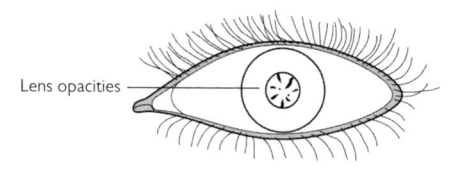

Lens opacities

(b) RETINOPATHY

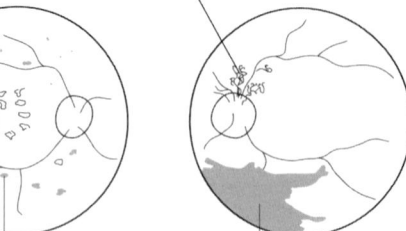

Exudates round macula

New vessels

Dot and blot haemorrhages

Vitreous haemorrhages

Fig. 14.1 Diabetic eye problems: (a) cataract; (b) retinopathy.

Treatment of diabetic retinopathy and maculopathy

Support and patient education

Any suggestion of possible or actual visual loss is terrifying. Depression is common, and quality of life is impaired in those with visual loss. Provide accurate information (in large print) and education about what can be done by patient and professionals to treat the problem and/or reduce the risk of progression. There is considerable benefit in careful risk factor reduction. RNIB has a website and helpline for those with visual impairment. ℞ <http://www.rnib.org.uk>

Laser photocoagulation

Used for proliferative retinopathy to reduce the stimulus to neo-vascularization by producing tiny retinal burns. The aim is to induce regression of new vessels and sometimes to seal leaking new vessels. It is also used to treat maculopathy. There are different kinds of laser. Laser treatment prevents severe visual impairment in the majority of patients, although the results for maculopathy are less predictable because treatment is close to the macula. Patients should understand that laser treatment may not improve vision but it should stop major deterioration. The treatment is usually given in one or more 30–60 min sessions as an outpatient. Modern equipment is quicker than this. Local anaesthetic and dilating eye drops are used, and the patient has to remain still and concentrate while the treatment is given. Afterwards there is blurring of vision, photophobia, and sometimes eye discomfort or headache. Pain is commoner in those with previous laser photocoagulation. Patients who complain of severe pain should be referred to the eye emergency service.

Intravitreal anti-VEGF

RCOphth guidance (➔ p. 268) states 'intravitreal anti-VEGF treatment (with or without laser) achieves superior visual outcomes compared to laser treatment alone for patients with similar criteria to those involved in the clinical trials i.e. centre-involving DMO.' Ranibizumab is licensed in Europe for treating centre-involving diabetic macular oedema. NICE (TA 274) states 'Ranibizumab is recommended as an option for treating visual impairment due to diabetic macular oedema only if the eye has a central retinal thickness of 400 micrometres or more at the start of treatment.' Bevacizumab is not licensed for this indication but has also been shown in studies to be effective.

Hearing, smell, and taste

Hearing

A meta-analysis showed that people with diabetes were 2.15 times more likely to have hearing loss than those without. The odds ratio for people with diabetes aged ≤ 60 yrs was 2.61 vs 1.58 for those aged > 60 yrs (*J Clin Endocrinol Med* 2013; **98**:51–8; ℰ doi: http://dx.doi.org/10.1210/jc.2012-2119). An audiometric US study found low-/mid-frequency loss in 21.3 % of those with diabetes vs 9.4 % in those without. For high-frequency loss the figures were 54.1 % vs 32.0 %. (NHANES *Ann Int Med* 2008; **149**:1–10; doi:10.7326/0003-4819-149-1-200807010-00231). Hyperglycaemia, albuminuria and CRP were linked with high-frequency loss (*Diabetes Care* 2010; **33**:811–6; doi:10.2337/dc09-1193). The mechanisms probably include both circulatory and neural factors. Patients with auditory neuropathy may also have balance and coordination problems.

Some rarer forms of diabetes are associated with deafness:

- Maternally inherited mitochondrial DNA abnormality causing deafness and diabetes. Affects up to 1 % of the diabetic population. Associated with mitochondrial encephalomyopathy, lactic acidosis, and stroke-like episodes
- Congenital rubella syndrome (deafness, eye problems, congenital heart disease, learning difficulties, growth retardation)—rare since immunization introduced.
- Wolfram's syndrome (diabetes insipidus, diabetes mellitus, optic atrophy and deafness, DIDMOAD)—very rare.
- Alström's syndrome (diabetes mellitus, deafness, and problems with eyes, obesity, liver, kidney, bladder, bowel, and heart)—very rare.

Patients with hearing loss should always have a formal auditory assessment. Consider rare syndromes in younger patients. Stop smoking. Ensure that blood glucose balance and other risk factor control is good.

Some patients will require a sign language interpreter in clinic. Record this need in their notes and give these patients the time they need to understand their condition. Profoundly deaf people with diabetes often know very little about their diabetes and how to stay well. Diabetes UK has produced a video: ℰ <http://www.diabetes.org.uk/Other_languages/Information-in-British-Sign-Language/>

Smell

The sense of smell may be diminished in diabetes. This appears to be associated with age and complications such as vasculopathy. (*Diabetes Care* 1993; **16**:934–7; doi:10.2337/diacare.16.6.934; *Physiol Behav* 1993; **53**:17–21; ℰ doi: http://dx.doi.org/10.1016/0031-9384(93)90005-Z.) This is an under-researched area as is taste.

Taste

A few studies have reported reduction in taste in people with diabetes. Impaired taste was found in 73 % of patients with type 1 diabetes vs 16 % of the non-diabetic controls in a French study (a tenth had no sense of taste at all). Hypoguesia appeared linked with peripheral neuropathy and particularly applied to sucrose or similar tastes. (*Diabetes Care* 1989; **12**:173–8; doi:10.2337/diacare.12.3.173).

Kidneys

More than 70 % of people with diabetes have some evidence of nephropathy (Table 14.3). Renal failure is the cause of death in 10–20 % of people with type 1 diabetes, but only 1–2 % of those with type 2 diabetes. There is considerable scope for preventing nephropathy.

The main cause is glomerulosclerosis but recurrent UTIs, renal papillary necrosis, and perinephric abscess are commoner in people with diabetes than those without.

Preventing or slowing renal impairment (➲ pp. 36–42)

Hyperglycaemia (➲ pp. 201–12)

Persistent hyperglycaemia is strongly linked with increased likelihood of developing nephropathy. Near-normalization of the blood glucose slows the rate of deterioration of renal function. ⚠ Insulin is cleared by the kidneys so there is a high risk of hypoglycaemia in patients with reduced eGFR who should do frequent SMBG. Those not on insulin are likely to need it ultimately. Care should be taken with non-insulin drugs, some of which are contraindicated in severe renal failure (➲ pp. 118–19). Most type 2 patients will end up on insulin. Half of all people with diabetes who develop end-stage renal failure have type 2 diabetes.

Hypertension (➲ pp. 257–8)

Tight control of hypertension slows deterioration of renal function in nephropaths. This means treating people whose BP would not normally fall into the treatment range for non-diabetic people. In patients with known diabetic kidney disease the aim is to keep BP 120–129/75–80 but be careful to avoid dizziness and falls in patients with severe postural hypotension due to autonomic neuropathy. Start with ACE inhibitors or ARBs. Check U&E + creatinine before starting, after 2 wks, and after changing dose. Other hypotensive drugs can be used (e.g. amlodipine, which does not need reduction in renal impairment).

Treat microalbuminuria (➲ p. 38)

ACE inhibitors (captopril, ramipril, lisinopril) and ARBs (irbesartan, losartan) are licensed to slow the progression of diabetic nephropathy if initiated when persistent microalbuminuria is detected. Test for ACR annually. If the ratio is raised in two of three samples collected consecutively within 1 mth, prescribe an ACE inhibitor and increase to maximal tolerated dose.

Low-salt diet

Reduced sodium chloride intake may help control hypertension and reduce fluid retention. Once the patient has significant renal impairment, a low protein and/or low phosphate diet may help. Seek a renal physician's advice before prescribing such diets via a dietitian.

Stop smoking (➲ p. 36)

Screening—kidneys

- Screen every patient at diagnosis of diabetes and annually thereafter.
- Screen by measuring laboratory urinary microalbumin:creatinine ratio, even in patients with known albuminuria/proteinuria (to measure effect of treatment) (➔ p. 92).
- Measure plasma creatinine concentrations and calculate eGFR.

Warning symptoms or signs

- None: in most cases, by the time symptoms and signs develop, severe renal impairment is present
- Hypoglycaemia or falling insulin or non-insulin hypoglycaemic dose
- Rising BP
- Oedema
- Frothy urine in patients with severe proteinuria, e.g. nephrotic syndrome

Diabetic nephropathy

It may take several years for microalbuminuria to progress to overt albuminuria and for other signs of renal impairment to develop. The rate of deterioration of renal function can be slowed down. If eGFR is reduced, the Renal Association recommend repeating it in 2 wks, and if stable then, repeat in 90 days.

Evidence of nephropathy

- Raised ACR (> 3.5 mg/mmol in men, > 2.5 mg/mmol in women)
- Dipstick proteinuria—some patients develop nephrotic syndrome
- Haematuria:
  - microscopic—rare in purely diabetic nephropathy, seek other cause;
  - macroscopic—exclude menstruation, refer to urology
- Low eGFR (see Table 14.3)

If nephropathy check:

- Personal history of renal or urinary disease (e.g. recurrent UTIs)
- Family history of renal disease or rare syndrome
- BP (lying and standing)
- Heart (high cardiovascular risk)
- PAD (severe PAD increases likelihood of renal artery stenosis)
- Fundi (if no retinopathy seek non-diabetic causes of nephropathy)
- Urine microscopy and culture
- Laboratory ACR annually (protein:creatinine ratio (PCR) is sometimes used in patients with heavy proteinuria; 24-hr urine protein collections are no longer recommended)
- Blood U&E, creatinine, eGFR, lipids, calcium, albumin, phosphate, FBC, HbA$_{1c}$—if fasting sample used tell patient to drink plenty of water but avoid food—risk of dehydration and worsening CKD
- Renal ultrasound if CKD 3+
- Appropriate tests if non-diabetic cause suspected

Action

- See Table 14.3.
- Consider referral to the diabetes team.

Table 14.3 Stages and management of chronic kidney disease

CKD stage	eGFR ml/min/1.73m²	NDA* 2011/12	Kidney function	Management Check your local referral guidelines
No CKD	> 90	24.9 %	Normal ACR/PCR normal	Annual review of creatinine and ACR
1	> 90	5.1 %	Normal but urine abnormality including ACR/PCR > 3.5 mg/mmol men, > 2.5 mg/mmol women or structural abnormality or genetic trait renal disease	Monitor Refer diabetes team? BP 120–129/75–80 if safe HbA$_{1c}$ 6.0–6.5 % if safe. Avoid hypoglycaemia Cholesterol < 4 mmol/l ACE I or ARB titrate to full dose Statin Aspirin 75 mg once daily Stop smoking *Renal referral if:* ACR > 30 mg/mmol + microscopic haematuria ACR > 70 mg/mmol despite treatment Suspected renal artery stenosis BP not controlled despite four drugs Possible rare cause CKD
2	60–89	42.9 %	Mildly reduced kidney function + above (but eGFR calculation less accurate in this zone, so repeat with patient well hydrated)	As CKD 1 Refer diabetes team?

(Continued)

Table 14.3 (Cont.)

CKD stage	eGFR ml/min/1.73m²	NDA* 2011/12	Kidney function	Management Check your local referral guidelines
3	30–59	16.4 %	Moderately reduced kidney function	As CKD 1, but HbA$_{1c}$ 6.5–7.3 % Check for sepsis, CCF, big bladder Renal ultrasound Refer diabetes team *Renal referral if:* Rapid fall in eGFR (> 5/yr or 10/5 yrs) Microscopic haematuria ACR > 70 mg/mmol or PCR > 100 mg/mmol Unexplained anaemia Abnormal potassium, calcium, or phosphate Suspected systemic illness Uncontrolled BP (> 150/90 on three agents)
4	15–29	1.3 %	Severely reduced renal function	As CKD3 + urgent renal referral
5	< 15	0.5 %	End-stage/ established kidney failure	As CKD3 + same-day renal referral

*National Diabetes Audit: percentage of people with diabetes experiencing CKD. Results unknown in 8.9 %.

⬧ <http://www.hqip.org.uk/assets/NCAPOP-Library/NCAPOP-2013-14/NDA2011-2012Report2ComplicationsMortalityINTERACTIVEPDF26-11-13.pdf>

Source data from Renal Association guidelines: ⬧ < http://www.renal.org/guidelines/modules/detection-monitoring-and-care-of-patients-with-ckd#sthash.IqixhfwZ.dpbs>, and NICE CG 73.

- Vigorous renal and cardiovascular risk reduction:
  - ACE or ARB first line to maximal tolerated licensed antihypertensive dose unless hypotension (captopril, ramipril, losartan, irbesartan)—watch for ↑potassium, renal function
  - diuretic—thiazide CKD 1 + 2; loop diuretic CKD 3–5 (beware dehydration); watch for ↓potassium, check renal function
  - amlodipine: beware oedema
- Early, vigorous, and careful glucose control: risk of hypoglycaemia with worsening eGFR—SMBG four times daily
- Weight loss if needed, with appropriately increased exercise
- Statin if not on it and no contraindications
- Hepatitis B immunization if not already done
- Avoid NSAIDs and other nephrotoxins
- Check Renal Association website: ♫ <http://www.renal.org>
- Keep monitoring ACR long term

Patients with CKD 3+ should usually be seen by a diabetologist and also referred to a renal physician (see Table 14.3). Several centres now have joint renal diabetes clinics. Patients may need haemodialysis. Continuous ambulatory peritoneal dialysis (CAPD) is still used sometimes. Insulin can be given intraperitoneally. Nowadays nephrologists are moving towards early kidney transplant as this produces better outcomes than dialysis. Diabetes specialist input to glucose management in diabetic patients on dialysis is essential. CAPD has a 60 % 3-yr survival rate in diabetes.

Patients with diabetic nephropathy always have retinopathy and often have foot problems, neuropathy, vascular disease, and ischaemic heart disease. Many die from the latter rather than from their renal impairment. Renal Registry data shows that, among people aged ≥65 yrs starting renal replacement treatment there is little difference in survival between those with or without diabetes. However 5-yr survival of people aged 18–44 yrs was 70 % for those with diabetes vs 89 % of people without diabetes. ♫ <http://www.renalreg.com/Reports/2013.html>

Overall, 5-yr survival of patients (with and without diabetes) post transplant from a deceased donor is 87 % in the UK. Of all patients entering the UK renal transplant programme in 2007–12, 15 % had diabetes. Post transplant their renal function deteriorated more rapidly than in non-diabetic recipients. People with type 1 diabetes who require renal transplant should be offered a simultaneous pancreatic transplant (SPK) (➲ p. 180). Kidney transplant patients may be eligible for islet cell transplants (➲ p. 180).

Diabetic neuropathy

Diabetes can damage any nerve and produce virtually any sensory, motor, or autonomic neurological deficit or combinations of these. Measurement is difficult so its frequency is unclear. It may affect up to 50 % of people with diabetes. After 20 yrs of diabetes most people have evidence of impaired nerve function on detailed testing. About one in 12 people with newly diagnosed type 2 diabetes have clinically detectable neuropathy.

There are several classifications of diabetic neuropathy. One classification is:

- Rapidly reversible hyperglycaemic neuropathy
- Generalized symmetrical polyneuropathies (chronic sensorimotor, acute sensory, autonomic)
- Focal and multifocal neuropathy (cranial, thoracolumbar radiculopathy, focal limb, proximal motor (amyotrophy))
- Superimposed chronic inflammatory demyelinating neuropathy (*Diabetes Care* 2004; **27**:1458–86; doi:10.2337/diacare.27.6.1458)

In practice, the different variants may not be clearly definable. From the patient's point of view it is important to know if any sensory modality is missing so as to be careful to avoid injury, if it hurts or feels peculiar, or if a muscle is weak or does not work. The commonest forms are chronic sensory distal peripheral neuropathy and autonomic neuropathy. Most neuropathic patients will have other diabetic tissue damage (e.g. retinopathy or nephropathy) so seek this.

Screening for neuropathy

- Screen every patient at diagnosis of diabetes and annually thereafter
- Symptoms: none, or numbness, tingling, weakness, postural dizziness
- Examination:
  - Muscle wasting
  - Muscle weakness (if symptoms/wasting)
  - Feet: light touch—cotton wool or Ipswich touch test (➋ p. 305)
  - Pressure—monofilament (≤ 10 g is normal). Test multiple sites— see: ⌨ <http://www.nhshighland.scot.nhs.uk/YourHealth/ Diabetes/Documents/Use%20of%2010g%20monofilament.pdf>
  - Pin-prick—Neurotips® (Owen Mumford) (do not use needles!)
  - Vibration—tuning fork (128 Hz pitch) or neurothesiometer
  - Position sense
  - Tendon reflexes—ankle, knee
  - BP: lying and standing
- Electrophysiological or nerve conduction testing is rarely needed
- Single use devices are best if possible. Remember to clean multiple-use equipment

Check for non-diabetic causes of neuropathy

Diabetic neuropathy is a diagnosis by exclusion. One in 10 diabetic patients with neuropathy has another cause which may be treatable, e.g.:

- vitamin B12 deficiency (may be low on metformin (➋ p. 76)
- vitamin B$_6$ deficiency

- alcohol excess
- drugs (e.g. isoniazid, chemotherapy)
- uraemia
- HIV or its treatment
- collagen-vascular disease
- monoclonal gammopathy
- neoplasia (do CXR)

Neuropathies

Hyperglycaemic neuropathy

Uncommon, this occurs in newly diagnosed patients, or those who have had a period of very high glucose. It usually comes on rapidly, produces peripheral symptoms, sometimes painful, with or without signs, and clears with good glucose control.

Sensory peripheral neuropathy ('glove and stocking')

The most common form of neuropathy is symmetrical loss or blunting of sensation in a 'sock' and/or sometimes 'glove' distribution. Different modalities may be differently affected. Problems that arise are:
- numbness so that rubbing or injury is not noticed
- loss of temperature discrimination with a risk of burning
- loss of position sense—walking or balance may be affected
- loss of vibration sense
- tingling or pain (➔ p. 284)

Mononeuropathy(ies)

Single-nerve lesions, with or without entrapment, are quite common. They include median (carpal tunnel syndrome), ulnar nerves, common peroneal nerve (foot drop), lateral femoral cutaneous nerve, those serving eye movement (➔ p. 270)and facial nerve (Bell's palsy). Several single nerves in different parts of the body may be affected in one patient. Encourage weight loss in those who need it. Avoid surgery if possible—results are variable. Acute Bell's palsy is often treated with steroids (treat hyperglycaemia).

Truncal radicular neuropathy affects one or both sides of the thorax or abdomen, often with pain, and, rarely, muscle impairment.

Neuropathic muscle weakness

Muscle weakness may be secondary to an individual nerve lesion or more diffuse and symmetrical.

Diabetic amyotrophy can affect the thighs with marked wasting, weakness, and pain. It is rare but distressing and disabling. Refer promptly to a diabetologist. There is thought to be a vasculitic component. Improve glucose control and relieve pain (➔ p. 284).

Symptoms of neuropathy (or not)

Many patients are unaware of the extent of their neuropathy until they are affected by one of its consequences, such as a foot ulcer at the site of an unnoticed injury.

As many as 16–20 % of people with diabetes experience painful neuropathy. Refer such patients to a diabetologist. If patients have severe pain, it limits them in any way, or their underlying condition has worsened, refer them to a pain clinic too (➔ p. 284).

⚠ *Warning for patients with sensory neuropathy*
- Never walk barefoot
- Check shoes and socks for foreign bodies every time you put them on
- Never use a hot water bottle
- Check the bathwater temperature with a bath thermometer
- Wear gloves for washing up
- Use a long wrist-protecting oven glove
- Protect hands, arms, legs, feet during work or hobbies (e.g. gardening) where scratches, burns, or injuries may occur
- Inspect your feet every day
- Check your shoes every day, inside and out

Diabetic autonomic neuropathy (DAN)

(*Diabetes Care* 2003; **26**:1553–79; doi:10.2337/diacare.26.5.1553)
DAN is present in 7 % of patients with newly diagnosed type 1 diabetes. This can be found on specific testing in most patients with long duration of diabetes. Symptoms are relatively uncommon. If the patient does have symptoms, they may be unpleasant and the prognosis is poor. Of all type 1 patients with asymptomatic DAN, 27 % will be dead within 5 yrs (vs 8 % if autonomic function tests are normal) (*Q J Med* 1991; **79**:495–502).

Symptoms include:
- postural dizziness or fainting
- exercise intolerance
- difficulty swallowing (➲ p. 286)
- gastric fullness or vomiting (➲ p. 287)
- diarrhoea or constipation; faecal leakage (➲ pp. 288–9)
- urinary retention, urinary frequency
- sexual dysfunction in men and women (➲ pp. 353–5)
- altered sweating
- loss of hypoglycaemia warning (➲ p. 186)
- sudden death

Refer all patients with symptomatic DAN to a consultant diabetologist who may liaise with a neurologist specializing in autonomic neuropathy. Investigation and treatment are complex, and these patients have multiple complications.

Cardiovascular autonomic neuropathy

⚠ *Sudden death*
May occur at any time. People with DAN are at especial risk of sudden death if they become hypoxic, during anaesthesia or situations where there are circulatory changes (e.g. trauma). Always tell the anaesthetist that the patient has DAN. Anaesthesia should be performed only in a hospital with full resuscitation and medical support.

Postural hypotension
- May be severe, even on sitting up in bed
- May be immediate on rising or delayed for some minutes

- Symptoms:
  - none
  - dizziness or faintness
  - confusion
  - sudden collapse
  - falls in elderly
- Worsened by:
  - fluid depletion
  - excessive treatment of hypertension
  - diuretics
  - nitrates and other vasodilators
  - psychotropic/pain-relieving drugs (such as tricyclics)
- Management
  - seek non-diabetic + diabetic causes
  - ensure adequate hydration and salt intake
  - remove or reduce drugs worsening hypotension
  - consider compression stockings (check arterial circulation, sensation)
  - consider fludrocortisone (beware oedema)
  - flurbiprofen, ephedrine, and midodrine have been used in specialist services (off licence—see BNF)
  - warn patient to get up slowly and exercise calf muscles before walking

Exercise intolerance

During exercise, heart rate and blood pressure cannot increase appropriately and cardiac output is insufficient, limiting patient activities. Silent myocardial ischaemia may be more likely in these patients.

Altered sweating

Patients may sweat less on the feet but more in the upper half of the body. This may cause dry skin and cracking—advise emollient cream but not between the toes.

Gustatory sweating is facial sweating precipitated by spicy or highly flavoured foods. Avoiding these foods may help and antimuscarinic drugs (e.g. propantheline) are sometimes used.

Urinary retention

Symptoms of bladder dysfunction occur in up to half of all people with diabetes, and more may show this on testing. Patients may have urinary frequency. The bladder slowly enlarges. An increasing post-micturition volume forming a reservoir for infection. Regular urination with suprapubic pressure may help. Prophylactic antibiotics such as trimethoprim may be required for recurrent UTIs. Exclude other causes of urinary retention, such as prostatism. They may coexist.

Screening—autonomic neuropathy: symptomatic patients

Apart from BP, tests for autonomic neuropathy are usually reserved for symptomatic patients. Definitions vary. Some tests are complex and require specialist testing. The following can be done with a mobile patient, a sphygmomanometer, an ECG machine, and this paper which provides age-banded results: *Diabetic Med* 1992; **9**:166–75; doi: 10.1111/j.1464-5491.1992.tb01754.x.

- Lying and standing systolic BP. Check at 2 min. Postural hypotension ↓BP by > 20 mm Hg systolic (NICE 2014).
- Heart rate during and after Valsalva manoeuvre. Do not do this in people with proliferative retinopathy.
- Heart rate after standing ('30:15 test').
- These tests are fraught with practical difficulties (patients who find it hard to stand up, ECG leads fall off, etc.).

Preventing or treating neuropathy—general

Glucose control

People with persistently high blood glucose levels are more likely to have peripheral neuropathy than those with normal glucose levels. Near-normalization of the glucose concentration (some authorities believe insulin should be used) may relieve severe pain or abnormal feelings in neuropathy. Returning the glucose to normal slows worsening peripheral neuropathy, and may also improve it. DCCT showed that intensive glucose-lowering therapy slowed development and progression of abnormal autonomic function tests but with increased hypoglycaemic unawareness (*Diabetologia* 1998; **41**:416–23; doi: 10.1007/s001250050924. Weight loss will help glucose control and may improve some improve entrapment syndromes.

Medications and other treatments

There is, as yet, no licensed treatment for loss of sensation or motor function. Aldose reductase inhibitors have shown promise (*Diabetes Care* 2006; **29**:1538–44; doi:10.2337/dc05-2370). The NHANES study found a link between low vitamin D levels and self-reported neuropathy (*Diabet Med* 2012; **29**:50–5; doi: 10.1111/j.1464-5491.2011.03379.x), but studies of vitamin D replacement are awaited. For general health reasons, it seems sensible to check vitamin D and replace it if low (➲ p. 76).

Painful neuropathy can be very distressing whether or not there is clinical evidence of nerve damage on examination. (see NICE CG 173). Provide supportive assessment of physical and emotional health. Clarify the symptoms and their impact, and discuss the pros and cons of amitriptyline, duloxetine, gabapentin, or pregabalin as initial treatment for neuropathic pain (NICE CG 173). Gabapentin and duloxetine mention diabetes in their SPCs. Capsaicin cream can be used for localized neuropathic pain or in patients for whom the other drugs are inappropriate or not wanted. Minor analgesics are not usually effective (many neuropathic patients will have nephropathy in which NSAIDs must be avoided), and tramadol should be used only for acute rescue.

Gastrointestinal problems

Mouth

Diabetes is associated with an increased likelihood of both oral and dental problems (Box 14.3). Most of these conditions are more likely with smoking ± hyperglycaemia (*Clin Diabetes* 2005; **23**:171–8; doi:10.2337/diaclin.23.4.171).

Oral problems
- Dry mouth—lack of saliva. More likely with hyperglycaemia, and with neuropathy. Worsens other oral/dental problems. Advise saliva substitute or stimulant.
- Parotid enlargement found in 25 % of diabetic patients.
- Bad breath—periodontal disease, oral hygiene problems.
- Oral candida—risk 2–5 times, particularly with dentures. Treat with improved oral hygiene and nystatin or fluconazole (beware interactions).
- Tongue—glossitis, atrophic patches, fissures.
- Angular cheilosis.
- Denture stomatitis.
- Lichen planus—risk of cancer and candida. May need steroid treatment.
- Poor wound healing in mouth.
- Burning mouth syndrome.
- Fibromas.

Box 14.3 Recommendations for oral health
- Ask people with diabetes about their oral health, specifically if they have noticed any signs of infection, bad breath, or a bad taste in their mouth, or if they have any other symptoms.
- Ask about the last dental check-up.
- Remind all diabetic patients to register with a dentist.
- Remind diabetic patients to have dental and periodontal check-ups every 6 mths or more frequently if needed.
- Tell patients to see their dentist straightaway if they notice signs of infection such as sore, swollen, or bleeding gums, loose teeth, mouth ulcers, or pain.
- Look in their mouth—soft tissues and teeth.
- Advise regular tooth brushing and flossing. An electric oscillating toothbrush may clean teeth better—ask the dentist.
- Regular mouthwash (e.g. chlorhexidine) may help—ask the dentist.
- Stop smoking.
- Keep HbA$_{1c}$ 48–58 mmol/mol (6.5–7.5 %) if safe.

Adapted from American Diabetes Association guidelines. *Clin Diabetes* 2005; **23**:171–8;doi: 10.2337/diabclin.23.4.171

Dental problems

- Periodontal disease. This infection is especially linked with hyperglycaemia. Treatment of periodontal disease with antibiotics (e.g. amoxicillin) may improve glucose balance. Mouthwashes such as Listerine® or chlorhexidine may prevent periodontal disease. Some authors suggest that periodontal disease increases the risk of atherosclerosis.
- Gingivitis—plaque irritates the gums. Good tooth brushing to remove plaque reduces the risk. Symptoms are red, swollen, painful, and bleeding gums.
- Dental caries—painful, damaged teeth impair healthy eating.
- Loss of teeth.

Practical and financial issues

Every diabetic patient should have regular dental checks. Some patients cannot afford dental care. Some patients with diabetes have severe oral and dental disease which worsens their glucose balance and can seriously risk their general health.

Gastrointestinal symptoms

The multiple GI problems in people with diabetes are often unrecognized yet impact significantly on quality of life and diabetes management. DAN may not be the only cause; myopathy may contribute. GI symptoms are commoner in people with diabetes than those without, especially in those with poor glucose control. (Arch Intern Med. 2001; **161**:1989–96; doi:10.1001/archinte.161.16.1989): odds ratios: oesophageal 1.44, upper dysmotility 1.75, any bowel symptom 1.84, diarrhoea 2.06, constipation 1.54. GI symptoms were found in 87 % of Swedish patients on questionnaire on attending routine clinic (*Rev Diab Stud* 2011;**8**:268–75; doi: 10.1900/RDS.2011.8.268). Patients with diabetic GI problems should be reviewed by a diabetologist as well as a gastroenterologist. They are likely to have multiple diabetic tissue damage.

Remember that all non-insulin hypoglycaemic drugs can have GI side effects, especially metformin, DPP-4 inhibitors and GLP-1 agonists.

Stomach and oesophagus

Oesophageal dysmotility

- Oesophageal dysmotility was reported in 63 % of Swedish patients
- More likely with greater duration of diabetes
- Retinopathy may be present
- Abnormal oesophageal motility may impair swallowing
- Other symptoms include meal-related cough and regurgitation
- Must exclude other causes
- Metoclopramide or proton pump inhibitors may help reflux symptoms (but the latter slow gastric emptying)
- Erythromycin may help (*J Diabetes Complications* 2003; **17**:141–4; doi:10.1016/S1056-8727(02)00168-X)
- Drink fluids after oral medications
- Refer patients with swallowing problems to gastroenterology

Diabetic gastroparesis
- Measurable gastroparesis was reported in 13 % of Swedish patients.
- Mainly in type 1 diabetes
- Gastroenteritis is a more common cause of vomiting than gastropathy. Exclude DKA in a vomiting, insulin-treated patient (⮎ pp. 216–19)
- Stomach emptying may be delayed for ≥ 12 hrs (e.g. breakfast vomited in evening)
- Symptoms include:
  - feeling full early
  - abdominal discomfort or pain (gastric distension)
  - nausea
  - vomiting—may be debilitating and require hospital admission
  - bloating, belching
  - hypoglycaemia—insulin arrives in bloodstream before food
  - failure to recover from hypoglycaemia (oral glucose remains in stomach and so is not absorbed)
- Investigation
  - seek non-diabetic + diabetic causes (e.g. drugs such as opiates, calcium blockers), alcohol, smoking, hypothyroidism, renal impairment, electrolyte impairment, high glucose)
  - upper GI endoscopy in all—strict 8-hr fast; if food found, diagnosis confirmed—may need other tests via specialist (e.g. gastric emptying scintigraphy)
  - check for *Helicobacter pylorii* and treat it
  - refer to gastroenterology
- Treatment
  - difficult—share care with gastroenterology
  - it may improve over months or years
  - frequent small meals—solid food may pass more readily than liquids (counter-intuitive) – but maintain adequate fluid intake (non-fizzy)
  - avoid incretin-effect enhancers and acarbose
  - metoclopramide or domperidone; erythromycin (*Am J Gastroenterol* 2013; **108**:18–37; doi: 10.1038/ajg.2012.373)
  - optimize glucose balance
  - very careful insulin therapy—do *not* use rapid-acting insulin analogues (arrive in bloodstream long before food does); CSII can improve glycaemic balance (*Diabetologia* 2011; **54**:2768–70; doi: 10.1007/s00125-011-2282-6)
  - tricyclic antidepressants may help
  - pancreatic enzyme supplements (worth a trial even if no proof of malabsorption)
  - electrical stimulation (gastric pacing) may be used for intractable vomiting (NICE Interventional Procedure Guidance 103)
  - in severe cases percutaneous jejunal feeding may be required
  - surgical options include: gastrostomy, pyloroplasty, or gastroenterostomy

Atrophic gastritis

Atrophic gastritis may occur in patients with autoimmune diabetes and is associated with iron and vitamin B12 deficiency. Parietal cell antibodies are found in 15–25 % type 1 diabetic patients (*Diabetes Care*, 2000; **23**;1384–8; doi:10.2337/diacare.23.9.1384).

Helicobacter pylorii

Patients with H. pylorii are more likely to have diabetes than those without. More common in diabetic patients than in non-diabetics (*Diabetes Res Clin Pract* 2013; **99**:200–8; doi:10.1016/j.diabres.2012.11.012). Seek it and treat it.

Bowels

Diarrhoea

The most common causes of diarrhoea in diabetic patients are metformin or gastroenteritis.

Diarrhoea and constipation due to bowel dysmotility may alternate in the same patient, making treatment hard. Hyperglycaemia may contribute.

- Symptoms of diabetic diarrhoea:
  - may be sudden with urgency
  - may cause faecal incontinence
  - often nocturnal or early morning
  - may come in bouts of days or weeks
  - may seriously limit going out
- Causes and investigation
  - Is the patient on metformin or other non-insulins with GI side effects? If so, stop it and use another agent. Review the patient 2 wks after stopping to check symptoms have settled.
  - Consider coeliac disease, pancreatic insufficiency, thyrotoxicosis.
  - Investigate as for non-diabetic patients. Refer to gastroenterology.
  - Colonoscopy—colorectal cancer is more common in diabetic patients than in non-diabetics.
- Treatment
  - Joint care by diabetologist and gastroenterologist is helpful.
  - Avoid metformin (or try modified release preparation), incretin-effect enhancers and acarbose.
  - BNF advises tetracycline (unlicensed). Erythromycin has been used to eradicate bacterial overgrowth and improve motility.
  - Soluble fibre may help.
  - Anticholinergics, colestyramine, pancreatic enzymes have been tried, as have octreotide (beware hypertensive crisis), and clonidine (beware worsening postural hypotension).
  - Risk of toxic megacolon.

Constipation

- Common—up to 60 % of patients.
- Often due to dehydration from hyperglycaemia (e.g. prediagnosis).
- DAN is a less common cause than dehydration.
- Prevalence of diabetic constipation increases with duration of diabetes.
- Management
  - Investigate as for non-diabetic patients.
  - Consider hypothyroidism and analgesics, or drugs used for painful peripheral neuropathy.
  - Consider colon and pancreatic cancer.
  - Consider gastroenterology referral.
  - Colonoscopy: N.B. will need careful bowel preparation for good view without hypoglycaemia—discuss with gastroenterology team first. This also applies to radiological investigations (e.g. CT pneumocolon).
  - High-fibre diet and bulking compounds, e.g. ispaghula (not if gastroparesis).
  - Metformin for glucose control.
  - Laxatives, e.g. lactulose (a non-absorbed osmotic laxative).
  - Care with stimulant laxatives.

Anal or rectal problems

Anorectal problems—faecal incontinence or anal blockage are also associated with DAN and cause much distress. Seek symptoms, and if present seek expert advice (NICE CG 49). Loperamide may reduce incontinence.

Liver

Type 2 diabetes—see *Diabetes Care* 2007; **30**:734–43; doi:10.2337/dc06-1539.

Liver problems associated with diabetes or more prevalent in diabetic patients include the following:

- Elevated liver enzymes (LFTs) (mostly due to NAFLD)
- Non-alcoholic fatty liver disease (NAFLD)
  - non-alcoholic steatohepatitis (NASH)
  - cirrhosis (N.B. 30 % of patients with cirrhosis have diabetes)
  - hepatocellular carcinoma
  - liver failure
- Hepatitis B and/or C
- Adverse reactions to hypoglycaemic drugs (rare)

Also, patients with liver disease often have diabetes (12–57 %). Cirrhosis is associated with insulin resistance.

Raised liver enzymes

Raised LFTs (ALT, AST) are found in 2–24 % of type 2 diabetic patients, depending on the inclusion or exclusion of patients with known liver disease (about 5 %). Liver disease, usually NAFLD or chronic hepatitis, is present in 98 % of type 2 diabetic patients with raised liver enzymes.

NAFLD and NASH

Diabetes is now the most common cause of liver disease in the USA. Diabetes and metabolic syndrome are associated with the development of NAFLD. Prevalence estimates vary (34–74 %) but 100 % of obese type 2 diabetic patients have some evidence of NAFLD. Insulin resistance increases lipolysis and fat is deposited in the liver. In some, but not all, patients this leads to liver cell damage and fibrosis (NASH). This process may then continue to cirrhosis and liver failure. It may progress to cancer. Hepatocellular carcinoma is four times more common in people with diabetes than in non-diabetics.

In one study of NAFLD, 40 % of NASH patients had progressive fibrosis. Progression was more likely with weight gain. End-stage liver disease was found in 5 %, and half of these had hepatocellular carcinoma. The presence of NASH reduced survival. The absence of periportal fibrosis on liver biopsy indicated low risk of liver complications. Most patients with NAFLD who are not diabetic initially will become so with time. (*Hepatology* 2006; **44**:865–73; doi: 10.1002/hep.21327).

Hepatitis C

Hepatitis C infection is three to four times more common in the diabetic population than in non-diabetic people. An Italian study found that 76 % of patients with type 2 diabetes and abnormal LFTs tested positive for hepatitis B or C or both (24 % neither B nor C, 25 % B only, 29 % C only, and 17 % B and C) (*Diab Res Clin Prac* 2000; **48**:147–51).

Management of liver abnormalities in diabetes

Local diabetologists should agree guidelines with their local hepatologist/gastroenterologist and radiologist. Suggestions for the management of raised LFTs in diabetic patients are as follows.

Tests
- Check for non-diabetic causes (e.g. alcohol, drugs, gall bladder disease, viruses)
- Blood (fasting):
  - ALT, alkaline phosphatase, bilirubin, albumin, INR
  - lipids—for triglyceride
  - ferritin (haemochromatosis)
  - hepatitis A, B, C screen
  - HbA$_{1c}$ if not done in last 2 mths
  - tests for non-diabetes-related causes.
- Liver ultrasound
- Liver biopsy (specialist service only)

Treatment
Treat non-NAFLD causes as usual. Drug management of NAFLD is controversial so emphasize careful weight loss and glucose control, which improves NASH and many other adverse consequences of diabetes.
- Monitor LFTs regularly
- If BMI > 25 kg/m², diet and exercise to lose weight gradually. Weight loss is important
- If HbA$_{1c}$ > 58 mmol/mol (7.5 %) (or above patient target) control glucose. Avoid hypoglycaemia—high risk in severe liver disease—and use glucose not glucagon to treat hypoglycaemia (→ p. 190). Use metformin unless there is a risk of liver decompensation and lactic acidosis. Pioglitazone improves some pathological features of NAFLD, including fibrosis, but can also cause liver toxicity. Nateglinide may improve LFTs (but can worsen them). Acarbose has been shown to improve glucose control and reduce ammonia levels in NAFLD-cirrhosis (*Diabetes Obes Metab* 2001; **3**:33–40; doi: 10.1046/j.1463-1326.2001.00103.x.)
- Most patients do not need other treatment
- Atorvastatin or gemfibrozil have been used in NAFLD, but can have adverse liver effects
- Avoid alcohol completely
- NASH appears to improve after bariatric surgery (although rapid weight loss may have adverse effects on the liver)
- Type 1 diabetic liver transplant patients may be suitable for islet-cell transplant

Lungs

Diabetic microangiopathy can affect the lungs, causing thickening of basal lamina in all parts of the lung—diabetic pulmopathy. Also infection risk is greater and infections may be prolonged and severe. This can lead to residual damage.

Direct or indirect pulmonary complications

- Reduction in forced expiratory volume in 1 sec (FEV_1), forced vital capacity (FVC), vital capacity (VC), and peak expiratory flow (PEF) by about 10 % compared with non-diabetic population. All measures gradually worsen. 'Absolute measures continued to decline at an annual rate of 68, 71, and 84 ml/yr and 17 l/min for FVC, FEV_1, VC, and PEF, respectively' (*Diabetes Res Clin Pract* 2000; **50**:153–9; *Diabetes Care* 2004; **27**:752–7; doi:10.2337/diacare.27.3.752)
- Decline in pulmonary function could be predicted by poor glycaemic control
- Respiratory neuromuscular function is impaired in type 2 diabetic neuropaths (*Diabetologia* 2007; **51**:191–7; doi: 10.1007/s00125-007-0856-0)
- Decreased FEV_1 has been associated with increased mortality
- Reduced diffusing capacity in type 1 diabetes with less adverse effects on volume functions
- Bacterial lung infections are common
- Tuberculosis
- Fungal lung infections
- Pulmonary oedema (secondary to cardiac disease)
- Respiratory arrest
- Pneumothorax, pneumomediastinum, pneumopericardium (rare)
- Adult respiratory distress syndrome (ARDS)
- Aspiration of gastric contents (with gastroparesis)

Sleep-disordered breathing (SDB) / obstructive sleep apnoea (OSA)

℘ <http://www.idf.org/sleep-apnoea-and-type-2-diabetes>

- OSA is found in 23% of people who have diabetes,; 58 % have some form of SDB which is also associated with obesity, hypertension, CVD, and metabolic syndrome.
- Of those people with OSA, 40 % have diabetes.
- Features of SDB:
  - Snoring, sleep apnoea
  - Excessive daytime sleepiness/no energy
  - Poor memory
  - Irritability, depression, personality change
  - Morning headaches
  - Sexual dysfunction
  - Nocturia

- Seek the symptoms
- Management
  - Weight reduction
  - Treat comorbidities
  - Specialist referral: diagnosis of OSA has consequences
  - OSA: inform DVLA. 'Driving must cease until satisfactory control of symptoms has been attained'
  - Continuous positive airway pressure.

Chronic obstructive pulmonary disease

Type 2 diabetes is more common (RR 1.8) in people with chronic obstructive pulmonary disease (COPD) than those without, but not in asthma (*Diabetes Care* 2004; **27**:2478–84; doi:10.2337/diacare.27.10.2478). An Australian study found that 5.9 % of patients with diabetes newly given metformin or sulfonylurea had COPD. Those on high-dose steroids were more likely to be admitted to hospital. (*Diabetes Care* 2013; **36**:3009–14; doi:10.2337/dc12-2197). Any steroid dose may cause hyperglycaemia.

Cystic fibrosis (CF)

- Autosomal recessive, 1:2500 Caucasian incidence, less in other ethnic groups
- Defect in gene regulating salt and water balance in secretory tissues which causes thickened secretions
- Chronic suppurative lung disease
- Failure of pancreatic enzyme production (exocrine function)
- Severe pancreatic damage causing diabetes
- Liver disease
- Gastrointestinal bleeding
- Osteoporosis
- Infertility
- About half of all adults with CF have diabetes (usually diagnosed around age 18–21 yrs). Microvascular complications occur
- In CF diabetes basal insulin production is usually preserved but there is an impaired insulin release to food (so normal fasting, but raised post-prandial glucose)
- Glucose intolerance worsened by lung infections or other complications
- Check HbA$_{1c}$ annually (➔ p. 107). CF Trust advise annual OGTT which may still be needed if HbA1c is < 48 mmol/mol (6.5 %) or there are co-morbidities precluding use of HbA$_{1c}$
- Insulin is the preferred treatment
- Continue CF specialist dietetic advice (e.g. high-calorie diet)
- Cystic fibrosis-related diabetes is difficult to manage and every such patient should be referred to a specialist unit
- <https://cysticfibrosis.org.uk/media/82070/CD_Standards_of_Care_Dec_11.pdf>
- *Practical Diabetes* 2010; **27**:198–200; doi: 10.1002/pdi.1481

Diabetic skin and soft tissue problems

Infection

- Minor skin infection may be the first clue to diabetes, remains a problem, and can lead to fatal deep infections
- Boils, carbuncles, abscesses, necrotizing fasciitis (→ p. 335)
- Pustules (especially on the legs) may be staphylococcal
- Cellulitis, often streptococcal or staphylococcal, can spread very fast
- Paronychia, especially related to ingrowing toenails, is common
- Fungal infections, usually candida, affect the perineum and produce intertrigo in the groin and elsewhere in obese patients
- Overweight patients may develop chronic sweat gland infections, cavities, and scarring in axillae and groin (hidradenitis suppurativa)

⚠ Pressure ulcers

People with diabetes are at high risk because of neuropathy and/or PAD. Heel ulcers (→ p. 309) are an especial risk for patients on trolleys, operating tables or in bed. Always protect the heels and other pressure areas from the moment of lying down. Once established, pressure ulcers may become gangrenous and/or infected and can rapidly extend to bone or abscess formation.

Diabetic dermopathy

Shin spots are flat reddish-brown marks in the pretibial region in about 50 % of people with diabetes. They may follow trauma but can emerge spontaneously. They do not require treatment. Protect legs.

Necrobiosis lipoidica diabeticorum

Uncommon (0.3 % of diabetic patients, mainly type 1) and may occur in non-diabetics e.g. in rheumatoid arthritis. Usually pretibial. Disfiguring red plaques with purple edge and yellowish centre which gradually becomes atrophic. They may remit spontaneously. Lesions may become infected. Treatment is not always satisfactory. Steroids can be used on non-atrophic lesions. Many other drugs have been tried; include immunomodulation. Improve glucose control if necessary, provide emotional support, protect the legs and refer to a dermatologist. Patient information: ☞ <http://www.bad.org.uk>

Erythema. Periungual telangiectasia

Some people with diabetes have reddening of facial (diabetic rubeosis) or other skin. Transient erythema may be seen in hyperglycaemia (and occasionally in hypoglycaemia, which also causes pallor). About 50 % of people with diabetes have periungual telangiectasia and may also have red nail folds and sore fingertips.

Bullosa diabeticorum

Large painless blisters on legs or hands. Risk of infection. Settle in weeks.

Hand problems

The skin of people with diabetes is thicker than in non-diabetics, sometimes becoming sclerodermatous. Three-quarters of all people with diabetes > 65 yrs old have diabetic hand syndrome with thickening of skin on dorsum and around interphalangeal joints causing stiff, painful hands (as discussed shortly).

Itching (➔ p. 3)

Localized itching may occur with perineal candidiasis. Generalized itching may be due to uraemia or jaundice. Perforating collagenosis—itchy spots which may become infected—may occur in diabetic nephropathy.

Dry or wet skin

Neuropathy (➔ p. 283).

Associated skin problems

- Acanthosis nigricans in insulin-resistance syndromes— dark furring of skin on neck and in creases. See PCOS (➔ pp. 334–5).
- Lipodystrophy with insulin-resistance syndromes.
- Vitiligo with type 1 diabetes.
- Bronzing with haemochromatosis.
- Eruptive xanthomata with hypertriglyceridaemia.
- Sweating, skin tags and skin thickening with acromegaly.
- Thinning, striae, excess hair with Cushing's syndrome.

Diabetic mastopathy

Occurs in women with longstanding type 1 diabetes (less often with type 2) with long-term hyperglycaemia. A painless, irregular, hard breast lump can be felt which may be difficult to differentiate from cancer. These lumps consist of lympocytic infiltration and fibrous tissue on biopsy. Mastopathy is often bilateral and frequently recurs after surgery. It has been suggested that it should be followed by ultrasound with ultrasound-guided biopsies if required. Refer to breast clinic. A painful breast lump is probably infected.

Diabetic musculoskeletal problems

Ligaments

Skin thickening can occur in diabetes but connective tissue thickening is more obvious in ligaments. Diabetes is associated with the following.

- Dupuytren's contracture and similar problems in the feet
- Carpal tunnel syndrome (➲ p. 281)
- Cheiroarthropathy—tightening of the skin and tendons so that fingers no longer straighten when pressed flat (30–40 % type 1 patients)
- Limited joint mobility
- Frozen shoulder
- Trigger finger

Bones

Bone disease is common in people with diabetes so ensure normal dietary calcium intake and supplement vitamin D if required (➲ p. 76). Prevent falls from hypoglycaemia (➲ pp. 181–200) or postural hypotension (➲ pp. 282–3).

Osteopenia and osteoporosis

People with diabetes can develop marked osteopenia occurring in over half those with type 1 (*Diabetes Care* 2008; **31**:1729–35; doi: 10.2337/ dc07-2426; *J Endocrinol Invest* 2000; **23**(5):295–303). Osteopenia can be seen even in adolescents. Loss of bone density may be most evident in the first few years after diagnosis and seems to be linked to poor blood glucose balance—improve this. Treat as for non-diabetic patients. Patients with severe nephropathy may have renal bone disease.

Increased bone density

Patients with type 2 diabetes may show diffuse interstitial skeletal hyperostosis with osteophytes and new bone (e.g. in the vertebrae). Although they may have increased bone density in some areas, they also at risk of osteoporosis (*Clin Diabetes* 2002; **20**:153–7; doi:10.2337/diaclin.20.3.153).

Fractures

Fractures of the femur and proximal humerus are more common in people with diabetes than in those without. Hip fracture is particularly common in diabetic women (type 1 RR 6.9–12.3, type 2 RR 1.7–1.8) (*Diabetologia* 1999; **42**:920–5; doi: 10.1007/s001250051248; *Diabetes Care* 2001; **24**:1192–7; doi:10.2337/diacare.24.7.1192). Patients on insulin have more than double the risk of foot fractures compared with the non-diabetic population (*J Clin Endocrinol Metab* 2001; **86**:32–8). Fractures are also more common in patients on pioglitazone than other drugs—RR for hip fracture 1.18 per yr of exposure; 90-day mortality 15 % (*Diabetologia* 2012; **55**:2929–37; doi: 10.1007/s00125-012-2668-0).

Charcot joints

Severe neuropathy and trauma may cause bone destruction in feet and Charcot joints (➲ p. 303). Refer to orthopaedics and specialist podiatry.

Osteoarthritis (OA)

OA also appears to be more common in people with diabetes. Type 2 diabetes is a strong predictor of severe OA requiring arthroplasty (HR 2.1 vs non-diabetics; (*Diabetes Care* 2013; **36**:403–9; doi:10.2337/dc12-0924).

Rheumatoid arthritis

Type 1 diabetes was found in 13 % of the family members of patients with rheumatoid arthritis (*Ann Rheum Dis* 1983; **42**: 297–300; doi:10.1136/ard.42.3.297), but it is unclear if rheumatoid disease is commoner in those with diabetes. If patients have both, check glucose control with steroid treatment. Screen for hypothyroidism and B12 deficiency. Refer to podiatry for preventive foot care advice.

Cancer

Several studies have reviewed cancer incidence and prevalence in diabetes. Obesity is a risk factor for cancer so may confound results. A large prospective US study of about a million people with 16-yrs mortality follow-up showed an increased frequency of cancer in patients with any form of diabetes of colon, pancreas, female breast; and liver + bladder in men (*Am J Epidemiol* 2004; **159**:1160–7; doi:10.1093/aje/kwh161).

Patients with newly diagnosed diabetes have twice the risk of pancreatic cancer compared with non-diabetics, especially if young with gastrointestinal symptoms (*Clin Gastroenterol Hepatol* 2006; 4:1366–72; doi:10.1016/j.cgh.2006.06.024).

A Swedish study showed a 20 % increase in frequency of cancer in type 1 diabetes, with cancer of stomach, cervix, and endometrium being more common.

A US study found a 3× risk of pancreatic cancer and a 2× risk of gall bladder cancer (World J Gastroenterol 2009; 15(42): 5274–8).

The largest analysis was from the Emerging Risk Factors Collaboration (→ pp. 248–9). Results were corrected for age, sex, smoking, and BMI. There was a significant increase in the risk of death from the following cancers (HR with diabetes):

- Liver 2.16
- Pancreas 1.51
- Ovary 1.45
- Colorectum 1.40
- Bladder 1.40
- Lung 1.27
- Breast 1.25

There has been recent concern that some diabetes treatments may increase the risk of cancer.

A meta-analysis of controlled studies showed that pioglitazone use is associated with an increased risk of bladder cancer (HR 1.23 vs controls), with a risk of 20.8 cases per 100 000 person years (*Diabetic Med* 2013; 30:1026–32. doi: 10.1111/dme.12144). (→ p. 131)

Incretin-effect enhancers may increase the risk of pancreatic and neuroendocrine tumours. While 'an association exists . . . causality has not yet been proved' (BMJ 2013; 346:f3750) (→ pp. 134–8).

Concern was raised that Lantus® increases the risk of a cancer diagnosis. This was on the basis of observational studies and has not been proven (*Diabetologia* 2012; 55:51–62; doi: 10.1007/s00125-011-2312-4. *Diabetologia* 2012 55:7–9; doi: 10.1007/s00125-011-2352-9).

Metformin seems to be associated with a lower cancer risk than sulfonylureas or insulin (*Diabetologia* 2009; 52:1766-77; doi: 10.1007/s00125-009-1440-6).

People with newly diagnosed diabetes have a full clinical assessment which may reveal co-existing but hitherto undetected cancer. Studies confirm this. Patients have different combinations of different glucose-lowering treatments for differing durations in different environments with different forms of diabetes of different duration and complexity, so enormous studies are needed for any review to be sufficiently powered to answer the question of cancer risk conclusively for every diabetes treatment. It should be remembered that untreated diabetes causes disability and premature death. At present, a commonsense approach could be:

- assess newly-diagnosed diabetic patients thoroughly
- follow BNF guidance on prescribing
- keep up-to-date with hypoglycaemic drug warnings (e.g. MHRA)
- ensure your practice or clinic can readily find out which patient is on what drug for his/her diabetes
- ensure that smokers stop and non-smokers don't start
- ensure patients do not drink excessive alcohol
- help overweight patients lose weight
- identify and manage patients with NASH and NAFLD (➜ pp. 290–1)
- have a high level of alertness for the warning signs or symptoms of diabetes-associated cancers and investigate such patients promptly

Summary

- Diabetes is a multisystem disorder of which one manifestation is hyperglycaemia.
- Diabetic tissue damage is largely preventable. Every effort must be made to detect risk factors and management vigorously.
- If present, tissue damage can be treated, and its progress slowed. Look for it.
- Tissue damage can affect every part of the body—don't forget the less obvious complications.
- Assess diabetic patients fully at diagnosis and at least annually.
- Be alert for symptoms of tissue damage and remember that cancer is now regarded as a complication of diabetes.
- Don't forget diabetic foot disease (➜ pp. 301–4).
- Tissue damage has emotional consequences—look for them and provide support and treatment as needed.

Diabetic foot problems

Introduction

Foot problems have been given their own chapter because they are so common, so preventable, so distressing, so disabling, and, sadly, so often missed or mismanaged. Integrated multidisciplinary specialist care is vital—there is good evidence that it saves limbs. Introducing such a team in Ipswich showed a fall in amputation rates of 82 % (*Diabetes Care* 2008; **31**:99–101; doi:10.2337/dc07-1178). Every locality should have a multidisciplinary diabetes specialist footcare team (DSFT) either incorporating or linked to a foot protection team (FPT).

We bear our entire weight on our feet, subjecting their components to enormous stresses every day. Early warning of problems helps us to protect our feet.

Diabetic foot problems are largely preventable. Assal and colleagues (*Recent trends in diabetes research*, Bostrom ed., pp. 276–90. Stockholm: Almquist & Wiksell, 1982) dramatically reduced the amputation rate in a Swiss diabetes service by introducing an intensive patient education and foot care programme.

Current or past foot ulcers are present in 5–7% of people with diabetes. About one in 600 people with diabetes in England and Wales had a major amputation in 2010–12. The NDA showed that mortality for people with diabetes within 1 year of admission for major amputation was three times that of the general population. Five-year mortality after major amputation is 68–78 %. Diabetic foot problems cost the NHS £639–662 million in 2010/11 with considerable scope for financial savings (Kerr, M. Footcare for people with diabetes: the economic case for change, at:

  <http://www.diabetes.org.uk/Documents/nhs-diabetes/footcare/footcare-for-people-with-diabetes.pdf>

Why are the feet so vulnerable?

Neuropathy (⤵ p. 281)

Diabetic neuropathy reduces sensation of pain, touch, temperature, and position. Rubs, scrapes, and knocks are ignored because they cannot be felt. Patients may walk all day with a pebble in their shoe without realizing it. Skin may be burned by hot water with no sensation of heat or pain. If you do not know where your foot is in space, you cannot keep it in the best position for safe weight-bearing. Patients buy overtight shoes. Calluses can build up, e.g. under the metatarsal heads.

Microvascular disease (⤵ p. 246)

Small vessel disease may damage the healing response so that minor injuries are not repaired and infections may eventually spread to threaten the viability of deeper tissues.

Arterial disease (⤵ pp. 264–5)

Atheroma is common in diabetes, affecting not only large vessels but also smaller ones, e.g. those supplying the legs and feet, in which calcification may be seen on X-ray. PAD causes intermittent claudication, rest pain, and finally gangrene. It worsens other problems by depriving injured or infected areas of oxygen, slowing healing, and allowing anaerobic bacteria to flourish. Antibiotics may not reach the areas of infection in sufficient concentrations to be effective.

Deformity (⤵ p. 296)

Diabetes can cause ligamentous changes. In the feet this may lead to clawed or hammer toes. This causes further abnormalities of weight-bearing, and the curled toes may develop corns on top as they rub against shoes. Neuropathy, vasculopathy, and infection may cause damage leading to deformity, as can surgery. The foot then develops multiple pressure points and callus build-up.

Bones (⤵ pp. 296–7)

Bone density is reduced in people with diabetes, more so in those with type 1 than in type 2. Diabetic autonomic neuropathy intensifies this process in the feet with increased vascularity and shunting. When this is combined with peripheral neuropathy, small injuries can initiate bony destruction and distortion, which extends rapidly with continued weight-bearing or repeated injury. The bones and joints are gradually destroyed, causing Charcot joints.

Infection (⤵ pp. 427–8)

Hyperglycaemia reduces white cell mobility, and a poor blood supply slows delivery of white cells and nutrients, thereby impeding the body's defensive response to infection. Via areas of callus, pockets of infection can extend deep into the foot and thence into the tissue planes and bones. Infections there and elsewhere do not hurt and progress rapidly.

Other problems

If they cannot feel pain, even those who can see or smell a problem may not treat it with the seriousness it deserves: 'if it doesn't hurt it can't be too bad'; 'it can't be happening to me'. Those who are aware of the seriousness may be so frightened of losing their foot or leg that they conceal the problems. Partially sighted patients may not be able to see foot problems.

Les, with long-standing diabetes, attended between annual reviews. 'Are your feet all right?' asked the doctor. 'Yes, thanks', he replied. A month later he was admitted very ill with infected gangrene of his foot. At that point he confessed that he had gangrene at the time of the clinic visit but had been so terrified of being admitted to hospital that he had lied to the doctor.

Prevention of diabetic foot problems

Patient and staff education are crucial. Many people know that diabetes can lead to leg amputation, but patients may still fail to take the practical steps to prevent this. Healthcare professionals, whether in hospital or in general practice, fail to check patients' feet, and often fail to act sufficiently vigorously when patients present with what look like minor foot problems. A small blister on a little toe can ultimately lead to amputation.

Examine the feet

Examine every diabetic patient's feet on diagnosis, annually, and on hospital or care facility admission. Read 'Putting Feet First', ℘ <http://www.diabetes.org.uk/Documents/Professionals/Education%20and%20skills/Footcare-pathway.0212.pdf>. Print it out for all staff involved in caring for people with diabetes. Remove shoes, socks, or tights (warn patients to be ready for this) and check:

- skin: colour, ulcers, rubs, blisters, corns, calluses, etc.
- shape of feet and toes: hammer or claw toes, bunions, missing toes, surgery, deformities
- swelling
- pulses: anterior and posterior tibial
- sensation: light touch, monofilament, vibration
- hygiene
- shoes and hosiery

Determine risk status:

- Active foot problem (danger signs (➲) pp. 308–9)—refer to the multidisciplinary diabetes specialist foot care team (DSFT) within 24 hrs.
- High risk—previous ulcer or foot/leg surgery; or > 1 risk factor, e.g. neuropathy, or PAD with callus or deformity. Refer to FPT. They will determine frequency of monitoring. Each patient should have a coordinating key worker to avoid gaps in care and ensure good communication.
- Moderate risk—1 risk factor, e.g. sensory loss or PAD without callus or deformity—action as for high risk.
- Low risk—no risk factors—healthy feet. Annual review.
- Provide written and verbal education and information for all patients, including emergency phone numbers and when to use them. Patient leaflets (general guidance Table 15.1) tailored to risk are available at: ℘ <http://www.diabetes.org.uk/putting-feet-first>

At interim visits inspect moderate- and high-risk patients' feet. The Ipswich touch test can be used for rapid assessment of sensation and probable risk of ulceration (e.g. by nurses on patient arrival on their ward) but should not replace full initial and annual examination (*Diabetes Care* 2011; **34**:1517–18; doi:10.2337/dc11-0156).

Patients can also use a touch test. ℘ <http://www.diabetes.org.uk/Guide-to-diabetes/Complications/Feet/Touch-the-toes-test/>

All diabetic patients should have priority access to podiatry (chiropody) and those at risk should have regular podiatry with the FPT. Check your local arrangements and FPT/DSFT contact numbers before you need them.

Table 15.1 Look after your feet: guidelines for patients

1.	Look at your feet every day. Use a mirror or ask someone else to help if you have difficulty seeing
2.	If you have any of the following see your doctor (or chiropodist or diabetic clinic) within 24 hrs:
	any colour change
	any new pain or soreness or unusual feeling
	any corns, blisters, cracks, calluses, ulcers, bunions
	swelling anywhere
	any break in the skin (ulcers, cracks, blisters)
	a strange smell from your feet
3.	Treat any skin break by washing with dilute antiseptic (follow the instructions on the container). Dry gently with sterile gauze, and cover with a dry, sterile, non-adherent dressing. Use hypoallergenic tape and never wind it round a toe. Then contact help
4.	Wash your feet daily in lukewarm water. Dry carefully, especially between the toes
5.	If you have dry skin use a moisturizing cream or emollient lotion, but not between the toes
6.	Cut toenails in a gentle curve and file smooth without leaving sharp edges to dig into that or other toes
7.	Wear clean socks, stockings, or tights every day (no hard seams or elasticated tops)
8.	Buy shoes which do not squeeze your foot, and which do not hurt or rub anywhere the first time you try them on. Low-heeled lace-ups with plenty of toe room are best
9.	Do not walk bare foot
10.	Do not use corn cures, or cut corns or callus
11.	Do not use a hot water bottle
12.	Do not use vibrating foot massagers or baths
13.	Do not smoke
14.	See a state-registered chiropodist (SRCh) or podiatrist regularly

This table may be photocopied for use by patients only. ©2014 Dr Rowan Hillson.

Patient Other patient care leaflets are available at: ℛ <http://www.diabetes.org.uk/putting-feet-first>

Patient foot care advice leaflets in 30 languages can be printed out from ℛ <http://www.diabeticfoot.org.uk>

Assessment of diabetic patients with foot problems

Always remove dressings, having first warned the nursing staff that they will need to be redone (Figure 15.1). Use formal nursing wound management protocols i.e. dressing pack etc. Inspect the whole of both feet and legs.

The foot/leg

- Ensure that the patient and you are comfortable.
- Make sure you can see the whole foot in good light without contorting the patient or yourself.
- Listen to the clinical story. Check the social situation.

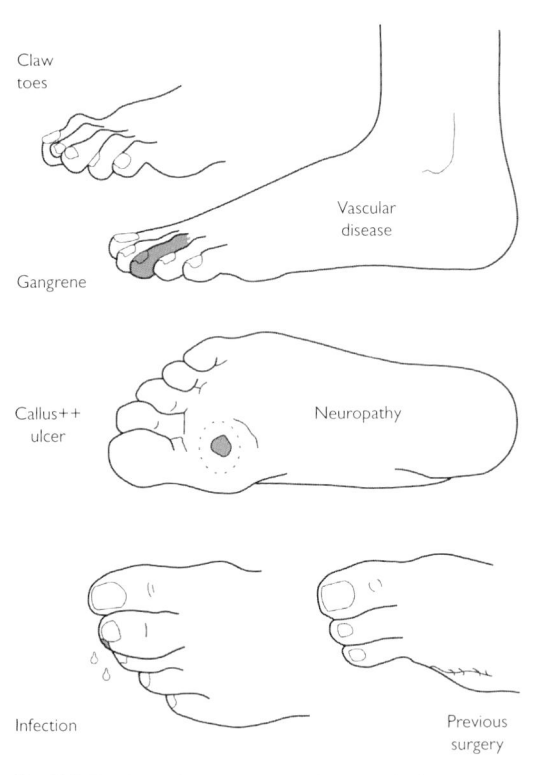

Fig. 15.1 The diabetic foot: warning signs during examination.

- Assess skin colour.
- Seek skin damage: rubs, blisters, scratches or ulcers, calluses.
- Fungal infections? Verrucas?
- Assess shape: deformities, scars, surgery, amputations.
- Oedema.
- Fluid? Clear ooze, pus, blood?
- Check for pressure discoloration or sores (if present on heels, check the sacral area).
- Look for gross distortion of foot anatomy with warmth, swelling, and neuropathy—Charcot foot, but these feet can also be infected.
- Note malodour—bad smell usually means anaerobes ± other organisms.
- Note dryness (neuropathy).
- Note heat or cold to touch.
- Measure monofilament sensation, light touch, vibration (and temperature with cold tuning fork), position sense, ankle and knee reflexes.
- Palpate peripheral pulses: dorsalis pedis and posterior tibial.
- Digital photograph of foot lesion with ruler (and patient consent).
- Wash hands before and after (and use gloves). Use appropriate sterile technique. Don't forget to clean multiple-use equipment—single-use is best.

The rest
- Review glucose control.
- Most patients with diabetic foot problems have diabetic tissue damage elsewhere—seek it.
- When admitting patients with foot problems, fully clerk patient including neurology (➲ pp. 280–4).

⚠ Danger signs = active foot problem
Patients with any of the following features should be referred to the DSFT for a full assessment within 24 hrs. They may need admission:
- Active ulceration
- Spreading infection (or failing to improve)
- Critical ischaemia
- Gangrene
- Red, hot, swollen foot
- Painful peripheral neuropathy
- Acute Charcot foot

Colour change
Refer to hospital and DFST same day.
- Red foot (infection or 'sunset' ischaemic foot)
- White (no circulation)
- Blue/black (gangrene)

Blisters/crepitus
Due to subcutaneous infection, oedema, or diabetic dermopathy. Crepitus (crackling feeling) indicates gas gangrene which is usually due to multiple organisms, but could be *Clostridium welchii*. Transfer to hospital 999 and contact DFST at the same time.

Infection

If you suspect any infection is major or extends below the immediate sub-cutaneous tissues, or if neuropathy or PAD are present, refer the patient to DFST and hospital immediately.

Superficial infected areas should be cleaned and dressed (➲ Table 15.1, p. 306) and seen daily by a nurse or doctor until healed. Any infection which is not healing in 3 days or spreads should be referred to the DFST. Refer patients with worsening foot or leg infection to the DFST immediately. N.B. Infected diabetic patients are often apyrexial.

Ulceration

- Clean punched-out ulcers are usually neuropathic but some will also have peripheral vascular disease.
- Irregular-edged ulcers are usually neuro-ischaemic (it is rare to find any purely vascular ulcers in diabetic patients. Cancer can be found in long-established ulcers—e.g. in 10 % of skin ulcers that had worsened despite 3 mths treatment in a general population (*Arch Dermatol* 2012; **148**:704–8. doi: 10.1001/archdermatol.2011.3362).
- Exudate or frank pus, odour, surrounding erythema, oedema, pain indicate infection.
- If you can probe to bone at the bottom, assume osteomyelitis (but not feeling bone does not exclude osteomyelitis).
- There may be a sinus.

Swelling

This may mean infection, autonomic neuropathy, Charcot joints, cardiac failure, or nephrotic syndrome. Swelling is usually a danger sign in people with diabetes. Consider referral to a diabetologist. If Charcot foot is sus-pected tell patient not to weight-bear until seen by the DSFT.

Pain

Pain requires urgent investigation. It may represent an easily treatable problem, or it may represent major trouble such as infection. Neuropathy may blunt pain but it can also cause pain. Always take new foot pain in a neuropathic patient seriously. Charcot joints develop in neuropathic limbs, but may be painful while evolving. Repeat X-rays in diabetic neuropathic patients with persistent pain, swelling, or heat after an injury.

Heat

A hot area may indicate infection or an active Charcot joint. Always inves-tigate 'hot spots'.

Cold

A cold foot or leg strongly suggests PAD. Rapidly developing coldness indi-cates acute vascular block and the need for immediate inpatient vascular care (➲ pp. 264–5).

Absent foot pulses (➲ pp. 264–5) and/or neuropathy (➲ p. 281)

These patients are high risk and should be under the FPT's supervision.

Management of diabetic foot problems

⚠ Refer patients with active foot problems to the DSFT within 24 hrs. Personally confirm that they have received the referral and that they have taken over care (named consultant). All diabetic inpatients with foot or leg problems should be referred to the inpatient DSFT. This particularly includes those in care of elderly or rehabilitation/long-stay wards, and patients on vascular or orthopaedic wards. Follow their advice.

NICE CG 119 (2012) states:

'[e]ach hospital should have a care pathway for patients with diabetic foot problems who require inpatient care.

The multidisciplinary foot care team should consist of healthcare professionals with the specialist skills and competencies necessary to deliver inpatient care for patients with diabetic foot problems.

The multidisciplinary foot care team should normally include a diabetologist, a surgeon with the relevant expertise in managing diabetic foot problems, a diabetes nurse specialist, a podiatrist and a tissue viability nurse, and the team should have access to other specialist services required to deliver the care outlined in this guideline.'

All patients with active foot disease should be under the care of a DSFT. The following sections provide guidance for their investigation and care should such a team not be available. In that case, urgent consideration should be given to referring the patient to such a team in another hospital. Diabetic foot problems can worsen to the point of no return within days (sometimes hours) and no patient should lose his or her leg (or die) because of lack of local expertise.

Investigations

Blood tests
- Full blood count—white count may be normal despite infection
- C-reactive protein (CRP) —may be normal despite infection
- U&E
- LFT
- Calcium
- Thyroid function tests

Infection screen
- Ideally sample from ulcer base
- Ulcer/pus swabs, bone debris, slough—always send sample to microbiology in appropriate medium/container
- Remind surgical teams to send samples for microbiology, e.g. debridement, bone, or amputation specimens
- Blood culture
- MRSA screen

Cardiovascular
- ECG in all. Very high risk of coronary artery disease
- Echocardiogram if possible if cardiac failure and not done recently

- Ankle–brachial pressure index: measure this in all patients but remember that it can appear falsely normal as highly calcified blood vessels do not compress (➲ p. 264).
- Venous and/or arterial duplex scans: have a low threshold for requesting detailed vascular imaging. Patients with diabetes may have venous ulcers. PAD is very common.
- Angiography—after review by vascular team.

Radiology
- Tell the radiologist exactly where the ulcer or colour change is or draw a picture on the request form.
- Always X-ray the foot even though there may be little superficial evidence of problems. Patients with neuropathy can have multiple fractures with little or no pain. Osteomyelitis can lurk beneath subtle superficial change.
- Osteomyelitis is not excluded by negative X-rays—if suspected do MRI.
- Use white cell scans if MRI is contraindicated.
- Do not use bone scintigraphy (not helpful—NICE CG 119).

Treatment
- Review frequently (daily if inpatient).
- Pain relief is often needed, including in neuropathic patients. Critical ischaemic pain is agonizing and relentless. It prevents sleep. Such patients hang their foot out of bed for relief. Opiates are usually needed.
- Suspect infection in all patients. Treat if any evidence or strong clinical suspicion. Use your district or hospital antibiotic protocol for diabetic foot patients. Seek local microbiologist advice about individual patients within 24 hrs. Several organisms and anaerobes may often be present. Screen all diabetic foot patients for MRSA when first seen. Consider MRSA screening once or twice annually thereafter if recurrent infections. Many patients referred to hospital will already have failed to respond to one or more courses of oral antibiotic so consider IM or IV antibiotics, especially if osteomyelitis is present. As these patients may have significant neuropathy and slow gastric emptying, as well as poor circulation, the highest safe concentration of antibiotics should be sought. Many of these patients will have renal impairment and may need dose reduction. Patients with osteomyelitis may need several months of antibiotics (usually oral). Take great care to prevent MRSA or *Clostridium difficile* infection.
- Debridement/excision is essential if there is dead tissue or such grossly infected tissue that antibiotics will not penetrate. Podiatrists or nurses experienced in wound care will remove slough. Debridement must be thorough. More extensive surgical excision may also be needed. In patients with vascular disease perform angioplasty or vascular surgery promptly first.
- Larva therapy can be used to clean up sloughy ulcers.
- Avoid occlusive dressings—these can worsen diabetic ulcers.
- Avoid further pressure on the affected area(s). This may mean complete non-weight-bearing. A specialist total-contact cast or boot can remove

the pressure but allow walking. Ensure the cast/boot does not rub, especially in neuropathic patients.

- Elevation—unless there is severe arterial insufficiency, swollen feet or legs should be elevated to reduce fluid and aid healing. Be very careful to avoid heel pressure ulcers.
- Most hospitalized diabetic foot patients need thromboembolism protection with low molecular weight heparin. Thromboembolism prevention stockings are not a good idea unless one is certain that arterial function is reasonable, as ischaemia can ensue. Also, neuropathic patients may develop sores in the creases under such stockings.
- Good nutrition is essential. Many of these patients have not eaten properly for months and have lost weight. They may have vitamin deficiencies. Refer to the dietitian.
- Psychological support is essential. Depression and anxiety are common.
- Optimize glucose control.
- Reduce cardiovascular risk. A Scottish group reduced 5 yr mortality in diabetic foot ulcer patients from 48.0 % to 26.8 % with vigorous CVD risk-reduction therapy including high-dose statin (*Diabetes Care* 2008; **31**:2143–7; doi:10.2337/dc08-1242).
- Seek other complications and comorbidities and treat vigorously.
- Vascular treatment. Review arterial and venous circulation in all patients. All patients with any vasculopathy should be seen by the vascular team on the day of admission and urgent vascular investigations arranged. Check renal function, and stop metformin, ensuring that patients are well hydrated before angiograms. Monitor renal function in all patients after any contrast is used. If stenoses (above or below the knee) are amenable to angioplasty or surgery, this should be performed promptly, with referral to centres of expertise if necessary. Ensure that a senior anaesthetist assesses the patient. Warn of autonomic neuropathy (risk of cardiac arrest) if present (➲ p. 282). Regional blocks are often used.
- Amputation—nowadays we try and try to preserve limbs. However, this may mean months in hospital with deteriorating physical and emotional health. Patients with very severe infection or gangrene often do better with early rather than late amputation (after vascular intervention if appropriate). Address psychological problems before and after this mutilating surgery. Refer patients to the rehabilitation team before surgery.
- N.B. no decision should be made about amputation until the patient has seen a multidisciplinary specialist vascular team.

Preventing further diabetic foot problems

- The greatest risk factor for diabetic foot problems is a previous foot problem.
- Such patients must remain under specialist diabetes care.
- These patients should be monitored for life by a podiatrist experienced in complex diabetic foot care (FPT) as signs of early trouble may be subtle. Ideally, the same podiatrist should monitor the patient each visit.
- Refer to orthotics for made-to-measure footwear with insoles if appropriate. This should be checked at each visit to ensure that the foot shape or gait has not changed—beware rubbing. New shoes may be needed.
- Patient education for self-care.
- Diabetic foot patients may have problems with concordance with healthcare and should be included in community case management systems if locally available. Liaise with social support if needed.
- Healthcare staff education for foot and general diabetes care of *this* patient.
- Work with the patient to reduce all risk factors for diabetic glucose instability and tissue damage.
- Reassess the whole patient for tissue damage regularly (➲ p. 249).
- React fast if any further foot problems appear (same day referral to diabetic foot team).
- Local commissioners should ensure that diabetes services participate in the National Diabetes Foot care Audit (starting 2014) as part of the NDA suite. ℘ <http://www.hscic.gov.uk/footcare>

Summary

- Diabetes foot problems are preventable.
- The consequence may be amputation.
- Educate the patient about daily foot care.
- Take a personal interest in their feet. Check at least annually.
- Examine high-risk feet at every visit.
- Respond urgently to any foot problems. A small ulcer may eventually kill the patient.
- Refer all patients with diabetic foot problems to the DSFT.
- Institute full risk factor preventive care.
- Be alert for other diabetic tissue damage.
- Audit care.

Diabetes in young people

Diabetes in young people

This chapter is about teens to early twenties—adolescence. While most teenagers are now managed in paediatric services, some will be in adult clinics and many in transition. 'Current provision of care for children and young people is variable and does not always meet national standards. The experience of service users is not always positive.' This statement was made in 2007 in 'Making every young person with diabetes matter'.

℘ <http://www.diabetes.org.uk/Documents/Reports/ MakingEveryYoungPersonMatter.pdf> It could still be said today. The National Paediatric Diabetes Audit (NPDA) 2011/12 showed that of young people aged 12 ≥ yrs and diagnosed diabetic for at least a year only 6.7 % had received all recommended care processes. Those aged > 15 yrs were less likely to have had an HbA_{1c} done. Of the whole NPDA, 82.6 % had an HbA_{1c} ≥ 58 mmol/l (7.5 %). ℘ <http://www.rcpch. ac.uk/improving-child-health/quality-improvement-and-clinical-audit/ national-paediatric-diabetes-audit-n-0>

Pre-teens (not included in this book) should be cared for by specialist paediatric diabetes teams which should continue to provide care throughout their teens, in liaison with adult specialist diabetes services. All those providing care should have specific training in the management of diabetes in adolescence. Great efforts should be made to avoid 'losing' the patient in clinical service or geographical moves, or by failing to respond appropriately to disengagement.

In England, under Payment by Results, there is now a Best Practice Tariff for paediatric diabetes which requires detailed specialist care for those < 19 yrs. ℘ <http://www.gov.uk/government/uploads/system/uploads/attachment_ data/file/214902/PbR-Guidance-2013-14.pdf> Regional Paediatric Diabetes Networks help to deliver this.

Diabetes will be affected by, or will influence, most other physical and emotional healthcare issues. Diabetes may also have a major effect upon the young person's parents and siblings, and vice versa. Communication between the services involved (often many) must remain good at all times.

Adult thought processes and behaviours begin to develop in the teens, but progress to full maturity varies widely. Assume that all young people wish to be fully involved in their own care and have their views properly heard, and their confidentiality and personal privacy respected. Follow your profession's guidance. GMC guidance is in '0–18 years'.

℘ <http://www.gmc-uk.org/guidance/ethical_guidance/children_ guidance_42_43_principles_of_confidentiality.asp>

Health professionals caring for patients < 18 yrs old should be aware of responsibilities and procedures for child protection should concerns arise.

Presentation and assessment

Presentation

Most patients with new diabetes under the age of 30 yrs will have type 1 diabetes. However, variants of type 2 diabetes are becoming more frequent, especially among patients of South Asian and African–Caribbean origin, particularly if overweight. In the USA nearly half the diabetes in young people is now type 2. Diabetes presents with the same symptoms as in adults (➔ pp. 2–3). Additional features may include growth retardation, difficulties at school, behavioural problems, and bed-wetting (even in teenagers). Weight loss can be dramatic. In type 2 diabetes more gradual symptoms and onset may lead to delayed diagnosis and symptoms not being taken seriously.

⚠ Contact specialist paediatric/adult diabetes team same day.

Diagnosis

See Chapter 1, particularly Figure 1.1 (➔ p. 11).

Assessment of newly diabetic young people (➔ pp. 23–30)

- Full history and examination.
- Height and weight—plot on centile chart.
- Pubertal stage.
- General clinical state—ill or not? Admission required?
- Is diabetes the only problem? Has the presentation been triggered by infection?
- Remember that diabetes is more frequent in a variety of chromosomal disorders, and in other conditions such as cystic fibrosis. About 4 % of patients with coeliac disease have diabetes.
- Family history. Could this be MODY or MIDD?
- Investigations as for adults including tissue transglutaminase, islet cell, and antiGAD antibodies.

Management

Treatment

What type of diabetes is it? (➲ pp. 16–20)
Definition can be difficult. The following are practical suggestions. Seek expert specialist advice same day. If in doubt as to whether type 1 or 2 diabetes use insulin and monitor very carefully until expert help arrives. I would now advise sending blood for islet cell and antiGAD antibodies on all newly diagnosed diabetic patients < 20 yrs of age. Only a positive result is really helpful. Negative results do not disprove a diagnosis of type 1 diabetes, they merely make it less likely.

- Ill ± severe symptoms ± ketones present (≥ 1mmol/l in blood or > + in urine) ± venous bicarbonate < 15 mmol/l = type 1 diabetes—needs insulin. ?DKA (➲ pp. 216–19).
- Not 'ill' ± milder symptoms ± minimal ketones (< 1mmol/l in blood or ≤ + in urine) ± overweight ± South Asian or African–Caribbean origins ± strong family history of diabetes = type 2 diabetes. May manage with tablets (or may be early type 1 and actually need insulin).

Most young people now start treatment at home with specialist support and without hospital admission. Some centres still admit type 1 patients for a few days. The home start approach can be achieved only by a DSN supported by a diabetologist. Other members of the team may be seen at the hospital or at home. The patient and their family are visited once or twice a day until they are confident in insulin injection technique and diet. A 24-hr telephone diabetes helpline is essential.

Insulin
Basal–bolus regimens are first choice (➲ p. 174) because of flexibility of control. CSII works well for motivated young patients (➲ pp. 164–8). Young people will have diabetes for the rest of their lives with high risk of tissue damage so must be encouraged to aim for good glucose control from the start. It is *not* kind to undertreat them. It is difficult to achieve good control. Young people are as capable of injecting insulin as adults, but also have the same range of anxiety about injections. Encourage them to do their own injections from the start—overprotection by staff or parents is not helpful. 'Pinch and prick' techniques are best to avoid IM injections in slim patients. The Novopen® Junior or HumaPen® Luxura™ HD, which give half units, may be needed for smaller or more active patients. The lunchtime injection is problematic in patients who are unable or unwilling to give it themselves. Young people usually feel embarrassed about injecting insulin at school, and this may be difficult to arrange. Schools or colleges should provide a room in which this can be done. Patients and parents need to be warned about the honeymoon period of diabetes (➲ p. 177). Seek lipohypertrophy which is common, especially abdominal. Avoid injections in these lumps (➲ p. 173).

Non-insulin treatments

Most pharmaceutical manufacturers have not caught up with the increasing need for treatment for type 2 diabetes in young people. The relevant SPCs state the following.

- Metformin. 'In children from 10 yrs of age and adolescents, Glucophage® film-coated tablets may be used as monotherapy or in combination with insulin.'
- Slow-release metformin: 'In the absence of available data, Glucophage® SR should not be used in children.' The same applies to Glucient® SR.
- Sulfonylureas. The SPCs do not recommend use in children. BNF for Children (BNFC) states they can be used second line, e.g. tolbutamide, or gliclazide (which is often used to treat MODY ➲ p. 17).
- Repaglinide. Contraindicated in children < 12 yrs of age. SPC.
- Nateglinide. 'There are no data available on the use of nateglinide in patients under 18 yrs of age, and therefore its use in this age group is not recommended.' SPC.
- Pioglitazone: 'There are no data available on the use of pioglitazone in patients under 18 yrs of age, and therefore its use is not recommended in this age group.' SPC.
- Incretin effect enhancers should not be used in children
- Dapagliflozin and canagliflozin: The safety and efficacy of these agents in children aged 0–< 18 yrs has not yet been established. SPCs.
- Paediatricians are less familiar with oral hypoglycaemic agents than adult diabetologists—another reason for joint clinics for diabetic teenagers.

Diet

Refer all young people with diabetes to a dietitian used to caring for this age group. Advise a healthy diet which everyone should follow (➲ pp. 67–86). It helps if the whole family has the same diet. Quantities should be enough to maintain appropriate weight for height and continued normal growth and development.

Food is the most common battleground between the diabetic teenager and his/her parents. Teenagers like to 'graze', and formal family mealtimes are increasingly uncommon. Chocolate, crisps, and burgers are often what their peer group eats. Banning sweets at home increases secret outside consumption. It is better to include sugar/chocolate as part of meals; this will reduce its impact on the blood glucose and reduce the desire for guilty extras. Young people need to eat enough to grow properly—the 'diet' must not be interpreted as weight restricting unless the child is actually obese. Teenage boys need to eat a lot (> 3000 cals a day), and those who play a lot of sport will need more. There is no place for 'diabetic' foods. Discourage fatty and salty foods. Introduce the new diet gradually and help the child to learn about different types of food and how they might affect diabetes. For patients and families who wish, carbohydrate counting (➲ p. 72) makes insulin adjustment easier long term and helps to improve glucose balance.

The patient must carry glucose if on insulin or sulfonylureas, and have snacks immediately available (agreed beforehand with the school or college if necessary). School lunches can be prepacked if that is what peers do. If lunch is provided, encourage healthy options. However, once out of parental view teenagers will eat what they want. The patient may need to 'jump the queue' for food to avoid hypoglycaemia—risking embarrassment.

By the end of the school day a teenager often arrives home hungry, and possibly hypoglycaemic leading to a large snack, followed by the full evening meal later. An extra dose of insulin may be needed to cover the snack to avoid high glucose levels later.

Teach teenagers how to shop economically for healthy food before they go away to university or college. Basic nutritional principles and cooking skills are also essential.

Weight and body image

Obesity

More than one in four < 16-yr-olds in the UK are overweight. This has contributed to the increase in type 2 diabetes in young people and to adult obesity. Young people reflect family lifestyles, health beliefs, and eating patterns. Obese teenagers are often bullied and may be depressed. A prolonged combined psychological, family, and dietetic approach is needed. Set realistic goals—first, not gaining more weight. Diet and exercise are both important.

Weight loss or limitation

Some authors suggest an increased frequency of eating disorders in diabetes (these can affect adults too). Both anorexia nervosa and bulimia occur, and may explain bizarre fluctuations in blood glucose control (especially the latter). Laxative abuse also occurs and can cause dangerous hypokalaemia in insulin-deficient patients.

A more common form of self-abuse, usually in girls (up to one in three), is insulin omission as chronically high glucose levels cause weight loss (diabulimia ⊃ p. 414). Suspect this in slim girls with persistently high HbA$_{1c}$.

Any eating disorder or deliberate insulin omission needs specialist psychological and psychiatric advice from multidisciplinary teams familiar with caring for such patients and their families (Community Adolescent Mental Health Services). A first step is to elicit the problem non-judgmentally (e.g. 'Lots of people worry about their weight. Sometimes they cut their food or their insulin. Have you ever thought about doing that?'). Show that it is safe to talk about it. Discourage parental nagging which is understandable but counter-productive.

All these patients are at increased risk of diabetic tissue damage (e.g. retinopathy) and must be monitored closely. See NICE 2004 guidance for eating disorders ⌕ <http://www.nice.org.uk/guidance/CG9>

Exercise

Increasing time on smart phones or online and less time in physical activity may lead to reduced face-to-face friendship, but intense electronic communication. It reduces overall fitness and may cause repetitive strain injury in hands/wrists. School sports and gym can help maintain exercise, but these activities have been reduced in some schools. Obese young people feel embarrassed in sports or swimming kit and try to avoid activities. Encourage any safe physical activity which the young person is happy to do.

Even walking further from the parental car to the school gate can help. The paediatric DSN can talk to the physical education teacher at school. Those who enjoyed sport at school may find that they have no time or opportunity for this at university. Encourage them to find a practical physical activity which fits their new timetable.

Check SMBG before and after a sports session. Follow the rules for exercise (→ p. 237). The physical education teacher or trainer should carry glucose tablets or glucose drink and know how to recognize and treat hypoglycaemia.

Home blood glucose monitoring (SMBG)

- SMBG is often more unpopular than the insulin injections.
- Find the finger-pricking system and part of finger which hurts least. Consider needle-less methods.
- Safety tests (before bed, before sport, when ill) should be insisted upon.
- Ideally the tests should be more frequent to allow insulin and dietary adjustment.
- New meters and 'cool' electronics are popular, and may improve testing.

Diabetes kit

- Small bag/bum bag/pocket bag
- Fast-acting insulin pen (also for pump patients in case of pump failure)
- Insulin pump if used
- Compact glucose meter with integral strips
- Small finger-pricker
- Glucose tablets ± glucose gel
- Durable snack
- Diabetic card/ID

Complications start in childhood

It is not true that only diabetes after puberty 'counts' towards the development of diabetic tissue damage. This dangerous myth led to undertreatment of childhood diabetes for years. Children as young as 10 yrs old can develop retinopathy.

Researchers followed 527 children with diabetes diagnosed at mean age 8.8 yrs for 9.8 yrs. Cumulative prevalence of microalbuminuria was 25.7 % at 10 yrs and 50.7 % after 19 yrs. Cumulative prevalence of progression to macroalbuminuria was 13.9 % at a mean age of 18.5 yrs. High HbA_{1c} predicted progression (*Br Med J* 2008; **336**:697; doi: http://dx.doi.org/10.1136/bmj.39478.378241.BE).   ACE   inhibitor   treatment induces remission of microalbuminuria (*Diabetes Care* 2011; **34**:424–9. doi:10.2337/dc10-1177). We must improve diabetes care in children and teenagers. Failure to do so may seriously impair quality and quantity of life. This requires intensive patient and parent education and support, with good access to out-of-hours help. Sadly, adult diabetes services still see 20 yr olds with multiple diabetic tissue damage.

Microvascular disease (retinopathy or nephropathy) is the most likely complication, but hypertension and macrovascular disease occur in young people. Even young diabetic children may have abnormal vascular resistance. The accepted limits for blood pressure readings in those <15 yrs old (systolic is thought to be most reliable) are <95 centile for gender, age, and height; checked on three occasions. (*J Hypertension*:2009; **27**:1719–42; doi: 10.1097/HJH.0b013e32832f4f6b)

The Diabetes NSF advises digital photographic retinal screening for children > 12 yrs old. Retinopathy can occur at younger ages. Microalbuminuria should be screened annually, as for adults (➋ p. 92).

For microalbuminuria and hypertension in young people reduce dietary salt and tighten blood glucose control. Many snacks (e.g. crisps) are high in salt. Weight normalization is also important.

In those > 16 yrs treat persistent microalbuminuria or hypertension as for adults. There is no consensus about treatment for those < 16 yrs but ACE inhibitors have been used (BNFC). Girls past menarche are often sexually active and at risk of pregnancy (➋ pp. 336–7).

Lipids are not routinely measured in paediatric diabetic clinics, yet this will identify those with concomitant familial hyperlipidaemia who are then at much increased risk of cardiovascular disease. They should be monitored in adolescents. Treat young patients with significant hyperlipidaemia as for adults (➋ pp. 261–3). Seek specialist advice. Do not give statins to girls at risk of pregnancy.

Growth

- All diabetic young people < 20 yrs old should have a growth chart (height and weight) in their hospital and GP records. Mark parental heights on the chart. Use age-related BMI charts as well.
- Note menarche and pubertal staging.
- The Royal College of Paediatrics and Child Health (RCPCH) provides growth charts: ☞ <http://www.rcpch.ac.uk/child-health/research-projects/uk-who-growth-charts/uk-who-growth-chart-resources/uk-who-growth-ch-0>
- High glucose levels suppress growth hormone release and stunt growth. Improve glucose control to avoid permanent shortness.
- Normoglycaemia with a healthy diet containing sufficient calories is essential for normal growth.
- Obesity is increasing. About a million children < 16 yrs in the UK are obese, and about one in four of children aged 2–15 yrs are overweight.
- If weight starts to rise inappropriately, ask the patient 'to get back to the right weight for your height' with the dietitian's help. Do *not* just say 'lose weight' as this may fuel an eating disorder.

Puberty and sex

Puberty, with its changing hormonal balance and metabolic demands, usually needs insulin dose increases. Blood glucose balance may become erratic. Food intake usually increases around puberty. Beware excessive insulin fuelling hunger and excessive eating.

Follow RCPCH advice about assessing pubertal stage. Many young patients find genital assessment embarrassing. A self-reporting system is available.

Menstruation (median onset of menarche is 13 yrs (range 7–20 yrs) in UK non-diabetic girls) can cause cyclical hyperglycaemia (sometimes hypoglycaemia). Menarche may be delayed in girls with diabetes. When periods start ensure that diabetic girls know about sexual intercourse, the possibility of pregnancy, and the need for family planning in diabetes. Parental presence may sometimes inhibit discussions about sexual issues, although many parents are supportive. Even nowadays sex education and knowledge vary. Everyone thinks 'it won't happen to me!' An unsuspected pregnancy can precipitate DKA, and it is particularly important to avoid unwanted pregnancy in diabetic girls. Remind both genders of the need for protection from sexually transmitted diseases (including HIV). Partners can be very supportive in diabetes self-care and some young patients bring them to clinic.

The Family Planning Association has leaflets for young people (➲ pp. 336–7) ☞ <http://www.fpa.org.uk/information/>

Parents and siblings

Diabetes is a frightening condition. Some parents with diabetes will be consumed by guilt—'I gave it to him!' Healthcare staff do not have to live with the child and his diabetes every day. No-one wants their child to have injections. Many parents are so frightened of possible adverse consequences that they adhere rigidly to the guidelines they were given on diagnosis without realizing that some flexibility is possible. Many need a lot of support in introducing flexibility. The paediatric DSN's role is crucial. Parents may be terrified of hypoglycaemia and so run the glucose too high. Conversely, anxieties about tissue damage may lead to over-stringent glucose control and hypoglycaemia. Siblings may receive less attention that the person with diabetes, causing jealousy—but they may also be frightened that their brother or sister may die.

When children are young, consultations are predominantly with their parents. Adult consultations are usually with the patient. Both young people and their parents may find this transition difficult. Some young people find being asked direct medical questions threatening and clam up. Give them time and have a more general discussion first. Ensure that they have enough opportunity to ask questions. The need to allow a teenager to speak to the doctor or nurse on his or her own may make the parent feel excluded and angry. Listen to parents too.

Alcohol and recreational drugs

Alcohol

Alcohol is cheap and readily available. Most teenagers start drinking before the legal age and many drink to excess by their teens. This exposes them to the risk of injury and unwise sexual behaviour. Remind them of the law, but make sure that they are aware of advice for safe drinking for people with diabetes (➲ p. 77) as they are likely to ignore your advice to drink only legally.

Alcohol poisoning can cause ketosis and may mimic DKA.

Recreational drugs

In one study 28 % of diabetic patients aged 16–30 yrs said they had tried or were using recreational drugs (*Diabetic Med*, 2004; **21**: 295; doi: 10.1046/j.1464-5491.2003.01092.x). Ask all young patients about recreational drug use (parental presence may inhibit reliable answers). Ensure that your patients know that recreational drugs are dangerous in anyone, but especially so if one has diabetes.

Recreational drugs can have direct effects on glucose control or impede ability to self-care. Cannabis causes mood change which may mask hypoglycaemia, although the 'munchies' it induces may raise glucose. Ecstasy reduces urinary water loss and could worsen the hyponatraemia associated with high glucose, especially if a lot of water is drunk. Both cocaine and amphetamines can raise glucose. Opiates may affect insulin and glucagon release. Drug use may precipitate DKA and should be sought in the history.

Psychological issues

Psychiatric disorders are two to three times more common in diabetic adolescents than in their peers. In one study 37 % adolescents met criteria for formal psychiatric diagnosis, particularly young women. Psychiatric disorders were present in half those with a history of poor diabetes control vs a quarter of well-controlled patients. Those with poor glucose control were more likely to have had pre-diabetic behaviour problems (*Diabetic Med* 2005; **22**:152–7; doi: 10.1111/j.1464–5491.2004.01370.x). Bullying (including electronic) is common and can cause great distress and even suicide.

Many adolescent patients are anxious. Patients may seize on a small comment in clinic and worry about it for months. Specifically seek worries in each consultation.

⚠ Depression is common among young people. Believe them when they say that they are depressed or have considered suicide. Sadly, people may think they are exaggerating because they are teenagers. They are not.

Seek expert help immediately if the patient is depressed. Suicidal ideation requires an immediate phone call to your local mental health service for young people.

Unfortunately, specialist adolescent mental health services may be difficult to access in some areas. Young people may be too old for children's mental health services and too young for adult services. Clarify local arrangements for adolescents before they are needed. Websites for young people with diabetes include:
- ✆ <http://www.youthhealthtalk.org>
- ✆ <http://www.diabetes.org.uk/Guide-to-diabetes/My-life/>

Transition

The transition from paediatric to adult diabetes services is a potentially dangerous time when patients can become lost. Young patients are asserting their independence. They may be studying away from home. Furthermore, adult and paediatric services may be in separate hospitals or even in separate geographical or health service areas. Rigid organizational boundaries can greatly impede care.

'Join us on our journey' studied how best to deliver 'Making every young person with diabetes matter'. The project reported:

'[p]articipants did not necessarily know what transition meant and when they were in transition they were often unaware of what was happening and why. Transition was regarded as a vital time in respect of a young person's diabetes journey and had important implications for the ways in which young people continued to manage their condition. Differences in record-keeping between paediatric and adult diabetes services region-wide had important implications for continuity of care.

Participants who attended the paediatric diabetes service were happy with the care they received. Young adults who accessed the adult diabetes service were less positive. Staff attendance at clinic and discontinuity in care were the main concerns raised. Access to 24-hour diabetes specialist care was not always available. Allocated clinic sessions and appointments were often too short. Diabetes teams had taken steps to improve clinic, but many aspects of clinic organisation were beyond their control.' ℘ <http://webarchive.nationalarchives.gov.uk/20130513172055/http://www.diabetes.nhs.uk/about_us/research_and_evaluation/join_us_on_our_journey/#>

Patients of all ages would benefit from improving some of these concerns. Clinics should be organized for patients not the system.

- Prepare children and parents for transition
- Pay care attention to practicalities, e.g. travel
- Ensure good and continued liaison between paediatric and adult services
- Ensure transfer of records
- Ensure continued support and unbroken 24-hr access to advice
- Provide continuity of staffing in young adult or adult services
- Establish robust call and recall systems. Seek out young people who do not attend
- Listen to the patient—services should work for him/her

Brittle diabetes

Brittle diabetes is defined as metabolic instability sufficient to disrupt the patient's life but is usually interpreted as meaning apparently irresolvable instability. There may be hypoglycaemia and/or hyperglycaemia. Whilst one must always recognize the impact of psychological factors on health it is essential systematically to seek out and treat other causes of recurrent glucose instability (➲ pp. 196–7, pp. 203–4). Admission may be triggered by infection on top of persistent hyperglycaemia caused by prolonged insulin omission for psychological reasons.

One young woman with brittle diabetes can generate multiple admissions for DKA and/or hypoglycaemia and massive hospital records, and engage the attentions of the diabetes team, every on-take medical team in the hospital, mental health teams, social services, GP, and practice staff. Her parents may require psychiatric and medical help, and some staff may need psychological support. Although this dramatic behaviour is memorable and time-consuming, remember that there are few such patients in most districts.

Most of these patients have complex psychological ± diabetes education issues. ⚠ They are at risk of early death. They must remain under diabetologist care with a clear communication plan and management strategy. If problems arise, contact the diabetes team immediately to reduce duplication and manipulation. One member of the diabetes team (e.g. DSN) should coordinate care, but will need back-up as caring for such patients can be emotionally draining.

Concordance vs non-concordance

Adolescence is a time of experimentation with one's personality, sexuality, family, and the outside world. It is often 'make or break' time—examination results determine further training, apprenticeships further careers, marriage partners may be chosen. Boundaries are tested—parental authority, school or college rules, health and fitness, relationships. Parents must start handing over diabetes care to their children, if they have not already done so. This can be difficult. The worries that parents experience waiting for a child to come home from a late-night party are compounded when that child has diabetes. Has she eaten enough? Drunk too much? If late, has she gone hypo? It is hard to relinquish care of a potentially dangerous disorder when a young person is rebelling against authority and appears least capable of taking care of themselves.

Health professionals' and parents' views of the aims of diabetes care do not always match the patient's. Teenagers want to hide their diabetes. They often run a high glucose because hypoglycaemia is frightening, and they want to avoid embarrassment in front of their friends. Clarification of the patient's goals can help acceptance of overall care.

Many adolescent diabetes clinics have a 25 % non-attendance rate. Phone calls, texts, e-mails, letters have all been tried and work for some. The DSN is most likely to succeed in re-establishing contact. For the young patient clinics may be frightening, boring, and confusing places that smell of hospitals, where you are told off for not doing something, and asked embarrassing questions in front of your parents by a doctor you have never seen before who behaves like a policeman. The following steps may help.

- Try to maintain continuity of care from the same individual staff.
- Train all staff in working with young people.
- Maintain contact with the patient in whatever way works for them and however 'difficult' the patient's behaviour.
- Listen properly. Respect the patient's opinions. Be non-judgemental.
- Ensure that patients know that rescue will always be provided (and how to access it) if the glucose goes badly wrong (e.g. DKA).
- If the 'lost sheep' returns, give him or her a friendly welcome, manage emergencies swiftly, then negotiate future improvements in care. The key is maintaining contact.
- Seek depression or anxiety, or other psychological issues.
- It is very important for young people to 'save face'.
- Don't underestimate fears of being 'different' or peer pressure.
- Insulin may be genuinely or deliberately forgotten. Any insulin injections are helpful; the right injections at the right time are excellent. Ask 'how are the insulin injections going?'
- Provide opportunities to admit lapses: 'Are you managing to do any blood tests?' Any blood glucose tests are helpful; the right tests at the right time are excellent.
- Encourage the use of glucose meters from which results can be downloaded onto a computer.
- Teenagers hate writing down glucose results. Ask them to bring the meter to the clinic and download it there.
- Tell the patient about diabetes apps (➔ p. 101).

- Faked blood test results are common, as is omission of high readings. If suspected try: 'lots of people forget to write all their sugars down and try to remember them later. Does that ever happen with you?' Or 'I don't quite understand this result—might it be a mistake?'
- New gadgets and technology may encourage more tests and more injections.
- Concordance may improve when a driving licence application is needed.

Education and diabetes

Young people spend much of their time at school or in further education. Schools often have rigid rules and staff may not understand the needs of diabetic teenagers. There is no coordinated training for teachers and school staff about diabetes and there is considerable individual variation in the way in which young people with diabetes are supported at school. DSNs will teach staff about diabetes and the needs of individual students. Nowadays teachers may not be allowed to assist with medical care and there may be no school nurse or first-aider. Less support is provided in secondary schools than in primary schools. Diabetes UK has clear guidance for parents and schools. Essex County Council has produced guidance for school staff about supporting pupils with diabetes in Essex schools.

    ℘ <http://www.diabetes.org.uk/Documents/Professionals/Essex%20Diabetes%20Guidance%20for%20Schools%20Updated%20Amendments%20Diabetes%20UK%2005%2002%2011.pdf>

Areas of self-care which can make diabetes easier to manage at school are dietary knowledge, blood glucose testing, awareness of the symptoms of hypoglycaemia and how to treat them, and knowledge of how to cope with exercise. Self-injection means that the child can go on school trips. Everyone (including fellow pupils) should be aware that he/she has diabetes, otherwise there may be accusations of drug abuse if injections or blood tests are observed. Remember bullying occurs.

Time off school/college should be rare. Repeated absences because of diabetes must be investigated promptly so that diabetes care can be improved. There is a complex interrelationship between poor glycaemic balance, the psychological effects of diabetes, academic work, and behaviour. Resolution may require the combined efforts of parents, teachers, child psychologist, paediatrician, diabetologist, diabetes team, and GP—clear communication is vital. Most diabetic students do as well as their non-diabetic peers academically, and there is some suggestion that they may do better, perhaps because of greater pressure to succeed.

Most young people complete their training unimpeded by their diabetes. Occasionally diabetes develops around examination time or interferes with a crucial time at school or university. Prompt diagnosis and treatment focused on a return to academic or practical activities as soon as possible can minimize the damage. Rarely, the young person may be unable to perform up to their usual standard for a few weeks or occasionally months. A formal doctor's letter to academic or training authorities may be needed to help the patient to gain another chance.

Leaving home

This section relates to any move from home. Going to university is the most common—exciting but worrying for students and parents.

- Students should locate and inform university medical services about their diabetes.
- Visit the medical centre and doctor on arrival—most will require students to register with them.
- It may be best to remain with the familiar home diabetes clinic but the student should be provided with a letter for the university's local diabetes specialist team. Liaise with these specialist diabetes services if the student is likely to require their care.
- Book holiday visits to the home diabetic clinic.
- Tell students they can still phone/text/e-mail their usual DSN if necessary.
- Ensure sufficient supplies (and spare) of insulin, testing strips, etc.
- Ascertain arrangements for re-supply while at university.
- Teach self-catering and economical shopping (family and dietitian).
- Take a mobile phone with unlimited calls.
- Ensure accommodation is clean, warm, and secure
- Find a secure place for back-up diabetic kit.
- Carry daily diabetic kit around.
- Tell personal tutors about the diabetes.
- Tell new friends about the diabetes.
- Ask the DSN and diabetologist about adjusting diabetes treatment to new way of life.

Summary: issues to consider when caring for young people with diabetes

- What the patient wants and fears
- How best to stay in touch—phone/text/e-mail/letter
- Family (parents—together or not, siblings, others)
- Friends and partners
- Home environment—emotional and physical
- School or further education
- Hobbies
- Sports
- Career planning—diabetes precludes some careers (➜ pp. 384–5)
- Work (➜ pp. 383–92)
- Learning to drive/driving (➜ pp. 395–400)
- Financial issues
- Emotions—look out for depression or anxiety (➜ pp. 409–16)
- Alcohol
- Recreational drugs
- Sex
- Anything which may require Child Protection investigation
- Growth and pubertal development
- What type of diabetes do they have?
- Home blood glucose testing
- Diabetes treatment—insulin or non-insulin
- Food—home, school, eating out
- Exercise (➜ pp. 233–43)
- Diabetic tissue damage—prevention, detection, and treatment (➜ pp. 245–9, pp. 301–4)
- Other health problems
- Clinic attendance
- Transition

Diabetes in women

Check BNF, NICE and other national guidance regularly as guidance on the use of drugs in pregnancy may change (pp. 113, 147).

Effects of diabetes in women

All the changes of womanhood can influence, and be influenced by, diabetes.

Menstruation

Menarche may be delayed if diabetes is diagnosed before puberty. About one in three diabetic women experience some menstrual abnormalities, most commonly infrequent or irregular periods. This is thought to be due to hypothalamic dysfunction.

The hormonal changes before and during menstruation can cause both hypoglycaemia and hyperglycaemia in different individuals. The most frequent change is hyperglycaemia on the last day or so premenstrually or, most often, during the first 2 days of bleeding. Some women are hypoglycaemic premenstrually or as bleeding subsides. Others have unpredictable oscillations in glycaemic balance, and a few may develop DKA at this time. Women with predictable glucose rises before or during menstruation can increase their insulin during this time. Hyperglycaemia can cause menstrual irregularity or amenorrhoea, especially in untreated diabetes.

Polycystic ovary syndrome (PCOS)

- PCOS is common
- Symptoms and signs
  - overweight
  - irregular or absent periods
  - anovulatory infertility
  - acne
  - hirsutism (or thinning head hair)
  - acanthosis nigricans
  - depression or mood change may also occur
- Glucose intolerance in up to a third of PCOS patients—the greater the BMI, the more likely the glucose intolerance
- Type 2 diabetes—2–4 times more likely than in general population
- Hyperinsulinaemia
- Increased cardiovascular risk
- Increased risk of uterine cancer
- Assuming other causes of hyperandrogenism or menstrual problems have been excluded, a diagnosis of PCOS requires two of:
  - infrequent or no ovulation (usually shown by infrequent or absent menstruation)
  - evidence of hyperandrogenism—hirsutism, male head hair loss, acne, or raised testosterone
  - polycystic ovaries on ultrasound
- Note that actual ovarian cysts are not essential for the diagnosis

Treatment

- Weight loss is the key treatment to improve clinical features.
- Use metformin to control glucose.
- Metformin has been used off-licence in PCOS without diabetes (see BNF) as it may aid weight loss in conjunction with dietary advice, improve ovulation and menstrual regularity, and reduce hirsutism.

Not all studies showed these effects with metformin, and weight loss alone may be as effective. Some patients had side effects (➲ p. 122). Some authors advise using it only in PCOS with glucose intolerance or diabetes.

Infections

- Diabetic women may not mention 'trouble down below'. This may be the cause of raised glucose levels. Ask.
- Thrush (candida albicans or glabrata)—may be a presenting feature of diabetes. Combining single-dose oral fluconazole or itraconazole (check BNF) and vaginal imidazole creams or pessaries may provide cure and comfort more reliably. Diabetes predisposes to recurrent thrush so treat promptly and effectively. Send fungal samples—glabrata is commoner in diabetes. Improve glucose control. For recurrent infection or candida glabrata (often azole resistant) seek genitourinary clinic advice.
- Urinary tract infection is common. Use antibiotics from local guidelines. Check clearance with a urine dipstick for blood, protein, nitrite, and leucocytes a week after antibiotics finish.
- Pyelonephritis may be severe in diabetic patients.
- Vulval or groin abscess may precipitate DKA. Groin or genital infections can precipitate multiple organism necrotizing fasciitis which, albeit rare, is more common in people with diabetes than in non-diabetic patients and often fatal.
- Seek genitourinary clinic advice for the following which are more common in women with diabetes than in non-diabetic women:
  - herpes simplex
  - vaginal warts

Fertility and contraception

Fertility

Diabetic women can conceive but may have reduced fertility in some situations. Factors which affect fertility are:

- late menarche
- menstrual irregularity
- PCOS
- increased risk of primary ovarian failure (and other autoimmune conditions in type 1 diabetes)

Diabetes duration increases the risk of complications so women with diabetes are advised not to delay pregnancy if health and circumstances permit this.

Contraception

Consider each patient's needs individually. Diabetic women should use the most reliable form of contraception that is safe for them. Check BNF for up-to-date advice.

Hormonal contraceptive drugs

Hormonal contraceptive drugs are very effective. WHO and the Faculty of Sexual and Reproductive Healthcare, RCOG, provide guidance on their use <http://www.fsrh.org/pdfs/UKMEC2009.pdf>

- History of gestational diabetes: no restriction on use.
- Non-vascular disease and type 1 or type 2 diabetes: the advantages of using the method generally outweigh the theoretical or proven risks.
- Diabetic nephropathy, retinopathy, or neuropathy, other vascular disease: the theoretical or proven risks usually outweigh the advantages of using the method.

WHO also assumes that women with diabetes > 20 yrs duration should be treated as those who have complications. However, all these women are also at greater risk of complications of pregnancy. Balance the risks.

The combined oral contraceptive pill (OCP) has a pregnancy rate of < 1/100 woman-yrs if used properly. Advise current first-choice OCPs for the general population. Monitor blood pressure, glucose control, and lipids which may all rise, and increase alertness for both venous and arterial thrombo-embolic diagnoses.

A combined oestrogen–progestogen patch has the same risks as the OCP but can be removed if the patient has an adverse reaction. Patches are changed once a week. Some patients find these easier to remember than daily pills. Used properly the pregnancy rate is the same as an OCP but patches may fall off.

A combined oestrogen–progestogen vaginal ring also has the same risks as the OCP but can be removed if adverse effects occur.

Some centres advocate progesterone-only contraception for diabetic women as there is less effect upon lipids and thrombosis risk. There may be irregular or unexpected 'periods'. Pregnancy rate is 1/100 women-yrs. Depot contraception implants can be used which can be removed if adverse effects occur or the patient develops diabetic complications.

The RCOG advice is:
- History of gestational diabetes: no restriction on use.
- Non-vascular disease and type 1 or type 2 diabetes: the advantages of using the method generally outweigh the theoretical or proven risks.
- Diabetic nephropathy, retinopathy, or neuropathy, other vascular disease:
  - for progesterone-only pills and implants: the advantages of using the method generally outweigh the theoretical or proven risks.
  - for progestogen-only injectables (depot medroxyprogesterone and norethisterone enantate): the theoretical or proven risks usually outweigh the advantages of using the method.

Intra-uterine contraceptive devices (IUCDs) have a pregnancy rate of < 1/100 women-yrs. RCOG notes that for copper-bearing devices there is no restriction in use for women with diabetes. For levonorgestrel-releasing devices the advantages of using the method generally outweigh the theoretical or proven risks.

In any woman there is a risk of pelvic infection, rarely leading to infertility. This risk is greater in women with diabetes because of their propensity to infection generally.

Barrier methods have no metabolic or thrombotic sequelae but have a greater failure rate than the methods discussed (pregnancy rates: male condoms, 2/100 women-yrs; female condoms 5/100 women-yrs). They are also harder to use properly. The addition of a spermicide which does not damage the condom improves contraceptive effect. Condoms protect from sexually transmitted diseases. They are readily available. A diaphragm or cap requires gynaecological assessment for fitting and there may be an increased risk of vaginal and urinary infection. Pregnancy rate is 4–8/100 women-yrs.

All barrier methods are useless if not used properly, and planned conception and the avoidance of unwanted pregnancy are particularly important in women with diabetes. Some patients, especially those with multiple sexual partners, use both an OCP and a condom.

The rhythm method and withdrawal are not effective and cannot be recommended for diabetic women.

Emergency contraception using oral medication or a copper IUCD can be used after unprotected intercourse. Emergency contraceptive pills can be purchased from a pharmacist in the UK. An IUCD is more effective but requires medical input which may deter some patients.

The Family Planning Association website provides information for girls and women: ✆ <http://www.fpa.org.uk>.

Pre-pregnancy counselling

⚠ Refer all diabetic patients planning pregnancy to a specialist pre-conception diabetic clinic promptly. Delay may mean that the woman arrives at the clinic already pregnant!

Advise teenage diabetic girls and women of childbearing potential to plan pregnancy when they do decide to have a family, and to use contraception, if necessary, until then. Find out their wishes about having a family and about contraception. Explain that good glucose control pre-conception and during pregnancy reduces the risk of miscarriage, congenital malformation, still birth and neonatal death, although these risks can never be fully eliminated in any pregnancy.

All health professionals, especially GPs and practice nurses, should consider the possibility that every girl or woman with diabetes of childbearing potential might become pregnant. This includes women with type 2 as well as type 1 diabetes. Discuss contraception or pregnancy plans with women at annual review, and at other visits if their wishes are not yet clear.

Half the pregnant women in pregnant diabetic clinics in London have type 2 diabetes, and half of those are from non-white ethnic backgrounds. A high proportion of type 2 diabetic pregnant patients live in areas with high social deprivation. CEMACH 2007 audited pregnancies in diabetic women and noted that fewer than half the women surveyed had had pre-pregnancy counselling, under half had been given folic acid, and a third had had no measure of glucose control in the 6 months antepartum. Two-thirds had evidence of poor glucose control antenatally or during the first trimester. Suboptimal glucose care was linked with poor pregnancy outcome, as was suboptimal antenatal care. Half the women had suboptimal post-natal diabetes care. 29 % of babies had a congenital anomaly. ℘ <http://www.hqip.org.uk/cmace-reports> lists the series of diabetes reports>.

A review of pregnancies in women with pre-existing diabetes in Northern England in 1997–2008 found that increasing periconception HbA$_{1c}$ concentration > 49 mmol/mol (6.6 %), prepregnancy retinopathy, and lack of prepregnancy folic acid consumption were all independently associated with increased odds of fetal and infant death (*Diabetologia* 2014; **57**:285–94. doi: 10.1007/s00125-013-3108-5). Regrettably, much still needs to be done to improve safety of pregnancy in women with pre-existing diabetes and their unborn children.

The National Pregnancy in Diabetes audit was established to support clinical teams to deliver better care and outcomes (➲ pp. 460–2). ℘ <http://www.hscic.gov.uk/npid>

Congenital malformations are most likely if women are hyperglycaemic in the first 8 weeks of pregnancy. Strict normoglycaemia pre-conception dramatically reduces the likelihood of congenital malformation to near that of the non-diabetic population (Figure 17.1).

As few women know when they conceive, the usual advice is to maintain contraception, adjust treatment to achieve normoglycaemia, and then stop the contraception. It is easier to use barrier methods as menstrual cycles may be erratic after stopping OCPs so women may not realize they are pregnant. Normoglycaemia is continued until after the baby is born. It is hard work and means 4–7 finger-prick glucose tests daily, sometimes for

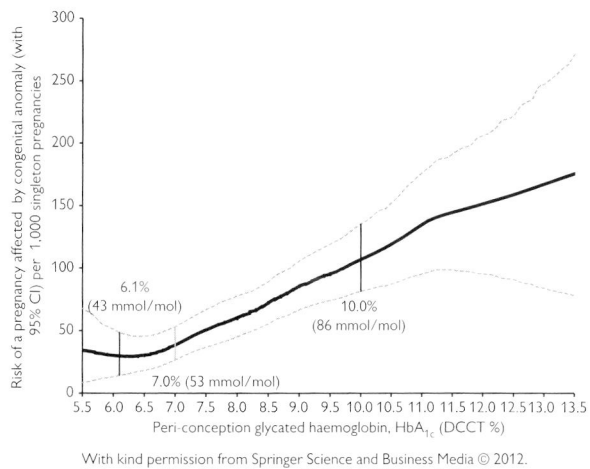

With kind permission from Springer Science and Business Media © 2012. *Diabetologia* 2012; 55:936–947; doi 10.1007/s00125-012-2455-y For conversion of HbA1c to mmol/mol ➲ Table 7.5, p.109

Fig. 17.1 Association between peri-conception HbA$_{1c}$ in women with pre-existing diabetes and the risk (with 95% confidence intervals) of a pregnancy affected by major congenital abnormality.

years if conception is slow to occur. Many women find this stressful and can blame themselves if problems do arise during pregnancy. Beware, and warn of, the high risk of hypoglycaemia, particularly nocturnal. Type 1 women should be warned specifically about DKA and given blood ketone strips and taught when and how to use them and what to do about the results (➲ p. 110).

Medication (check in current BNF)

Hypoglycaemic therapy

NICE CG63 2008 states that '[w]omen with diabetes may be advised to use metformin as an adjunct or alternative to insulin in the preconception period and during pregnancy, when the likely benefits from improved glycaemic control outweigh the potential for harm. All other oral hypoglycaemic agents should be discontinued before pregnancy and insulin substituted.' NICE also points out that '[m]etformin is used in UK clinical practice in the management of diabetes in pregnancy and lactation. There is strong evidence for its effectiveness and safety. This evidence is not currently reflected in the SPC. The SPC advises that when a patient plans to become pregnant and during pregnancy, diabetes should not be treated with metformin but insulin should be used to maintain blood glucose levels. Informed consent on the use of metformin in these situations should be obtained and documented.' The UK Teratology Information Service (UKTIS) states in 2011 '[t]he available data does not show an increased risk of congenital malformations or other adverse pregnancy outcomes. Where clinically indicated, use of metformin at any stage of pregnancy may be considered.' ℗ <http://www.uktis.org/>

Glibenclamide has been used in pregnancy (again, off licence) and is included as an option for oral treatment in pregnancy in NICE CG63. However, it is not often used in the UK due to concerns that it may cross the placenta. UKTIS (2011) states: '[u]se of glibenclamide may be considered in pregnancy where clinically indicated, however experience of use within the first trimester is currently too limited to rule out any possibility of an increased risk of adverse pregnancy outcome.'

Insulin has been used in pregnancy for many years. NICE notes that Novorapid®, Humulin® S, and Isophane (NPH) have not shown adverse effects in pregnancy. The FDA has approved the use of Levemir® in pregnancy. Observational studies have not shown adverse fetal effects from Lantus®. Consider the possible harm from unstable glucose control when changing from the insulin on which a patient is well-controlled to new regimen.

Folic acid

Prescribe folic acid 5 mg daily for diabetic women planning pregnancy and continue until 12 weeks' gestation (note the dose is higher than for non-diabetic women). Check B12, especially in South Asian women or those on metformin.

Vitamin D

Check levels and replace if low (➥ pp. 76, 342).

Other drugs

NICE CG107 (updated) states: '[t]ell women who take angiotensin-converting enzyme (ACE) inhibitors or angiotensin II receptor blockers (ARBs):

• that there is an increased risk of congenital abnormalities if these drugs are taken during pregnancy
• to discuss other antihypertensive treatment with the healthcare professional responsible for managing their hypertension, if they are planning pregnancy

Stop antihypertensive treatment in women taking ACE inhibitors or ARBs if they become pregnant (preferably within 2 working days of notification of pregnancy) and offer alternatives.

Tell women who take chlorothiazide:

• that there may be an increased risk of congenital abnormality and neonatal complications if these drugs are taken during pregnancy
• to discuss other antihypertensive treatment with the healthcare professional responsible for managing their hypertension, if they are planning pregnancy.

Tell women who take antihypertensive treatments other than ACE inhibitors, ARBs or chlorothiazide that the limited evidence available has not shown an increased risk of congenital malformation with such treatments.'

Labetalol is licensed for the treatment of hypertension in pregnancy. Methyldopa is often used but note the side-effect profile in BNF. Patients usually continue methyldopa until pregnancy and breastfeeding are complete and contraception is in use. The BNF states '[l]abetalol is widely used for treating hypertension in pregnancy. Methyldopa is considered safe for use in pregnancy. Modified-release preparations of nifedipine [unlicensed] are also used' but 'may inhibit labour; manufacturer advises avoid before week 20; risk to fetus should be balanced against risk of uncontrolled maternal hypertension; use only if other treatment options are not indicated or have failed'. Elsewhere the BNF also indicates caution with using labetalol in the first trimester.

Statins are teratogenic and must be stopped 3 months before trying to conceive. Do not restart until breastfeeding is finished and contraception is in use.

Overall fitness for pregnancy

The woman's fitness to withstand pregnancy and her prospects of healthy survival to care for her child until grown up must also be considered. Nowadays, women with severe tissue damage are surviving pregnancy with normal infants, but this requires very intensive effort for months to years until a child is born.

Retinopathy can worsen in pregnancy, and digital photographic screening should be part of the pre-pregnancy screen (p. 269) as should assessment of renal function. Renal failure may also worsen considerably during pregnancy, and such women should be managed jointly by obstetrician, renal physician, and diabetologist from pre-pregnancy onwards.

Pre-menopausal diabetic women may have cardiovascular disease. If there is any suggestion of this refer the patient for formal cardiological assessment.

Education

Provide structured diabetes education for women planning pregnancy. Diabetes UK has information at: <http://www.diabetes.org.uk/Guide-to-diabetes/Living_with_diabetes/Pregnancy/>

Pregnancy

- If pregnancy is suspected, proceed as if the patient is pregnant.
- Patients attending a pre-conception clinic should contact their diabetes team the same day if they suspect pregnancy (individual discussion is required for those with irregular periods).
- Send a blood sample for quantitative beta human chorionic gonadotrophin analysis. Often the patient has made the diagnosis herself using over-the-counter tests.
- Refer pregnant diabetic women the same day by telephone to the diabetologist and obstetrician who provide joint care (most diabetologists will contact the obstetric services themselves). An urgent fax with full details is very helpful.
- Prescribe folic acid 5 mg daily until 12 weeks' gestation (some clinics say longer). Check B12 in South Asian women or those on metformin.
- The RCOG states 'In general, vitamin D 10 micrograms (400 units) a day is recommended for all pregnant women in accord with the national guidance…This should be available through the Healthy Start programme… High-risk women are advised to take at least 1000 units a day (women with increased skin pigmentation, reduced exposure to sunlight, or those who are socially excluded or obese).' (→ p. 76)

℘ <http://www.rcog.org.uk/globalassets/documents/guidelines/scientific-impact-papers/vitamin_d_sip43_june14.pdf>

- In the joint diabetic–obstetric clinic.
  - Full clinical assessment, including BP check and renal function
  - Arrange formal ophthalmological review
  - SMBG before and 1 hr after each meal, and occasionally during the night
  - Basal–bolus insulin regimens or CSII are best in those needing insulin
  - Adjust insulin to achieve blood glucose concentrations if safe:
    - 3.5–5.9 mmol /l fasting
    - 4.0–7.7 mmol /l 1 hr after meals
    - ≥ 6 mmol/ at bedtime to reduce the risk of hypoglycaemia
  - HbA$_{1c}$ 20–42 mmol/mol (4–6 %) if safe
  - Prescribe glucagon and show her partner/others close to her how to use it
  - ⚠ Hypoglycaemia is common as patients strive for normoglycaemia and patients and their partners must be warned of this. The patient should always carry glucose on her person and needs to be particularly careful to avoid hypoglycaemia if she is already caring for small children
  - Insulin dose rises during pregnancy and may have more than doubled by term
  - Near term hypoglycaemia and the need to reduce insulin dose may indicate placental underfunction—review immediately for possible admission

- Re-educate each type 1 diabetic woman about DKA and provide blood ketone testing strips with instructions about when to use them and what to do about the results (➲ p. 110)
- A dietitian and DSN or midwife trained in diabetes care should see the patient. The diabetes specialist nurse or midwife can also see her at home
- Obstetric care will comprise very frequent checks as detailed in NICE CG63 with serial ultrasound scans, including examination for cardiac anomalies
- Additional diabetes discussions (e.g. phone calls or visits) are usually needed to discuss glucose balance
- Women with complications (e.g. retinal, renal) will also need review by the relevant specialty.
- Many obstetricians deliver diabetic women at 38 weeks and may have a low threshold for Caesarian section.
- Uterine contractions may be weaker in women with diabetes.
- Cover Caesarian section with prophylactic antibiotics as there is high risk of infection.
- During labour and delivery, insulin and glucose need to be infused intravenously according to a sliding scale.
- Within hours of delivery the insulin requirements will fall to the pre-pregnant dose. In women with established diabetes using insulin pre-pregnancy, reduce insulin dose immediately after birth. Monitor SMBG closely.
- Check thyroid function 2 mths post-partum.
- Do not use HbA_{1c} to monitor glucose control until at least 2 mths post-partum.
- If routine medication was changed for pregnancy, check to see if previous medication should be restored.
- The intensive healthcare, travel and expense required during pregnancy is stressful. Patients can spend a lot of time in clinic. Care should be organized to reduce pressures on the patient (e.g. using telephone calls to discuss diabetes care if appropriate).

Risks in pregnancies of diabetic women

Most complications of pregnancy are increased for mother and fetus in diabetic women. They include:
- pregnancy-induced hypertension
- polyhydramnios
- ketoacidosis
- fetal malformation
- poor fetal growth
- macrosomia
- sudden intra-uterine death
- respiratory distress syndrome
- post-partum hypoglycaemia (mother and fetus)

These complications can be reduced by intensive diabetes and obstetric management, but some women who have been normoglycaemic throughout pregnancy still have macrosomic babies. NICE CG63 (2008 being revised) reviews this.

Don't delay care!

Many of the problems for diabetic women during pregnancy could be avoided or greatly reduced by optimal pre-conception diabetes care and patient education.

The most important factor before and during pregnancy is frequent care by a specialist diabetes and obstetric team experienced in the management of diabetes in pregnancy, with very close attention to detail. There should be 24 hr availability of immediate help (by telephone or in person) if problems arise.

Gestational diabetes (GDM) or hyperglycaemia in pregnancy

Pregnancy may be the first time a woman sees her GP for years. Consider checking such women for established diabetes straightaway if they have the characteristics listed in Box 1.3 (➜ p. 6). It is worth doing an HbA$_{1c}$ straightaway—if it is ≥ 48 mmol/mol (6.5 %) diabetes is highly likely as pregnancy lowers the HbA$_{1c}$. Note that an HbA$_{1c}$ < 48 mmol/mol (6.5 %) does not exclude diabetes (➜ p. 107). Also note that this suggestion does not conform to NICE CG63 although it does follow IADPSG guidance and ADA guidance. Diabetic results in the first trimester indicate established diabetes.

Diabetes may arise during pregnancy, especially in the third trimester. The HAPO study confirms that GDM increases the risk of having pre-eclampsia, a large baby, and primary Caesarian section. The higher the maternal glucose, the greater the risk of adverse outcomes. Obesity independently increases these risks and adds to the adverse effect of GDM. Babies of obese women with GDM are more likely to have shoulder dystocia. (*Diabetes Care* 2012; **35**:780–6; doi:10.2337/dc11-1790).

In the past there was debate about whether treatment of GDM was of benefit. We now know that it is. The ACHOIS study confirmed that treatment of GDM with diet, and insulin adjusted according to SMBG, greatly reduces perinatal complications (*N Engl J Med* 2005; **352**:2477–86; doi: 10.1056/NEJMoa042973). The study also suggested that this treatment improved the women's quality of life.

This led the International Association of Diabetes and Pregnancy Study Groups (IADPSG) to produce consensus recommendations for the diagnosis of hyperglycaemia in pregnancy (*Diabetes Care* 2010; **33**:676–82; doi:10.2337/dc09-1848).

Screening for GDM

NICE CG 63 (2008) (currently under review) advocates identifying patients at booking for subsequent GDM screening. They specify later 75 g OGTT (➜ p. 13) but no other glucose test. This guidance could miss patients with established but undiagnosed diabetes. NICE advises that the following patients be identified at booking:
- Previous GDM (offer SMBG or OGTT at 14–16 wks gestation)
- Others offer OGTT at 24–28 wks gestation):
  - South Asian, Black Caribbean, or Middle Eastern family origin
  - previous big baby (> 4.5 kg)
  - first-degree family history of diabetes
- Screen by performing a formal 75 g OGTT(➜ p. 13). Diagnostic values are in Table 17.1.
- Once diagnosed, women with gestational diabetes are treated like any other pregnant diabetic woman.

WHO (2013) has published new international criteria and classification of hyperglycaemia first detected in pregnancy. ✍ <http://apps.who.int/iris/bitstream/10665/85975/1/WHO_NMH_MND_13.2_eng.pdf> This advocates using the IAPSG cut-offs.

Table 17.1 75 g oral glucose tolerance test in pregnancy

	Venous plasma glucose concentration (mmol/l)	
	Fasting	2 hrs after glucose load
Diabetes (If glucose normalizes post-partum off treatment it was GDM)	≥ 7.0 *And/or*	≥ 11.1
NICE CG63 2008* based on 1999 WHO guidance:		
GDM	≥ 7.0 *And/or*	≥ 7.8
WHO 2013** & IADPSG:		
GDM	5.1–6.9 *And/or*	8.5–11.0

* ℘ <http://publications.nice.org.uk/diabetes-in-pregnancy-cg63/guidance#gestational-diabetes> (under revision)

** ℘ <http://apps.who.int/iris/bitstream/10665/85975/1/WHO_NMH_MND_13.2_eng.pdf>

International discussions about the precise cut-offs continue.

Post-partum care in patients with GDM

After delivery, glucose tolerance may revert to normal, or remain impaired. In GDM it is usual to stop insulin treatment immediately post-partum. Continue SMBG for 2 days post-partum and contact the diabetes team if it remains high. Check a fasting glucose 6 weeks post-partum (NICE CG63). Some clinics do a formal OGTT at 6 weeks but NICE does not advise this.

Over a third of women with gestational diabetes will eventually develop permanent diabetes. This is especially likely in Asian women. The maintenance of a diabetic diet and regular exercise (➲ p. 451) may delay or prevent the reappearance of diabetes. There is a high likelihood of gestational diabetes in further pregnancies.

A fasting glucose once a year (NICE CG63), or opportunistic screening when the patient attends the GP, will provide earlier diagnosis of diabetes in these women. Nowadays HbA$_{1c}$ is being used increasingly as the annual test, especially as it does not require fasting and can be done straightaway. However, a Spanish study showed that fasting glucose was a better predictor of abnormal glucose metabolism (as shown by OGTT) 1 yr post-partum (*Diabetes Care* 2012; **35**:1648–53; doi: 10.2337/dc11-2111). These women frequently get lost to follow-up (about two-thirds of the Spanish women did) and may reappear pregnant with frank diabetes so ensure a robust recall system.

Breastfeeding

Diabetic women can breastfeed. They may need to eat more carbohydrate (about 100 g more a day) and reduce their insulin dose according to blood glucose levels. They should snack before feeding and drink more fluid (e.g. milk). With disturbed nights and erratic exercise patterns, there is a risk of hypoglycaemia. Aim for higher SMBG levels during this time. Restart contraception unless further pregnancies are planned.

All non-insulin hypoglycaemic drugs are contraindicated while breastfeeding. See SPCs. However, NICE CG 63 says that metformin and glibenclamide can be used if patient consent is obtained as for their use in pregnancy.

Motherhood

Women sometimes forget about themselves as they rush around, cooking, cleaning, picking Danny up from nursery school, delivering Sue to her friend's house, and more. It is even harder work if the woman has an additional paid job. The diabetes can be the last item on the agenda, and the aim may be seen as 'keeping a little sugary to avoid hypoglycaemia and not testing too much because I'm busy'. The diet may be erratic, including remnants from the children's plates. 'I know what I ought to do. I'll focus on the diabetes when the children are older.' A family of two can occupy a woman for 18–20 years, long enough to develop all the complications of diabetes. Mothers should be encouraged to give themselves some time for daily body maintenance, perhaps when their partner is at home and can look after the children. The GP and practice nurse can keep an eye on the way in which the patient is coping with her diabetes when she attends with her children, as well as ensuring that she attends for her own check-ups.

Menopause and hormone replacement therapy

Blood glucose balance occasionally becomes erratic during the menopause although afterwards insulin requirement may fall. This may not apply if the woman is given hormone replacement therapy (HRT).

The MHRA (2007) states: 'use of HRT increases the risk of breast cancer, endometrial cancer and ovarian cancer in a duration-dependent manner. There is no evidence for a beneficial effect of HRT on cardiovascular disease—in fact HRT has been shown to increase the risk of myocardial infarction and venous thromboembolism, especially in the first year of use, and to increase the risk of ischaemic stroke. The risk of most of these conditions increases with age, therefore increasing the overall risks the longer HRT is taken.' The MHRA concluded:

- 'for the treatment of menopausal symptoms, HRT is beneficial for the majority of women in the short-term;
- when used in the long-term the balance of risks and benefits of HRT is such that it should be restricted to second-line therapy for the prevention of osteoporosis.

The decision to use HRT should take into consideration a woman's age, history, risk factors, and personal preferences, and for all women the minimum effective dose should be used for the shortest duration. Continued use of HRT should be regularly re-assessed (e.g. at least annually).'

Diabetes increases the risk of cardiovascular disease and thus HRT should be used with particular caution.

A Cochrane review concluded that there was a lack of evidence about the use of HRT in women with type 1 diabetes (doi: 10.1002/14651858. CD008613.pub2).

Summary

- All the changes of womanhood can influence, and be influenced by, diabetes.
- Menstrual irregularity is common.
- Glucose control may vary around period time.
- Diabetes is common in PCOS.
- PCOS is common in overweight diabetic women.
- Use the best contraception for each individual. OCPs can be used in diabetic women after risk assessment.
- Fertility may be impaired in some diabetic women.
- Pre-pregnancy counselling and care is essential to reduce the risk of congenital malformation.
- Diabetic pregnancy is associated with increased risk of most complications for mother and fetus.
- Normoglycaemia and very careful glucose monitoring avoiding hypoglycaemia is crucial.
- Diabetic pregnant women should be cared for only by specialist diabetic–obstetric services.
- Screening for GDM is essential as treatment is proven to reduce maternal and fetal risk.
- GDM may persist as diabetes post-partum, and increases long-term diabetes risk. These patients should have diet and exercise advice and be followed up.
- Glucose levels may alter around and after menopause.
- HRT is more risky in diabetic patients than in non-diabetic women and MHRA advice should be followed.

Further reading

NICE CG 63 <http://www.nice.org.uk/guidance/cg63>
Reviews of current thinking about diabetes and pregnancy: *Diabetic Medicine* 2014; **31** (whole issue 3)

Diabetes in men

Fatherhood

The diabetic father is under many of the same pressures as the diabetic mother. He may be the one looking after the children. In many cases, he may be the breadwinner. He may worry that his diabetes is going to stop him working and make him let his family down. As with working women, he may be working so hard that he neglects himself and his diabetes. He may ignore check-ups because he does not wish to take time off work. Working men or women may be difficult to contact—text or e-mail may help. People don't want to take time off work but they may be prepared to attend an evening or Saturday clinic. Being self-employed can be particularly stressful.

Infections

Diabetic men may develop candidal balanitis. Treat with antifungals as in women (● p. 335). Consider treating the partner. Seek advice early if the balanitis does not resolve. As in women, the critical factor is returning the blood glucose toward normal.

Fertility

There are conflicting reports about whether or not diabetes alters sperm quality, quantity, or motility. Obesity may be a confounding factor. Some diabetic men may have retrograde ejaculation. Fertility does not appear to be impaired unless there is significant erectile dysfunction. There appears to be no problem for the fetus if the father is hyperglycaemic at conception.

Libido

Untreated diabetes or hyperglycaemia can temporarily reduce libido. The psychological stress and distress of the new diagnosis and subsequent difficulties may also reduce libido.

Erectile dysfunction

Of all men with diabetes, 30–50 % may experience erectile dysfunction (ED), either temporarily or permanently. ED may be under-reported as the ambience of many diabetic clinics or busy surgeries is not always conducive to such sensitive discussions. Bearing in mind that it may have taken considerable courage on the patient's part to reveal this symptom, any mention of sexual difficulties should be followed up, if necessary at another appointment with appropriate privacy and time, and preferably with his partner. Remember that ED is a marker for cardiovascular disease and earlier mortality.

Define the patient's problem. ED is the inability to develop and maintain a penile erection sufficient for sexual performance. Although some men with diabetes do have permanent ED associated with diabetic tissue damage, many have reversible ED. Reversible factors or those suggesting another condition requiring investigation and treatment should be sought, but a final decision that the ED is due to diabetes does not mean that the patient and his partner cannot be helped.

Assessment of a man with ED

- Take a full history, including prescribed and non-prescribed drugs and alcohol.
- Examine the patient including genitals.
- Check for penile deformity which may make drug treatment of ED dangerous.
- Check for evidence of the causes of ED.
- Remember that ED is a marker for increased risk of CVD and premature death.
- Seek CVD and ensure full treatment of active CVD and risk factors.
- Consider referral for cardiac check if ED in < 50 yr olds.
- Seek evidence of vasculopathy and neuropathy in particular.
- Consider his emotional state.

Blood tests

- Testosterone before 11 a.m.
- Check with your local endocrinologist—free testosterone, if available, is more helpful (*J Urol* 2012; **187**:1369–73; doi:10.1016/j.juro.2011.11.095).
- If total testosterone < 12 nmol/l repeat with sex hormone-binding globulin (SHBG), LH, FSH, prolactin, and prostate-specific antigen (PSA).
- If total testosterone < 12 nmol/l consider specialist opinion.
- If LH or FSH are low or normal in the face of low testosterone (they should be raised in that case), seek specialist advice (probable pituitary disease).
- Usual annual review blood tests if not done recently.

Causes of erectile dysfunction in diabetic men
- Psychological, including anxiety and depression
- Drugs, including antihypertensives, antidepressants, fibrates, statins, NSAIDs, H_2 blockers, psychotropics, allopurinol
- Alcohol (acute or chronic intake)
- Neuropathy (peripheral and/or autonomic)
- Vascular disease
- Endocrine–hypogonadism

All patients will have some psychological problems either causing or due to the condition. ED due to psychological factors may start suddenly, be associated with reduced libido, and be patchy, i.e. present with one woman and not with another, or present during masturbation but not when intercourse is attempted. However, all these can apply to ED due to diabetic tissue damage.

Before considering treatment of ED ensure that all cardiovascular risk factors including obesity are being managed fully, bearing in mind that some of the drugs may be causing the ED. ARBs may improve ED. Stop smoking and reduce excess alcohol intake.

Evidence of diabetic tissue damage elsewhere, such as retinopathy, nephropathy, neuropathy, and PAD, make it more likely that the ED will be related to diabetic tissue damage. Improve blood glucose control as hyperglycaemia can cause non-specific malaise which may be associated with ED. An erectile response to alprostadil injection demonstrates adequate vascular supply (trained staff only, risk of priapism). In unresponsive patients angiography may identify treatable vascular disease. If autonomic neuropathy is evident elsewhere (e.g. with postural hypotension or problems with bladder emptying), the ED is likely to be neurogenic.

Endocrine causes can be suspected by finding other evidence of hypogonadism clinically. It is also more common in patients with other endocrine disorders.

More detailed studies can be undertaken in specialist centres, ideally, by a diabetologist or endocrinologist with a special interest in ED, or urology or genitourinary medicine. Check local arrangements.

Treatment of erectile dysfunction

Provide psychological support as needed. Some patients will need specialist psychosexual counselling. Some districts have psychologists trained in assessment and treatment of psychosexual problems. In the UK, men whose ED is due to diabetes are entitled to NHS prescriptions for drug treatment for this.

Phosphodiesterase type-5 inhibitors
Phosphodiesterase type-5 inhibitors (PDE5i) are the most popular. They include sildenafil, tadalafil and vardenafil.

Before prescription consider that sudden resumption of sexual activity may increase exertion (especially at night), causing hypoglycaemia, and may precipitate angina or a cardiac event in those with severe coronary atheroma.

Avoid these drugs in patients with:
- blood pressure < 90/50
- recent history of stroke
- ischaemic heart disease or cardiac failure
- severe hepatic failure
- renal failure—adjust the dose according to SPC
- known hereditary retinal degeneration
- non-arteritic anterior ischaemic optic neuropathy
- nitrates, doxazosin and other vasodilators, cimetidine, ketoconazole, and erythromycin

These drugs are effective in a high proportion of diabetic men. Tell patients that they work only after sexual stimulation. Side effects include headache, flushing, dizziness, dyspepsia, nasal congestion, and visual changes. See SPC or BNF for full list.

Alprostadil

There are two versions: an intra-urethral dose via an applicator and intra-cavernosal injection. The first dose of alprostadil should be given in the ED clinic. Teach the patient how to give it and to assess response.

Avoid in men with:
- penile deformities and those susceptible to priapism, e.g. sickle cell
- urethral infections, i.e. balanitis or urethritis (intra-urethral version)
- urethral abnormalities (intra-urethral version)

Warn all patients of the risk of priapism and provide written information to bring to their nearest A&E department. The BNF has specific guidance on the treatment of priapism. Other side effects include penile pain, bruising and scarring with injection, urethral burning, hypotension, dizziness, and headache.

Testosterone and androgen analogues

Testosterone treatment works only in patients with proven testosterone deficiency and should be started only by a specialist service (e.g. endocrinology). Do not give testosterone to patients who are not testosterone deficient, it will not help and may cause harm e.g. prostate problems or jaundice.

Summary

- Diabetic men and women may struggle to balance their responsibilities to work and family with their need to care properly for their diabetes.
- Diabetes does not appear to cause male infertility in the absence of ED.
- ED is common and multifactorial. Proper assessment to define cause is important.
- ED is a marker for risk of cardiovascular disease and premature death. Find and treat undiagnosed cardiovascular disease. Treat CVD risk factors in all ED patients.
- Control the blood glucose.
- Phosphodiesterase type-5 inhibitors are effective in many patients.
- Only prescribe testosterone in patients with proven deficiency.

Older people with diabetes

Introduction

Diabetes is predominantly a disease of older people in whom type 2 is much more common than type 1 (although this can present at any age). Don't miss LADA (➔ p. 16). Diabetes prevalence varies according to ethnic variation within a population and increases with age. In the UK diabetes is found in 20 % men and 14 % women aged ≥ 75 yrs (Health Survey for England, HSE, ✎ <http://www.hscic.gov.uk/catalogue/PUB09300/HSE2011-Ch4-Diabetes.pdf> (Figure 19.1). The combination of old age, diabetes, and diabetes tissue damage can require complex care from many agencies. The potential role of preventative care is considerable, but its delivery can be difficult. Patient education is as important in the elderly as in the young, but it may take longer. Make the time.

Factors for the increased frequency of diabetes in the elderly include increased insulin resistance and reduced glucose clearance, as well as obesity and lack of exercise. Thiazides, steroids, and other drugs are diabetogenic.

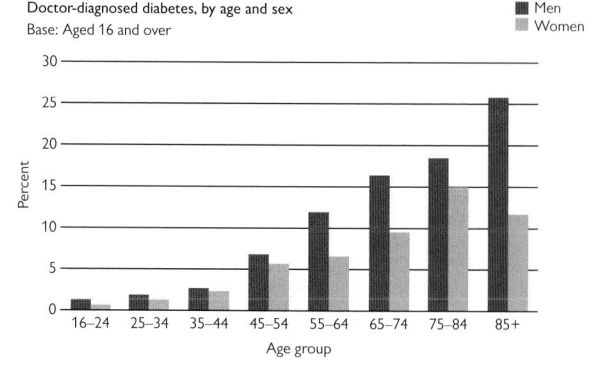

Fig. 19.1 Doctor-diagnosed diabetes in people aged ≥ 16 yrs (Health Survey of England 2011).

Presentation and assessment of diabetes in older people

Presentation

HSE found previously undiagnosed diabetes in 2.8 % of men, and 8.2 % of women aged ≥ 75 yrs. Check those at high risk of diabetes (Chapter 1 and Box 1.3, ⊃ p. 6), and also elderly patients if:

- unwell with no apparent cause
- thirst (but this lessens with age)
- polyuria, incontinence, or any urinary symptom
- cardiovascular disease
- ulcers or wounds
- recurrent infections or prolonged infections including tuberculosis
- falls
- confusion
- depression
- dementia
- 'off legs'
- difficulty coping
- repeated attendances (GP or hospital)

Assessment

It takes at least 40 mins fully to assess an older new diabetic patient. If the patient permits, see him/her with a partner or relative. Follow the assessment in Chapter 2 (⊃ pp. 23–30), with particular emphasis on a functional assessment. This includes ability to cope with activities of daily living, social support, accommodation, and careful drug history. Consider excess alcohol. Seek comorbidities. Assess vision, hearing, dexterity, mobility, and cognitive function. Review their health care arrangements. Who coordinates care? How easily is it accessed?

Management

Who supports the older diabetic patient?

- Most older diabetic patients function normally on their own.
- Older patients who have problems with self-care or are vulnerable may have a partner or caring relative or friend. If not who will provide care?
- Every older person should have a landline and/or mobile phone that they can use easily (big buttons, big on-screen font, audible).
- Vulnerable older diabetic patients who live alone should have a wrist band or pendant alarm (e.g. personal alarms: ℘ <http://www.ageuk.org.uk>)
- Advise wearing a diabetes/health warning pendant or bracelet (e.g. ℘ <http://www.medicalert.org.uk>). Is there a local 'message in a bottle' scheme to hold medical information? Some people just use an envelope attached to the fridge with a magnet.

Easy to read, easy to use, easy to access (?)

Written information

Most people find larger text easier to read as they get older. Many diabetic patients have visual impairment. This sentence is written in 8.5 point. It is too small for most older people to read easily. Use lower-case plain black font in 12–14 point aligned to the left margin on a plain white background. Use one font (not many) with bold for emphasis if needed. Use matt, not glossy, paper of ≥ 90 g weight. Note that current disability legislation requires that information provided for patients is easy to use.

If patients have difficulty seeing check for treatable causes (➡ pp. 268–73).

Easy to use

- Packs are harder to open if one has any upper limb, coordination, or visual problem. Childproof tablet bottles are a particular challenge. Provide easy access medications (store safely in homes with children). Consider pharmacy pre-packed daily dosage boxes or easy-open blisters.
- Electronic devices are often small and fiddly. Numbers are hard to read. So are instructions. Ensure that patients can actually use any devices (e.g. SMBG meters, insulin pens).
- Some older people find the electronic world difficult. A clear list of specific instructions may be needed for electronic equipment. Don't refer older patients to a website unless they are happy using the internet.

Easy to access

- Complex telephone answering systems, answer phones, busy receptionists, and complex appointment rules are barriers for all of us. Give vulnerable diabetic patients a direct line to someone who can deal with their concerns.
- Complex systems in the new NHS make it hard to understand who does what, when, and how in a patient's care. Provide the patient with a list in large print of who does what for him/her and how to contact them.
- Physical access to primary or secondary care is a huge issue. Plan how the patient is going to get to his/her diabetes appointments. Does transport need to be booked? Prepare the patient for possible long

journeys and waiting times if using NHS transport. He/she may miss meals. Patients should carry food, drink, and daytime medications to avoid hypoglycaemia or other glucose fluctuations.

- Can the patients hear? Remind them to bring their hearing aid—diabetes increases the risk of deafness (p. 274). If they need one and have not been assessed yet, arrange an assessment.
- Does the patient need an interpreter? If so, book one or bring one. Older patients from ethnic minority groups are less likely to speak English than their younger relatives.
- Don't waste the patient's time and effort. Combine appointments if possible—doctor, nurse, dietitian, podiatrist—but remember that older patients tire easily. Provide food and drink if they need it.
- A 15-min clinic visit, simple for the doctor, can be a whole-day nightmare for a disabled elderly person.
- Home visits are very helpful and provide much more information and educational opportunity than a clinic or practice appointment. Can the local DSN do one?

Diet

Diet is as important as in younger patients, but introduce change gradually. The patient has had many years on their previous diet and so is unlikely to want to change. One danger is of starvation because of over-strict interpretation of sucrose reduction or vague memories of the old low-carbohydrate diet. Sudden introduction of fibre can cause abdominal discomfort. Regular meals of sufficient calorie content but not too much sugar are the most important advice for thin, elderly people. Include snacks between meals. A practical weight-reducing diet with less fat and sugar is needed for overweight patients.

Ensure that the dietitian meets the person who does the shopping and cooking if this is not the patient. If the patient needs insulin (other than daily long-acting) the food must be linked with insulin injections which is hard when an outsider (e.g. the district nurse) is giving it.

Exercise

- Diabetes increases sarcopenia (loss of muscle mass with weakness)
- Keep the patient moving, even if limited by joint stiffness or pain
- Any exercise is helpful—walking, gardening, housework
- Patients can exercise while sitting
- Daily exercise is best
- Beware undue pressure on neuropathic feet
- Protect injury-prone areas—legs or hands
- Refer to physiotherapy if the patient has severe mobility problems
- Help carers to implement simple and appropriate exercise programmes

Medication review

- Review all medication
- Reduce polypharmacy where appropriate (you are about to add more drugs)
- Stop thiazides and replace with less diabetogenic agent
- Review steroids—are they really needed, and in that dose?
- Other glucose-affecting drugs (e.g. antidepressants)?

Glucose targets in older people
- As for younger people if safe and practical.
- If the patient lives alone, has problems with self-care, or if hypoglycaemia is a risk, aim for HbA$_{1c}$ 58–69 mmol/mol (7.5–8.5 %) or glucose levels 8–11 mmol/l.
- In frail elderly patients unable to maintain good glucose balance safely, the aim is symptom prevention without hypoglycaemia. This can be hard to achieve.

Non-insulin treatments in older patients (see Chapter 8, (➲ pp. 113–46))

Metformin
- Safe and practical for many elderly patients
- Long-acting preparation easier to remember and fewer side effects
- Monitor U&E regularly
- Rare risk of lactic acidosis in hypoxic patients or those with renal failure

Sulfonylureas
- All cause hypoglycaemia (➲ pp. 181–200)
- Long-acting drugs convenient but can cause prolonged hypoglycaemia
- Gliclazide M/R 30 mg initially with monthly increments if needed. No need for dose reduction in elderly
- Patients who eat at variable times might benefit from tolbutamide or glipizide (start treatment at a lower dose for both) with the meal
- Multiple drug interactions (➲ p. 127)
- Familiar to most doctors

Meglitinides
- Repaglinide could be useful with variable meal times and quantities
- SPC advices against use of repaglinide in patients > 75 yrs old as there have been no studies
- Nateglinide—experience in patients > 75 yrs old limited

Incretin-effect enhancers
- Linagliptin—no need for dosage adjustment but clinical experience in > 80 yrs is limited
- Saxagliptin and sitagliptin—no need for dosage adjustment but limited safety data in patients > 75 yrs old
- Vildagliptin—no dosage adjustment needed
- Exenatide—very limited experience in patients > 75 yrs old. Needs injection (easier than insulin pens for most patients)
- Liraglutide and lixisenatide—no dosage adjustment needed but limited experience in ≥ 75 yrs

SGLT2 inhibitors
- Dapagliflozin contraindicated > 75 yrs of age, more adverse reactions ≥ 65 yrs of age
- Canagliflozin—≥ 65 yrs of age—consider renal function and risk of volume depletion; ≥ 75 yrs more adverse effects.
- Empagliflozin—no dose adjustment for age, but beware volume depletion if >75 yrs old, and avoid if > 85 yrs old

Non-insulin treatments ineffective?
- Prescribe insulin. Persistent hyperglycaemia makes patients feel awful.
- Add insulin to oral agents where SPC allows.

Insulin in older patients (see Chapter 9, (⬅ p. 147–80))

Most older patients are completely capable of giving their own insulin and adjusting the dose according to blood glucose concentration.

Potential problems
- Visual impairment
- Reduced dexterity
- Cognitive impairment (which may vary)
- Erratic timing and quantity of meals eaten
- Risk of hypoglycaemia

Practical issues of insulin in older people
Type 1 diabetes, which may be slow onset, can occur in older patients (⬅ p. 16). They will be insulin-dependent.

Most patients needing insulin are type 2 and already on tablets. These should be continued as they may still be providing some glucose lowering. Adding Lantus®, Levimir®, or Tresiba® once daily may be sufficient to achieve glucose aims. When compared with Lantus®, Tresiba® appears less likely to cause hypoglycaemia in the elderly. Twice daily 30/70 analogue insulin mixtures before meals may be required in patients in whom once-daily insulin fails to cover post-prandial high glucose. Some patients may transfer to basal bolus regimens. District nurses are rarely able to provide more than twice-daily support.

If an insulin-treated patient has a very variable eating pattern, or refuses food, it can be extremely difficult to control their blood glucose. Carers can be given an insulin pen and a simple sliding scale and inject analogue insulin (e.g. Humalog® or Novorapid®) after food has been eaten. A single small dose of longer-acting insulin can be given in the morning if needed.
- Who is going to give the insulin? Patient? Carer? District nurse?
- If more than one person is caring for the patient do they all know about diabetes and how to manage the insulin?
- When is it going to be given?
- Who is going to buy and prepare the meals? Does the patient need Meals on Wheels or home-delivered foods?
- Is glucose available, e.g. easy-to-open glucose tablets or gel, Lucozade® (all may be hard to open)? A dish of sugar lumps/cubes may be simplest.
- Are carbohydrate snacks available? Easy to unwrap?
- Are the insulin and food going to coincide? District nurses have busy schedules and may not arrive at the patient's usual meal time.
- Where will the insulin be kept? If the patient is confused they should not be able to access the insulin.

Diabetes education in older people

'Does he take sugar?' was a BBC Radio 4 programme about disability broadcast in 1995. In diabetes this translates to 'he doesn't take sugar, does he?' Older diabetic people are often bypassed and patronized in this way. One 65-yr-old man told me he had been given a booklet about 'Mr Insulin and Mrs Sugar' at diagnosis.

The majority of older people with diabetes are fully able to run their own lives and manage their own care, and must be treated with courtesy and respect. Every patient with newly diagnosed diabetes should have an explanation in appropriate terminology (Chapter 4, ⊃ pp. 55–66). If the patient permits, include the partner, relative, or carer in the discussion.

Hypoglycaemia

See Chapter 10, ⊃ pp. 181–200)

Hypoglycaemia impairs cerebral function, which is what a person requires to recognize and treat it. Older diabetic patients often have cerebral atheroma and may find it hard to recognize hypoglycaemia, and even harder to initiate appropriate treatment. It takes about 45 mins for normal cerebral function to return after hypoglycaemia in younger people, but this time may be twice as long or even longer in the elderly. Features of hypoglycaemia in the elderly include:

- vagueness
- malaise
- confusion
- forgetfulness
- inactivity
- falls
- fractures
- sleepiness
- inattention
- being difficult to care for
- irritability or aggression
- paranoid behaviour
- coma
- cardiac arrhythmia or acute coronary event (which may be silent)
- apparent or actual stroke
- frequent admissions or GP call-outs
- hypothermia

Carers should have a high index of suspicion. If in doubt give oral glucose. Hypoglycaemia can kill elderly patients and must be avoided.

Tissue damage

No new symptom should be attributed to 'just old age'. Tissue damage is common in the elderly. Some patients have had decades of diabetes; others have had a long duration of diabetes pre-diagnosis. Seek tissue damage at diagnosis as most older patients will have some (Chapter 14, ➔ pp. 245–99).

Visual symptoms

Investigate. Cataract is common in the elderly and more so in diabetes. Cataract extraction can give a new lease of life. The retina cannot be assessed with severe cataracts, and so treatable retinopathy or macular degeneration may be missed (➔ pp. 268–73).

Hearing (➔ p. 274)

Deafness is common in the elderly and may act as a considerable barrier to care. Check for wax then refer for audiometry. Diabetes increases the risk of deafness.

Dexterity and mobility

Musculoskeletal damage (➔ pp. 296–7), and/or arthropathy limits dexterity and mobility. Clarify the problem and arrange orthopaedic or rheumatological referral if appropriate. Treat Dupuytren's contracture, trigger finger, and frozen shoulder—all complications of diabetes.

Type 2 diabetes is a disease of overweight sedentary people. Diabetes may limit mobility in many ways—stroke, foot problems, vascular disease, neuropathy, osteoarthritis, poor vision, or the breathlessness of cardiac disease.

Cardiac disease (➔ pp. 253–6)

Have a high index of suspicion for cardiac ischaemia, which may be difficult to detect in a diabetic elderly person in whom silent cardiac events are common.

The management of cardiac failure may be a balancing act between resolution of cardiac symptoms and biochemical derangement. Over-diuresis risks renal failure. Ankle oedema increases the risk of ulceration.

Nephropathy (➔ pp. 275–9)

Renal damage may develop insidiously, and the first sign may be hypoglycaemia. Diuretics, recurrent UTI, NSAIDs, dehydration, and hypertension may worsen the situation.

Postural hypotension(➔ p. 282)

Remember that autonomic neuropathy can cause postural hypotension and may precipitate falls. Hypotensive drugs can worsen this, so monitoring of blood pressure treatment in someone with diabetes should include lying and standing values. Modern target-oriented care with rewards for attaining a number may increase the risk of inadvertent over-medication and falls. Treat the patient not the target. (*JAMA Intern Med* 2014; **174**:588–95; doi:10.1001/jamainternmed.2013.14764).

Pressure sores

Sadly, these are common in the chair-bound or bed-bound diabetic patient and can rapidly turn into large holes. Any pressure sore is unacceptable. Major steps must be taken to prevent them by obtaining suitable seating or mattresses, and by teaching relatives or carers about pressure care. Hyperglycaemic urinary incontinence may contribute.

Feet

Foot care is vital. Most patients who need amputation are elderly. Diabetic patients > 60 yrs old should have regular chiropody/podiatry. Everyone caring for them should be taught about the risk of foot problems and how to prevent them. It is good practice for all healthcare professionals to look at the patient's feet on every visit (⊃ pp. 301–4).

Bladder and bowel problems (⊃ pp. 283, 288–9)

Bladder and bowel problems can be due to autonomic neuropathy or other factors. Incontinence may be precipitated by UTI. Thrush may cause severe perineal soreness. Urinary retention is less common, but diabetic neuropathy may add to the effects of prostatism. Constipation can be stubborn despite a high-fibre diet and may require laxatives or enemata. Diabetic neuropathic diarrhoea may cause urgency and faecal incontinence.

Risk factors for falls in diabetic patients

- Obese
- Sedentary
- Hypoglycaemia
- Visual problems:
  - retinopathy or maculopathy
  - cataract
  - laser treatment (reduced visual field and night vision)
- Neuropathy
  - peripheral sensory—painless (especially postural sensory loss) and painful
  - autonomic—postural hypotension
- Foot problems
  - ulceration
  - dressings or clumsy special boots or shoes
  - deformity
  - surgery (e.g. toe or limb amputation)
- Sarcopenia
- Hypertension—hence hypotensive therapy and postural drop
- Oedema (cardiac or renal) affecting walking
- Stroke
- Frequent urination and nocturia (high glucose, urinary tract infection)
- Dementia
- Diabetic diarrhoea and urgency (often early morning)

Diabetic patients are more likely to have osteoporosis than non-diabetic people (⊃ p. 296), more likely to fall, and more likely to sustain fractures. Women have about twice the risk of fractures of the hip, proximal humerus, and (if on insulin) foot (*J Clin Endocrinol Metab* 2001; **86**:32–8).

Mental effects

Cerebral atherosclerosis is more frequent in people with diabetes than in the general population. Patients may have one obvious stroke but multi-infarct dementia may be more common than is generally recognized.

Dementia is commoner in patients with diabetes than in the general population; relative risk Alzheimer's disease 1.46; vascular dementia 2.48; any dementia 1.51; mild cognitive impairment 1.21 (*Intern Med J* 2012; **42**:484–91. doi: 10.1111/j.1445-5994.2012.02758.x). It is more likely in those with micro- or macrovascular disease. Some patients have more than one form of dementia. Alzheimer's disease and diabetes have biochemical neuroendocrine similarities. Alzheimer's disease is sometimes called diabetes type 3. Note that memory problems may occur at a younger people with diabetes. Diabetes is common in those with dementia in whom it should be sought.

Carers may miss the transient cognitive problems of hypoglycaemia in patients known to be confused. Hypoglycaemia is more likely in patients with dementia especially if they miss meals and are on insulin or sulfonylureas. Occasionally, prolonged frequent hypoglycaemia can cause confusion or memory defects, or a state of paranoia which can be very hard to manage. Ensure carers know about hypoglycaemia and how to detect and treat it.

Depression is about twice as common in people with diabetes as in those without. The diagnosis may be less obvious in older patients and should be sought, particularly in those with poor glucose control or who are 'not coping'. Anxiety can also be an issue.

Principles of care for people with either dementia or diabetes or both:
- Aim for early detection of the secondary condition
- Prevent symptomatic hyperglycaemia
- Reduce the risk of distress in each patient
- Apply safe and effective medication management
- Prevent unnecessary hypoglycaemia
- Reduce the risk of further functional impairment and disability
- Reduce unnecessary hospitalisation
- Avoid institutionalisation
- Support and advise families and carers

See guidance: *Diabet Med* 2014; 31 (9):1024–1031. doi:10.1111/dme.12467.

Drugs in the elderly

Diuretics

Diuretic therapy can cause raised urea and may add to the effects of early nephropathy. Diuretics can also cause hyponatraemia and hypokalaemia. Thiazide-induced glucose intolerance, although minor in many patients, may be sufficient to cause failure of maximal oral therapy to control the blood glucose and an alternative diuretic or antihypertensive should be found. Loop diuretics can also impair glucose tolerance.

β-blockers

Loss of warning of hypoglycaemia can be a disaster at any age, but especially in the elderly. β-blockers can worsen the symptoms of peripheral arterial disease and must be used with care in cardiac failure. Don't forget that β-blockers in eye drops can be absorbed.

Vasodilators

Drugs such as nitrates and calcium-channel blockers can exacerbate postural hypotension, as can ganglion blockers, although these are less often used. The ankle swelling induced by nifedipine can be uncomfortable.

NSAIDs

These are one of the most commonly prescribed drugs in the elderly. They interact with sulfonylureas to cause hypoglycaemia. Aspirin also reduces mortality after coronary thrombosis and the likelihood of stroke in patients with transient ischaemic attack, and possibly slows the development of retinopathy. It can reduce the blood glucose but this is rarely clinically relevant. NSAIDs should not be used in patients with nephropathy as they may precipitate renal failure.

Carers and care homes

Often diabetes care in an elderly person is provided by a relative or professional carer. Therefore it is essential that they accompany the patient to the clinic or surgery. Provide diabetes education for both the patient and the carer. The combination of diabetes and old age can place great burdens on carers, and their health and well-being must also be considered. Ensure that they obtain appropriate attendance allowances if relevant. Carers must know what to do in diabetes emergencies such as hypoglycaemia or a foot infection, and whom to call in an emergency.

Up to a quarter of patients in care facilities have diabetes although a pilot audit found that homes had identified just 10 %. In care homes and other residential facilities:

- there should be a diabetes policy.
- staff should seek diabetes on admission and at 2-yrly intervals.
- people with diabetes should have a formal care plan agreed with the patient, diabetes team, and care staff.
- agree and provide appropriate glucose monitoring.
- people should be given medication as prescribed (check this in self-medicators).
- train staff to give insulin if required with safe use of insulin training (➡ pp. 157–60).
- train staff to know the signs of hypoglycaemia and how to treat it.
- provide a healthy diet in appropriate quantities, including snacks. Allow patients to choose their food if able.
- provide exercise options.
- patients should have at least annual formal diabetes checks by a doctor, DSN (preferably specializing in diabetes in older people) and dietitian.
- provide regular podiatry and appropriate protective footwear.
- protect pressure areas.
- ensure retinal screening.
- ensure access to DSN advice.

There is national guidance on good clinical practice guidelines for care home residents with diabetes.
  ℜ <http://www.diabetes.org.uk/Documents/About%20Us/Our%20 views/Care%20recs/Care-homes-0110.pdf>

An England-wide National Diabetes Care Home audit is planned. Care homes should audit their diabetes care.

Summary

- Diabetes is a common disease of the elderly.
- The presentation may be subtle.
- Perform a full assessment, including functional aspects.
- Check support.
- Ensure good access to information, help, and clinic/practice.
- Tailor the treatment to the person and safety needs.
- Encourage a healthy diabetic diet.
- Everyone can exercise in some way.
- Review medication.
- Use non-insulin treatments appropriately.
- Do not delay insulin if needed.
- Do not strive for normoglycaemia if this is going to be dangerous.
- Provide full diabetes education.
- Diabetes tissue damage is common in elderly people.
- Increased diabetic and non-diabetes-related health problems may hinder care and impair quality of life.
- Falls are common in diabetes and risk fracture.
- Dementia is more common in people with diabetes than in those without.
- Choose medication carefully.
- Provide carers with diabetes education.
- Ensure that care homes and residential facilities manage diabetes well.

Further reading

Sinclair A J (ed.) *Diabetes in old age* (3rd edn). Chichester: John Wiley, 2009
IDF, Managing Type 2 diabetes in older people
🔗 <http://www.idf.org/sites/default/files/IDF%20Guideline%20for%20Older%20People.pdf>

Chapter 20

Diabetes in different ethnic groups

Introduction

The International Diabetes Federation (IDF) estimates that the number of people with diabetes worldwide will increase from 382 million in 2013 to 592 million in 2035; see Atlas: ℗ <http://www.idf.org/diabetesatlas/download-book> The prevalence of diabetes varies according to ethnic background and the country in which the person is living. It also varies according to city and social situation. Inner-city communities have a higher prevalence than some more rural areas. This also applies to the UK. Changes in incidence and prevalence make it hard to plan health care. In the UK, diabetes is particularly common in the South Asian community and there is an increased frequency in the African–Caribbean and Chinese communities (Tables 20.1 and 20.2). NDIS provides information about diabetes prevalence and care by local authority or CCG. There are communities from many different backgrounds in the UK. People often come from countries with a high prevalence of diabetes (see IDF atlas). There are refugees from recent conflicts including people from Somalia and other African nations, Afghanistan, and Eastern Europe. Modern UK populations are mobile. This interrupts continuity of health care and people may 'fall through the gap'.

There are many different facets of the main religious groups. Religious beliefs and practice may vary by country of origin and current home, with further adaptations for different localities, forming very varied communities. Ask each individual about his/her personal health, religious, dietary, and other beliefs and practices as relevant to diabetes care.

Table 20.1 Prevalence of different ethnic groups among people with diabetes

	Census 2011* per cent	National Diabetes Audit 2011/12 per cent
White	87.2	79.0
Mixed	2.0	1.1
South Asian	6.2	12.4
Black	3.0	4.3
Other	1.6	3.3

* Source Mathur et al doi:10.1093/pubmed/fdt116

**NDA 2011/12 for patients in whom ethnicity was recorded.

Table 20.2 The risk of type 2 diabetes in different ethnic groups in the UK

	Men	Women
	Hazard ratios	
White/not recorded	1	1
Indian	1.71	1.93
Pakistani	2.15	2.54
Bangladeshi	4.07	4.53
Other Asian	1.26	1.89
Black Caribbean	0.80	0.96
Black African	0.81	1.70
Chinese	1.96	1.41

Data corrected for age, BMI, family history, and smoking status, and compared with the White community (including people whose ethnicity was not recorded).

BMJ 2009;**338**:b880; doi: http://dx.doi.org/10.1136/bmj.b880

Communication

Good communication is essential for good diabetes care. The patient must learn what diabetes is, how to care for him/herself, and how to stay fit. Communication can be difficult if the patient and the healthcare team have different ethnic and cultural backgrounds. Diabetes and its care are particularly influenced by cultural beliefs and practice. As in all interactions, healthcare professionals must ensure that they communicate in an appropriate way for that particular patient, enlisting help from interpreters as required, and providing educational material in appropriate media (e.g. written, pictorial, video, etc).

The treatment of diabetes is always tailored to the individual's needs. The patient must accept treatment for it to succeed. In a condition in which tissue damage develops silently until it is well advanced, it can be hard for any patient who feels well to understand the need for careful diet, regular medication, blood glucose testing, and regular self-care and health checks. A diabetes specialist nurse or practice nurse who speaks the patient's language can be of considerable help in teaching patients about their condition.

Information is available in a variety of languages, e.g.

- Diabetes UK ᨠ <http://www.diabetes.org.uk/Other_languages/>
- Foot care leaflets written by a podiatrist, Richard Hourston, are available in 30 languages at: ᨠ <http://www.diabeticfoot.org.uk>

Asian communities

In the UK diabetes is more common in the adult South Asian community than in the general population. In some communities up to one in four Asian people of working age have diabetes. The frequency increases with increasing age, and older Asian patients are up to seven times as likely to have diabetes as the general population. The likelihood of diabetes appears to vary according to the place of origin and other factors such as diet. Diabetes is also increasing in prevalence among Chinese people.

Most diabetes in Asian people is type 2. Type 1 diabetes is uncommon, although up to 50 % of patients with type 2 diabetes eventually need insulin to control their blood glucose level.

Diabetes may go undetected until the patient attends their doctor for another reason. A community nurse spent one day a week at an Asian day centre. Within a couple of months she had discovered previously unrecognized diabetes in 20 people.

It may be difficult for any patient to accept that he/she has a disease and should therefore modify his/her lifestyle and diet, or take medication when he/she does not feel unwell. Beliefs about the causation of diabetes vary but it is often thought to be outside the patient's control. Beliefs about behaviour and family pressures may counteract health advice. Clothing, modesty, local surroundings, and social pressure may limit exercise. Involvement of religious centres and leaders in helping local people to look after their diabetes is often helpful.

One study found that Bangladeshi people with diabetes believed that diabetes was inflicted from outside rather than within; that it was brought on by too much sugar, and was due to an imbalance between what is taken in and body fluids emitted (e.g. sweat or semen); that thin people were unhealthy; and that exercise could make illness worse. They did not always understand the concept of preventive care. (*Br Med J* 1998; **316**:978–83; doi: http://dx.doi.org/10.1136/bmj.316.7136.978).

Diet

People of Asian origin living in the UK eat a wide variety of diets. Many eat a Western diet which may contribute to the increased frequency of diabetes in this Asian population. Take a dietary history and talk with the person who actually does the cooking (often not the patient). Ideally, the dietitian should speak Asian languages and have a clear understanding of Asian diets.

The main CHOs in Asian diets are breads (nan, chapatti, bhatura), rice, and pulses such as lentils and beans. The breads can be made with wholemeal flour, and brown rice can be used, although this may be considered inferior. Butter or ghee is often used in breads, pilau rice, and curries. Patients may not count fat in cooking when trying to reduce dietary fat. Sugar is used in sweetmeats and festival foods (e.g. Mithai, Laddoo, Jalaibi, Gajer halwa, Karah parshad). Patients may not realize that ghor (brown sugar) needs to be included in sugar totals.

Suspicion that a food breaches religious rules may mean that the whole meal is discarded. Asian patients often prefer to eat food brought into hospital by their family. People vary in the strictness with which they observe religious rules, but their wishes must be respected. Vegetarians may be vegans who risk vitamin B12 deficiency. Other vegetarians eat dairy products. The use of ghee has religious significance. Different foods may have different significance under varied circumstances. Many foods are believed to cause allergies, and particular foods may be avoided in certain illnesses. Some foods are considered hot and others cold, and are taken to treat certain conditions. Some foods are regarded as 'strong' (e.g. sugar, ghee, beef, lamb). Raw foods and those which have been baked or grilled may be regarded as indigestible. In general, South Asian people eat less fruit and vegetables than other peoples. They may eat karela (➲ p. 378). Ensure adequate calcium and vitamin D intake (➲ p. 76).

Exercise

While South Asian patients may be aware that exercise will improve sugar control, many find it hard to include in everyday life. This especially applies to women. Reasons for not doing exercise include fulfilling family or work obligations, 'women cannot go out' but must cook and clean (of course, this includes physical activity), unused to going out and frightened, no chaperone, lack of single-sex facilities (*Health Ed Res* 2006; **21**:43–54).

See McAvoy B R and Donaldson L (eds). *Health Care for Asians*. Oxford: Oxford Medical Publications, 1990.

African and Caribbean communities

Diabetes is more common in this community than in White Europeans (see Tables 20.1 and 20.2). African Caribbean patients usually have type 2 diabetes. They are more often overweight and are more insulin-resistant than Europeans, but have a less unfavourable lipid profile than South Asian patients and are more physically active (*Int J Epidemiol* 2001; **30**:111–17; doi:10.1093/ije/30.1.111; *Int J Obesity Relat Metab Disorders* 1999; **23**:25–33; *Heart* 1997; **78**:555–63; doi:10.1136/hrt.78.6.555). Perhaps because of this they have a lower rate of coronary disease than one might expect, although they are prone to resistant hypertension.

People from African–Caribbean communities may mistrust advice, treatment, and services provided for diabetes care. The sun and general lifestyle in Africa or Caribbean countries is thought to be better for health than UK living. Medications and 'chemicals' may be mistrusted (*Br J Gen Pract* 2007; **57**:461–9).

Women from African communities, and some Middle Eastern or Asian communities, may have been subjected to female genital mutilation which can increase the risk of urinary infection and cause problems around pregnancy.

Diet

In some African cultures overweight people are viewed as more prosperous or more attractive. Feeding people is a sign of love in most cultures worldwide. Traditional foods may be very sweet, and many foods (e.g. jerk chicken or pineapple fritters) are fried. Salty foods (e.g. salt fish) are enjoyed. CHO foods include potato, sweet potato, yam, cassava, rice, cereals, breads, dumplings, beans (e.g. kidney beans), plantain, and noodles. Sauces may include coconut milk. Traditional foods are preferred and dietary advice that incorporates these is welcomed. Encourage a reduction in sugar and salt (e.g. using unsalted dried cod), and steaming, baking, or grilling rather than frying.

Patient advice can be found at: <http://www.diabetes.org.uk/Documents/catalogue/Living_Afro_Carribean.pdf>

Ketosis-prone type 2 diabetes

In the USA and increasingly in the UK a small proportion of patients with DKA have subsequently been found to be producing insulin long term (albeit suboptimally) and to be able to manage without insulin for some years, although they may ultimately require it. Most of these patients are African–Caribbean and half are overweight. There is often a family history of type 2 diabetes. This has been labelled type 1b diabetes (⊃ p. 16). It occurs in up to half of all African–Caribbean patients admitted with DKA (*Ann Int Med* 2006; **144**:350–7; doi:10.7326/0003-4819-144-5-200603070-00011; *Arch Int Med* 1999; **159**:2317–22; doi:10.1001/archinte.159.19.2317). Such patients must be assessed and monitored by the DST. Use diet, metformin, and sulfonylureas once the acute episode is over. Teach patients about the risk of further DKA, provide blood ketone strips and information about how to access help fast.

Complementary therapies

Patients in all cultures may add complementary or alternative treatments, prayer, or spiritual treatments to medical advice. Most of such therapies advocated for diabetes have not been assessed in formal clinical studies. A Google® search for 'herbal remedies for diabetes' found 18 million items. One author notes >30 Indian plants that may lower glucose, and multiple commercial preparations (*J Clin Biochem Nutr* 2007; **40**:163–73; doi: 10.3164/jcbn.40.163). Internationally, remedies include aloe vera, bilberries, bitter melon, cinnamon, chromium, coconut, fenugreek, garlic, ginger, ginseng, and honey. Bitter melon or karela is widely eaten across South Asia and it has been shown to lower glucose (*Br Med J* 1981; **282**:1823–4). So has cinnamon (*Diab Care* 2003;**26**: 3215–8; doi:10.2337/diacare.26.12.3215; *Ann Fam Med* 2013; **11**:452–9; doi:10.1370/afm.1517). Water drunk from vessels made of pterocarpus wood is believed to reduce glucose. The contents of many herbal remedies are unknown—some may be toxic, as may heavy-metal remedies. Homeopathic remedies are available. Patients also use acupuncture (e.g. for neuropathy). Colonic irrigation websites suggest this may help diabetes (unlikely).

Many Asian patients will consult an alternative practitioner. Western doctors should not take offence as alternative medicine is usual in the East and implies a 'belt-and-braces' approach to healthcare rather than lack of trust in a doctor's treatment. A variety of approaches include the advice of a hakim or vaid, Ayurvedic medicine, Hikmat, astrotherapy, urinotherapy (drinking urine is thought to help diabetes), herbal medicine, and homeopathy. Prayer is often used to support care.

African–Caribbean patients often use complementary remedies which may include teas (e.g. dandelion, a diuretic), lemon juice, or vinegar. They may take laxatives. Prayer can be particularly important—most patients will seek divine help for their illness. The support of a church or other religious group can be a great comfort.

Problems may arise when the alternative practitioner advises stopping the medical treatment or the physician stops the alternative therapy; or when the alternative therapy causes adverse effects or interacts with pharmaceuticals. Some 'herbal' remedies have been found to contain pharmaceuticals. Stopping insulin can kill patients with type 1 diabetes. Ask the patient what other treatment or advice he/she is using in an open way and discuss possible safety issues.

Patients who need insulin should be offered biosynthetic human insulin, as pork-derived or beef insulin may be against their religious beliefs. Even insulin itself may be viewed as inappropriate and stopped. This can lead to repeated admissions with severe hyperglycaemia as patients may not wish to upset the doctor by telling him that they have not taken the treatment.

Fasting

In addition to religious fasts, people may be trying to lose weight e.g. the '5:2' diet with five days eating and two fasting. Ask all patients specifically about any personal or religious rules about foods and about fasting.

Fasting

Many faiths require periods of fasting. In most cases, the local religious leader will advise people with diabetes that they do not need to do fast, but patients may still want to. Strict adherents may observe the following times of fasting:

- Bahá'i—in March
- Buddhists—afternoons
- Catholics—Ash Wednesday and Good Friday, with reduced food during Lent
- Eastern and Greek Orthodox—Lent, Holy Week, Nativity, Apostles, Dormition
- Hindus—varies, e.g. a specific day each week
- Jews—Yom Kippur, Tisha B'av, and other days
- Muslims—Ramadan, voluntary days

Ramadan

Ramadan is the month of fasting observed by Muslim communities. The timing varies each year by lunar calendar. Detailed advice can be found on ✆ <http://leicestershirediabetes.org.uk/searchresults.php?cat1=0&q=ramadan>, e.g. *BMJ* 2010; **340**:c3053; doi: http://dx.doi.org/10.1136/bmj.c3053. Ask Muslim patients if they are planning to fast and discuss potential risks with them. Advise pregnant women and patients with frequent hypoglycaemia or unawareness, hyperglycaemia or recent high-glucose emergencies, multiple complications, a very physical job, or acute illness not to fast, and caution should be advised in people on treatment that can cause hypoglycaemia.

Provide patient education well before Ramadan with dietetic support.

Food and fluid is permitted after sunset—the first meal is Iftar—and during the night. The last meal is Suhur (Sehur, Suhoor, or Sehri), just before sunrise, although in some communities Suhur is earlier in the night. In people with diabetes it is better just before sunrise.

Traditional foods for Iftar may contain high quantities of sugar and fat (fried food or oil added to cooked dishes). Advise patients to reduce these and eat more slow CHO—brown rice, chapatti, naan, and daal, with plenty of fruit and vegetables. Feasting follows during the celebrations on the first day of the next month—Eid ul-Fitr.

Patients on diet alone rarely have adverse sequelae from fasting. Nor do those on metformin, who should simply take this after the meal(s) if multiple dose (bigger dose after Iftar), or once after the largest meal if on the modified-release version.

Patients on sulfonylureas risk hypoglycaemia. They can be taken with the nocturnal meals but the dose taken at Suhur may need to be reduced. Modified-release gliclazide may be taken with Iftar. Meglitinides can be taken with meals, perhaps reducing the dose at Suhur. Glitazones can be taken once a day; it may be sensible to take them with Iftar. Exenatide must be taken close to a meal. DPP-4 inhibitors could be taken once daily as usual. Some evidence suggest incretin-effect enhancers given alone or with metformin do not cause problems during Ramadan.

Once-daily long-acting insulin may be continued, although the dose should be reduced depending on the usual level of glucose control. Multiple injections are more difficult. Analogue insulin can be taken with each meal during the night but care needs to be taken to avoid morning hypoglycaemia.

Patients should be aware that their insulin may need increasing if they are eating more during Eid ul-Fitr.

Exercise during the day can precipitate hypoglycaemia and patients who are observing the fast strictly may not treat it with oral glucose. This potential issue should be discussed beforehand. In this context glucose is an essential medicine (e.g. GlucoGel®).

Complications of diabetes

The NDA 2011/12 showed that 'when other factors, such as age, gender and type and duration of diabetes, were taken into account 'the eight reliable care processes were 7.1 per cent less likely to be recorded among patients with Asian ethnicity and 4.2 per cent less likely to be recorded for those with Black ethnicity than those with White ethnicity.' Patients must be checked for risk factors or the complications themselves to guide preventive care.

Ischaemic heart disease is common in Asian people. In a series followed for 11 yrs in Southall, the all-cause mortality of South Asians (242/730 died) aged 30–54 at baseline was 1.5 times that of the European cohort (172/304 died). The mortality ratio for circulatory disorders was 1.8 and that for heart disease was 2.02. In South Asians, circulatory disorders in total accounted for 77 % of deaths vs 46 % in Europeans (*Diabetic Med* 1998; **15**:53–9; doi: 10.1002/(SICI)1096-9136(199801)15:1<53::AID-DIA521>3.0.CO;2-V). South Asian people experience greater delays in obtaining appropriate specialist help and investigation for heart disease than Europeans, even though they are more likely to seek help for chest pain (*Lancet* 1997; **350**:1578–83). The increased risk of CVD was confirmed in the NDA 2010/11, which also showed that Black ethnic groups had a lower risk of CVD than White patients. Compared with Europeans, South Asian patients are more likely to be overweight and to have a high waist-to-hip ratio, unfavourable lipid profiles, and poorer glucose control.

In addition to greater cardiovascular risk, South Asian patients are more likely to develop microalbuminuria, and they are more likely to have retinopathy and hypertension (*Diabetic Med* 1998; **15**:672–7; doi: 10.1002/(SICI)1096-9136(199808)15:8<672::AID-DIA648>3.0.CO;2-3). Nephropathy occurs more often and earlier in South Asian diabetic patients, and they may need renal transplantation. Retinopathy and neuropathy are often severe when they are discovered, perhaps because there is a longer duration of diabetes before it is diagnosed. Foot problems do not seem as common as in other ethnic groups, possibly because of less constricting footwear and better personal foot care than other patients.

Both South Asian and African Caribbean patients are more likely to need renal replacement therapy (> 100 % more likely, NDA 2010/11) than the general population. They may form up to half of all patients requiring this in some clinics.

African–Caribbean-born patients with diabetes have a higher mortality from diabetes than the national rate (3.5× for men and 6× for women) (*BMJ* 1997; **314**:209–13; doi: http://dx.doi.org/10.1136/bmj.314.7075.209). The same applies for mortality from hypertension. Blood glucose control may be difficult in African–Caribbean patients, and they appear to have a greater risk of hyperosmolar non-ketotic hyperglycaemic states. They may have resistant hypertension which contributes to worsening their risk of endstage kidney disease. Calcium-channel antagonists appear particularly useful in this group, but multiple hypotensive agents are usually needed to improve blood pressure.

Foot ulcers are most common in White European diabetic patients 5.5/100 person-yrs vs 1.9 for South Asian and 2.7 for African–Caribbean (*Diabetes Care* 2005; **28**:1869–75; doi:10.2337/diacare.28.8.1869). This affects amputation rates too. The NDA found that White patients were more likely to be admitted with DKA than Asian patients.

Refugees

People from many nations seek asylum in the UK. They may have known diabetes or it may be diagnosed during health checks. Refugees have often fled atrocities and may have been badly injured, both physically and emotionally. They may have had minimal diabetes care in their country of origin—erratically available impure insulin of unknown type, dilute insulin (e.g. U40 i.e. 40 units/ml), infected or scarred injections sites, and no knowledge of diet or tissue damage. Some have extensive diabetic tissue damage. The new diagnosis of diabetes is yet another shock, as is the discovery of established tissue damage. Such patients may have little family or other support and be living in basic conditions. Their uncontrolled diabetes puts them at particular risk of infections such as tuberculosis, and injuries (gunshot, machete, torture) may not have healed properly. They may also have malaria, intestinal parasitaemia, HIV, and hepatitis B and C.

Find the right interpreter, perform a full assessment, treat any associated problems, and control the diabetes. Find and use local appropriate support groups. It is very rewarding to see someone who has never had proper diabetes care change from a terrified emaciated teenager into a smiling well-nourished healthy young woman.

Summary

- Good communication is essential for full diabetes education and care.
- Respect religious and cultural wishes.
- Diabetes is commoner in South Asian people, Chinese people, and Black African women compared with White European people.
- Reduce delays in diagnosis and appropriate treatment.
- Screen for, and treat, risk factors and tissue damage.
- South Asian patients are at increased risk of cardiovascular disease, retinopathy, hypertension, and nephropathy.
- African–Caribbean people are at increased risk of hypertension, nephropathy, and hyperosmolar non-ketotic hyperglycaemic states.
- White European patients have an increased risk of foot problems and DKA.
- Dietary advice must be tailored to the person's individual needs. Also talk to the person who prepares the food. Ask about fasting and provide safe education, dietary advice and support.
- Remember you may not be the patient's only health adviser.
- Refugees may have physical and emotional injuries and other health problems, often with poor previous diabetes care.
- Refugees may have continuing problems in obtaining proper diabetes care and appropriate standards of living.

Chapter 21

Work

Introduction

Diabetes is not a problem in most jobs. However, people with diabetes may experience difficulties at work. The job may make it hard to care for the diabetes optimally, or the diabetes may cause glucose or tissue complications which interfere with the job. Colleagues' and employers' attitudes vary widely and misunderstandings about diabetes and its effects can lead to problems.

Legal issues

In the UK it is illegal under the Equality Act 2010 for employers to discriminate against anyone because of disability. While people with diabetes may not think of themselves disabled they will often be considered so under the legislation (people with type 1 diabetes, and those with complicated type 2). The areas included are applications, interviews, aptitude tests, job offers, pay, terms of employment, training, discipline, promotion, dismissal, retirement, and redundancy. A person cannot be made redundant because he/she has become disabled. Recruiters can ask about health or disability to ensure that the interview and selection process comply as noted or to ensure that the person can do a task that is an essential part of the job. Employers must make 'reasonable adjustments' so that a person with diabetes is not disadvantaged compared with non-diabetic people at work. This could relate to hours of work. The Armed Forces are exempt from the Equality Act. <http://www.gov.uk/rights-disabled-person/employment>

These requirements are interpreted variably by different line managers or employers. Fear of difficulties may lead people with diabetes to conceal their condition. Concealment of a health issue that could interfere with how a job is done is likely to prevent any later claim against the employer under the Equality Act. If patients are on drugs which could cause hypoglycaemia, or have tissue damage which may impede their functioning, they should tell employers that they have diabetes, especially in any post in which hypoglycaemia or any disability from tissue damage could place them or others at risk. Diabetes treated solely by diet is not a barrier to employment unless the person has tissue damage which impedes function relevant to the job.

Practical issues

People with diabetes can apply for, and successfully perform, most jobs. The Equality Act protects them against discrimination in the workplace; however, each person with diabetes needs to make an individual decision about the job—whether it is the right post for them, and whether they can cope with it. Patients' abilities to manage their diabetes vary widely, and this will influence their job satisfaction and effectiveness. They will need to make their own balance between happiness, pay, and health.

Factors to consider are:
- the hours
- normal working day
- shifts—fixed or variable?
- journey to and from work
- travel for work
- physical activity

- working environment (e.g. temperature)
- clean or dirty job, and access to hand washing
- access to food and drinking water
- meal and snack breaks
- access to mobile or other telephone
- hazard to self or others
- responsibilities to and for organizations, things, people
- support at work
- colleagues at work
- access to help

Effects of the job on diabetes

Sedentary work

This poses few problems (other than lack of exercise). However, if the person is more active at home at weekends, he/she may need a different dose of glucose-lowering drugs for weekdays and weekends. If someone is normoglycaemic during a sedentary working day, unexpected exercise needs to be covered by extra carbohydrate. A change from an active to a sedentary job may need a reduction in food eaten and/or a reduction in hypoglycaemic treatment. Patients may need to guard against weight gain.

Physical work

The person needs to eat enough to fuel the work. This is not usually a problem, but some people with newly diagnosed diabetes are frightened of eating the wrong foods and they reduce their diet. Insulin-treated patients, and many on sulfonylureas, need regular snacks. People working on building sites and in similar industries must wear protective footwear, headwear, and gloves and have up-to-date tetanus immunization. Are they working at height, e.g. scaffolding, roof? If so, there must be no hypoglycaemia.

Shift work and hours

Shift work can be difficult for patients on insulin, and sometimes for those on sulfonylureas. They need to balance the timing of food intake, exertion, and insulin. One regimen is to have evenly spaced meals and snacks when awake, including one before going to sleep. A long-acting insulin is given every 24 hrs and analogue very-short-acting insulin is given before meals. Encourage patients to discuss their work pattern with their doctor—many do not and find it difficult to resolve their glucose balance. A Canadian study of people with type 1 diabetes found that those doing shift work had higher HbA$_{1c}$ than non-shift workers (*Occup Med (Lond)* 2013; **63**:70–2; doi: 10.1093/occmed/kqs176).

Working hours may influence diabetes control. A US study found that people with diabetes working > 40 hrs/wk had higher HbA$_{1c}$ than those working ≤ 20hrs/wk (*Am J Industrial Med* 2011; **54**:375–83; doi: 10.1002/ajim.20923).

Work risking infection or contamination

Many people with diabetes work in healthcare. They should have annual influenza immunization, a one-off pneumococcal immunization, and Hepatitis B immunization (➲ pp. 290, 402).

Many jobs involve dirt or grease, or infection risk (e.g. gardening, building). Finger-prick glucose testing may not be safe or feasible (ensure that tetanus immunization is up-to-date). Some patients find CGM helpful in this situation. Insulin injections may also be impossible, e.g. if impeded by protective clothing or dirt. CSII may be the answer. Glucose or food may be difficult to eat safely. Some glucose gels (e.g. GlucoGel®) can be ingested using a non-touch technique, but this is harder when someone is hypoglycaemic. Hand-washing facilities and a clean place to inject and eat food should be arranged.

Work involving driving or travelling

Driving, including PCV and LGV, is discussed in detail on (→ pp. 395–400). Any employee who drives in relation to his work must inform his employer of his diabetes. Failure to do so is likely to invalidate insurance cover. People with diabetes who drive for work must be prepared to keep meticulous SMBG and other health records. Patients must not become hypoglycaemic while driving. If long journeys are involved, insulin-treated patients should snack and test blood glucose at least every 2 hrs. If possible, the patient should take packed meals as it may be hard to find the components of a diabetes diet on the road. In any case, anyone who travels frequently or for long distances should carry sufficient carbohydrate for an emergency full meal in the car. Diabetes UK can provide advice about insurance.

The businessman or woman

Some of the hazards of the traditional business life are smoking, alcohol, and rich food. Smoking is now banned in UK workplaces and restaurants. People with diabetes can drink in moderation (1–2 units a day), but must never drink on an empty stomach. To reduce intake alcohol can be alternated with non-alcoholic drinks or diluted. Eating out may place a strain on the diabetes diet, but most restaurants will grill meat or fish and provide plain potatoes, rice, or pasta, with bread to top up. Salad or vegetables and fruit are usually available and there is no need to have butter, dressing, sugar, or cream.

Colleagues at work

People with diabetes on insulin or drugs which may cause hypoglycaemia should tell their work colleagues that they have diabetes. Insulin-treated patients should teach close colleagues what to do in the event of hypoglycaemia. Everyone on insulin should carry glucose, and a supply at work is essential. Some patients keep a supply of insulin and a blood-testing kit at work—this must be locked away. People who give insulin injections at work should do so openly in a clean environment with explanations to avoid stigmatization as a drug abuser. The same applies to SMBG. Many people do not test at work at all and miss essential information this way.

Effect of diabetes on the job

Glucose problems

High glucose levels may cause tiredness and lethargy, and increase urination. Risk of infection in small wounds increases.

Hypoglycaemia impairs concentration and may cause overt confusion and collapse. As well as endangering the patient and anyone for whom he/she is responsible, a severe hypoglycaemic attack alarms work colleagues and employers and may lead to job restriction or dismissal, although this can be challenged legally. Patients may forget or minimize hypoglycaemic episodes at work and fail to appreciate the effect they have on those at work. Urgently address prevention of hypoglycaemia.

An international questionnaire study found that non-severe hypoglycaemic events caused 8.3–15.9 hrs lost work each month, with most time lost after nocturnal hypos.

    🕮 <http://www.sciencedirect.com/science/article/pii/S1098301511001331>

Diabetic tissue damage

This may be present when a person applies for a job, or may develop during employment. People with diabetes may fail to appreciate the existence or significance of complications.

Visual loss from diabetic eye disease, retinopathy, or cataracts can obviously affect someone's job. Cataracts should be extracted promptly. Retinopathy or its treatment can cause visual loss: new vessels may cause vitreous haemorrhage, maculopathy can cause severe visual loss, and laser photocoagulation can reduce peripheral vision.

PAD may limit walking distance; cardiac disease may limit exertion. Neuropathy in the hands may limit jobs requiring fine finger work, and in the feet may cause problems for those relying on foot work. Diabetic foot problems may result in months taken off work and may be repeatedly exacerbated if, for example, the job involves standing all day. Amputation or the need for crutches or a wheelchair may limit where a patient can work and what he can do. Fears about work may delay a patient seeking or accepting treatment for foot disease and other complications.

Nephropathy may require time-consuming treatment. Autonomic neuropathy may be embarrassing (e.g. gustatory sweating or diabetic diarrhoea) or dangerous (e.g. postural hypotension which may limit where the person may work with safety).

Hazardous occupations

Diabetes UK has produced 'guidelines to help employers decide whether a person with diabetes can work safely in a hazardous occupation:

- You should be as physically and mentally fit as people without diabetes.
- You should visit your diabetes care team for regular (at least annual) check-ups.
- Your diabetes should be well controlled.
- You should test your blood glucose levels and be well informed and motivated to care for your condition.

- There should be no cases of disabling hypos and you should be aware of your own hypo warning signs.
- You should not have advanced diabetes-related eye disease (retinopathy), kidney disease (nephropathy), or severe nerve damage (neuropathy).
- You should have no significant circulation disorders of the heart (e.g. coronary heart disease), legs or brain.
- Your suitability for employment should be reviewed annually by both an occupational physician and a diabetes specialist. The review should be based on previous criteria.
- You may find that if you develop diabetes whilst in employment, the organization may change the nature of your job. This could be sensible and may be worth considering.'

🔖 <http://www.diabetes.org.uk/upload/Employment_factsheet_final3.pdf>

Limitations on employment

Uncomplicated diabetes controlled by diet alone should not be a barrier to any job. Potential barriers to employment are the use of medications that can cause hypoglycaemia (especially insulin) or the presence of complications that may impede the ability safely to do the job (e.g. visual loss). Failure to manage the diabetes responsibly and control blood glucose levels may also mean that a person is considered unsafe. Employers may need to modify the job if a person is diagnosed diabetic while employed, especially if he/she needs insulin.

In the past having diabetes requiring insulin treatment excluded people from some jobs. While this may still be the case in some situations, increasingly, the relevance of a job-seeker's diabetes is considered on an individual basis, for example in the police, fire or ambulance services. There will be particular concern if the person is working in a high-risk environment, e.g. underwater, handling fast vehicles or firearms; or directly responsible for other people's lives (e.g. a surgeon). These kinds of jobs, in which hypoglycaemia could be fatal or in which a hypoglycaemic person could be injured or cause injury, need careful consideration by a both a diabetologist and an occupational physician. The patient will have to prove that he/she is in full control of his/her condition, that there is no risk of hypoglycaemia at work, and that he/she has no tissue damage that limits relevant function. Such patients should be referred to a consultant diabetologist for assessment and monitored regularly. There should be good liaison with the occupational health physician. Sometimes patients face the dilemma of health or work.

> Bill was a diabetic bus driver. Oral hypoglycaemics were not sufficient to control his blood glucose. He was advised to start insulin treatment. He refused because he would lose his job. Over the next two years his hyperglycaemia increased. He steadfastly refused to consider insulin despite warnings that his health might be permanently damaged. He developed severe diabetic retinopathy, jeopardizing his vision.

A changing situation

The situation is changing as better methods for self-monitoring became more widely available and employers become better informed about diabetes. Cases must be assessed individually, and it is prudent to advise reassessment or regular checks as diabetes is a progressive disease. Advise patients to check with individual employers for up-to-date information.

Diabetes is a rapidly moving field and occupational physicians may not always be aware of the extent to which people with diabetes can now control their condition. A patient who is experiencing difficulties with gaining employment or with their employer should ensure that any medical officer appointed by the company communicates with his/her GP and with his/her consultant diabetologist. Diabetes UK provides an advocacy service for people with diabetes having difficulties with employment.

Work record and time off

Most studies have shown an increase in sick leave. Studies may be hampered by employees' reluctance to admit to having diabetes for fear of losing their job. A Finnish study (*Diabetic Med* 2007; **24**:1043–8; doi: 10.1111/j.1464-5491.2007.02216.x) found that diabetic employees had about double the risk of physician-certified sick leave of those without diabetes. They had 59 extra sickness absences per 100 person/yrs vs non-diabetic colleagues, equivalent to 4 days off sick per year. The excess was predominantly due to pre-existing non-cardiovascular diseases: asthma, chronic bronchitis, prolapsed intervertebral disc, osteo- and rheumatoid arthritis, peptic ulcer, fibromyalgia, depression, and other psychiatric disorders.

In a US survey of people aged ≥ 25 yrs, 6 mths work disability secondary to illness/disability occurred in 26 % of those with diabetes, and 8 % of those without. People with diabetes earned less than those without (*Diabetes Care* 1999; **22**:1105–9; doi:10.2337/diacare.22.7.1105). A study of French gas and electricity workers showed that those with diabetes were more likely to become disabled (Hazard Ratio, HR 1.7), retire (HR 1.6), or die (HR 7.3) than those without diabetes. Between age 35 and 60 yrs diabetic employees each lost 1.1 yrs in the workforce compared with non-diabetics (*Diabetes Care* 2011; **34**:1344–9; doi:10.2337/dc10-2225).

A Scandinavian study compared people with diabetes with those without diabetes but with either hypertension or musculoskeletal problems, and with people with no health problems. People with diabetes had lower incomes and were more likely to be on a disability pension than those with hypertension or no problems. Diabetic patients had more sick days and were more likely to have psychological problems than healthy people (*Scand J Soc Med* 1997; **25**:39–43).

Some people with diabetes with recurrent admissions for glycaemic instability or who develop major tissue damage (e.g. foot ulcers) may have prolonged sick leave. This may enhance an employer's negative image of diabetes.

Retirement, superannuation, and pensions

Retirement planning and pensions arrangements are complex and the situation is changeable. The Equality Act protects disabled people from pension discrimination. Patients may seek early retirement on health grounds. Diabetes may entitle patients to an enhanced annuity on health grounds. Remind patients that their GP and diabetes consultant can help by providing accurate up-to-date information about their health. They should also be aware that it is in their interests to shop around for insurance and pension schemes. Diabetes UK will provide up-to-date advice.

Summary

- Diabetes rarely impedes the opportunity or capacity for employment.
- Diabetes is a disability covered by Equality Act 2010 UK.
- Factors which do influence employability and safety are the risk of hypoglycaemia and its consequences, and tissue damage which may reduce function.
- People with diabetes have more sickness absence than those without. Diabetes-related issues may be improved by specialist care, but much of the excess absence is due to non-cardiovascular comorbidities.

Further reading

Palmer K T, Brown I, Hobson J (ed). *Fitness for work: the medical aspects* (5th edn). Oxford: Oxford University Press, 2013.

Travel

Walking

Increasing the walking done daily is the most accessible form of exercise for most patients, young or old (➔ pp. 233–43). This includes walking at home, to shops or work, and at work. This is a good form of exercise for elderly patients.

Patients on insulin or drugs that could cause hypoglycaemia should have glucose on their person. A longer or more vigorous walk than usual, or one in unfamiliar surroundings, should be preceded by either reduction in insulin or sulfonylurea/meglitinides (unless the glucose is high), or by eating a CHO snack.

Expeditions on foot (e.g. mountain walking) require a substantial insulin/sulfonylurea/meglitinide reduction (20–50 % of the daily dose) and huge amounts of CHO to fuel them A rule of thumb is to double the CHO in snacks and meals. For strenuous walking, advise two double snacks between each meal, and between the evening meal and bed. Nocturnal hypoglycaemia is a risk. An emergency meal should be carried. Mountain walkers should not go alone, and the group should file a route plan with a responsible person.

Good foot care is vital (➔ pp. 301–14). Any blister or rub should be treated immediately and protected from further damage. Patients with neuropathy or PAD are at particular risk.

Cycling

Cycling is increasingly popular. Many people now chose to cycle to work. It provides good exercise, sprint or endurance (➔ p. 237). Diabetic cyclists should not cycle on an empty stomach. Hypoglycaemia risks a road traffic accident, especially when cycling home from exercise (e.g. the gym) or work. Most cyclists will need to reduce their insulin—the short-acting with the previous meal may even need to be omitted, and for long rides, the basal dose may need reducing. Sulfonylurea/meglitinide may need reduction too. Cyclists should check their glucose before setting off—it should be at least > 6 mmol/l, and in most cases > 8 mmol/l. Again, easily accessible glucose must be carried. Long cycle trips should be treated like a mountain-walking expedition in terms of insulin and food. Liquid CHO is useful.

Driving

Hypoglycaemia is common. So is driving. A US study found that 52 % of drivers with type 1 diabetes had had at least one hypoglycaemia-related 'mishap' while driving in one year. These were linked to distance driven, history of severe hypoglycaemia and insulin pump use (*Diabetes Care* 2009; **32**:2177–80; doi:10.2337/dc08-1510). Such a study would be unlikely to achieve accurate figures in the UK these days. A recent unpublished survey by a diabetes charity showed that a substantial proportion of insulin-treated patients would not tell their doctor about hypoglycaemia for fear of losing their driving licence. This is dangerous for them and others.

Patients must satisfy the licensing requirements of the country in which they are driving. These vary. In the UK, the DVLA requires many people with diabetes holding any licence to inform it of their condition and treatment as described (the guidance is updated regularly, so check the website for current advice ⌖ <http://www.gov.uk/government/uploads/system/uploads/attachment_data/file/193489/INF188_2.pdf>). Document all advice you give about driving. The main issues are hypoglycaemia and disabling complications of diabetes (e.g. visual problems, neuropathy, foot problems, stroke, etc.). This book highlights the UK DVLA guidance which links to European guidance.

All drivers (Group 1—car or motor cycle)

All drivers (with or without diabetes) must meet visual field and acuity standards (⊃ pp. 398–9) and have no other disabling or other conditions that may affect safe driving.

Insulin-treated Group 1 entitlement (car or motorcycle)

- Must notify DVLA unless insulin treatment is for ≤ 3 mths (e.g. gestational diabetes).
- Must have awareness of hypoglycaemia. Impaired awareness is defined as 'an inability to detect the onset of hypoglycaemia because of a total absence of warning symptoms'.
- Must not have had >1 episode of hypoglycaemia requiring the help of another person in the preceding 12 mths.
- Must monitor blood glucose no more than 2 hrs before the start of the first journey and every 2 hrs while driving. May need to test more often if there is a greater risk of hypoglycaemia (e.g. after physical activity or an altered meal routine). This means that ALL insulin-treated drivers (whether they have type 1 or type 2 diabetes) must have sufficient blood glucose-testing strips to comply with DVLA rules.
- Must not be regarded as a likely source of danger to the public while driving.
- Drivers taking insulin for ≤ 3 mths may continue to drive providing they are under medical supervision and have not been told by their doctor that they are at risk of disabling hypoglycaemia. If they have disabling hypoglycaemia they must notify the DVLA. In any case they should follow the rules set for safe driving. If women need insulin for > 3 months after delivery they should notify DVLA.

Insulin-treated Group 2 entitlement (heavy goods vehicle, e.g. lorry; or passenger-carrying vehicle, e.g. bus)

Drivers on insulin may apply for a Group 2 licence lasting 1 yr if their condition has been stable for at least 1 mth. They are assessed by an independent consultant diabetologist initially and annually. In **addition** to the Group 1 rules they must:

- not have had **any** hypoglycaemia requiring the help of another person in the preceding 12 mths.
- have full awareness of hypoglycaemia and demonstrate that they understand the risks of hypoglycaemia.
- regularly monitor blood glucose at least twice a day using a glucose meter with a memory function to measure and record blood glucose levels.
- produce 3 mths worth of these readings at their annual independent review by a Consultant Diabetologist.
- sign an undertaking to comply with their diabetes doctor's directions and report any significant change in their condition immediately to the DLVA.

On tablets that risk hypoglycaemia, e.g. sulfonylureas or meglitinides, Group 1 entitlement

- Must not have had > 1 episode of hypoglycaemia requiring the help of another person in the preceding 12 mths.
- May need to monitor blood glucose regularly and at times relevant to driving.
- Must be under regular medical review.
- If all DVLA requirements are met (including those in Box 22.1) there is no need to notify DVLA.

Tablets that risk hypoglycaemia, e.g. sulfonylureas or meglitinides, Group 2 entitlement

- Must notify the DVLA.
- Must not have had **any** hypoglycaemia requiring the help of another person in the preceding 12 mths.
- Must have full awareness of hypoglycaemia
- Regularly monitor blood glucose at least twice a day and at times relevant to driving.
- Must demonstrate understanding of risks of hypoglycaemia.

On tablets that do not carry a risk of hypoglycaemia, non-insulin injectable treatment, Group 1 and 2

- If all DVLA requirements in Box 22.1 are met, and driver is under regular medical review, there is no need to notify DVLA unless conditions that require notification arise.

On diet alone

There is no need to notify DVLA unless conditions that require notification arise.

⚠ *Warn patients*

- Doctors and HCPs must warn ALL patients on glucose-lowering medication that can cause hypoglycaemia of this risk, and the possibility that it could occur while driving. Record your warning.
- Make patients aware of DVLA (or other national law). Record your warning.
- The DVLA receives 27 police notifications a month about driving incidents associated with hypoglycaemia. Drivers have received a custodial sentence for causing death whilst driving and hypoglycaemic on insulin.
- Motor insurance companies regard diabetes as a material fact. All diabetic drivers should notify them of their diagnosis and ascertain their rules for further notification. Failure to do so may mean that they are not covered if there is an accident.
- By law, all UK patients must inform the DVLA if they have impaired awareness of hypoglycaemia or > 1 episode requiring assistance in the past 12 mths. Group 2 drivers must report any such episode straightaway.
- Drivers must also report severe hypoglycaemia while driving.
- See INF188/2 (Box 22.1). 🖰 <http://www.gov.uk/government/uploads/system/uploads/attachment_data/file/193489/INF188_2.pdf>
- Seek evidence of hypoglycaemic episodes each time you review patients on medication that could cause this (check carefully in situations that increase the risk of hypoglycaemia (➲ pp. 194–5)).
- Warn drivers who have hypoglycaemic episodes of the risk that this may occur while driving and take steps to prevent hypoglycaemia.
- Warn patients with impairment of awareness of hypoglycaemia that they are at risk of hypoglycaemia while driving and take urgent steps to prevent future hypoglycaemia (Chapter 10). To be safe, all drivers must stop driving while their condition is being assessed.
- Frequent hypoglycaemia is likely to impair driving—STOP driving until satisfactory control re-established and confirmed by doctor.
- As these patients may be hypoglycaemic in clinic, check their finger-prick blood glucose and record it before telling them to stop driving. Write to them formally afterwards to reiterate this advice (copy to GP/other HCPs involved with the patient).
- Patients experiencing recurrent hypoglycaemia may become aggressive, especially if you tell them to stop driving.
- Fear of losing their driving licence may mean that patients deliberately conceal hypoglycaemic episodes from HCPs. Suspicion that this is happening should be handle sensitively. Most of us rely on our cars and this fear is understandable, but patients can be disabled or die from severe hypoglycaemia and may also harm others.

All diabetic patients—diabetic tissue damage

This often occurs gradually and patients may not realize that it could inter-fere with their ability to drive safely. Rules for Group 2 drivers are more stringent than those for Group 1. The following list applies to Group 1.

- Visual problems—must be able to read in good light (with glasses or contact lenses if worn) a car number plate at a distance of 20 m.

Box 22.1 DVLA guidance for patients

The applicant or licence holder must notify DVLA unless
stated otherwise in the text

INF188/2

Information for drivers with
Diabetes treated by non-insulin medication, diet or both

Please keep this leaflet safe so you can refer to it in the future.

Drivers do not need to tell DVLA if their diabetes is treated by tablets, diet or both and they are free of the complications listed below.

Some people with diabetes develop associated problems that may affect their driving.

Hypoglycaemia (low blood sugar)

Hypoglycaemia (also known as a hypo) is the medical term for a low blood glucose (sugar) level.

Severe hypoglycaemia means the assistance of another person is required.
 The risk of hypoglycaemia is the main danger to safe driving and can occur with diabetes treated with insulin or tablets or both. This may endanger your own life as well as that of other road users. Many of the accidents caused by hypoglycaemia are because drivers carry on driving even though they get warning symptoms of hypoglycaemia. If you get warning symptoms of hypoglycaemia while driving you must stop as soon as safely possible—**do not ignore the warning symptoms.**

EARLY SYMPTOMS OF HYPOGLYCAEMIA INCLUDE:

Sweating, shakiness or trembling, feeling hungry, fast pulse or palpitations, anxiety, tingling lips.
 If you don't treat this it may result in more severe symptoms such as: Slurred speech, difficulty concentrating, confusion, disorderly or irrational behaviour, which may be mistaken for drunkenness.
 If left untreated this may lead to unconsciousness.

What you need to tell us about

By law, you must tell us if any of the following applies:

- You suffer more than one episode of severe hypoglycaemia within the last 12 months. You must also tell us if you or your medical team feel you are at high risk of developing severe hypoglycaemia. For Group 2 drivers (bus/lorry), one episode of severe hypoglycaemia must be reported immediately.
- You develop impaired awareness of hypoglycaemia. (Difficulty in recognising the warning symptoms of low blood sugar).
- You suffer severe hypoglycaemia while driving.
- You need treatment with insulin.
- You need laser treatment to both eyes or in the remaining eye if you have sight in one eye only.
- You have problems with vision in both eyes, or in the remaining eye if you have sight in one eye only. By law, you must be able to read, with glasses or contact lenses if necessary, a car number plate in good

daylight at 20 metres (65 feet). In addition, the visual acuity (with the aid of glasses or contact lenses if worn) must be at least 6/12 (0.5 decimal) with both eyes open, or in the only eye if monocular.

- You develop any problems with the circulation or sensation in your legs or feet which make it necessary for you to drive certain types of vehicles only, for example automatic vehicles or vehicles with a hand-operated accelerator or brake. This must be shown on your driving licence.
- An existing medical condition gets worse or you develop any other condition that may affect your driving safely.

In the interests of road safety, you must be sure that you can safely control a vehicle at all times.

How to tell us:
If your doctor, specialist or optician tells you to report your condition to us, you need to fill in a Medical Questionnaire about diabetes (DIAB1). You can download this from ✆ <http://www.gov.uk/browse/driving>

Phone us on: 0300 790 6806
Write to: Driver's Medical Group, DVLA Swansea SA99 1TU

- Eye problems—cataract, retinopathy, maculopathy, glaucoma. The patient should ask the ophthalmologist about driving. Does visual acuity still comply with DVLA regulations? Has there been any laser therapy? DVLA notification may be required.
- Heart problems—DVLA guidance is very specific for each situation. Read it carefully. In general, STOP driving if there is a cardiac problem which could lead to collapse or distraction at the wheel. Treatment for this usually allows resumption of driving under cardiological guidance. This section includes implantable cardiac devices. Various periods without driving are advised after cardiac events or interventions.
- PAD does not usually require stopping driving or notification, but some aortic aneurysms do. Amputation—vehicle likely to need modification. Notify DVLA.
- Foot ulceration—patients must be able to use the pedals safely and promptly. They may be unable to drive until the ulcer has healed.
- Renal disease—no need for notification unless disabling symptoms, e.g. dizziness.
- Peripheral neuropathy—patients must be able to feel the controls (e.g. brake, clutch, accelerator) and operate them promptly and safely. If this is not possible, the vehicle must be modified and the DVLA notified.
- Stroke and TIA—STOP driving for a month and then review.

Vocational drivers

Fear of losing one's licence stops many patients starting much-needed insulin treatment.

- Vocational (Group 2) is for large goods vehicles (LGV) e.g. a lorry, or passenger-carrying vehicles (PCV). Insulin-treated patients may apply for Group 2 licences.
- Groups C1 (vehicles weighing 3.5–7.5 tonnes) and D1 (minibuses carrying < 16 people). People with diabetes on insulin can hold these categories if they apply for them as a Group 2 licence and meet the standards.
- Volunteers wishing to drive a minibus of < 16 seats may be able to do so without obtaining category D1 entitlement. They should contact DVLA.
- Taxi drivers are usually subject to Group 2 rules via their local licensing body.
- The DVLA does not recommend that people with diabetes on insulin drive emergency response vehicles e.g. police, ambulance, and healthcare drivers, but the decision rests with the relevant authority.

Advice for patients

- The GMC states that if 'a driving licence holder has a condition or is undergoing treatment that may now, or in the future, affect their safety as a driver. . . [t]he driver is legally responsible for informing the DVLA about such a condition or treatment. However, if a patient has such a condition, you should explain to the patient:
- (a) that the condition may affect their ability to drive (if the patient is incapable of understanding this advice, for example, because of dementia, you should inform the DVLA immediately), and
- (b) that they have a legal duty to inform the DVLA about the condition.' In rare cases, if a patient does not do this and continues to drive a doctor may need to inform the DVLA—see specific GMC guidance <http://www.gmc-uk.org/Confidentiality_reporting_concerns. pdf_55976735.pdf>

Pancreatic or islet cell transplant

For whole pancreas transplant '[a]s long as not on insulin, driving may continue provided the driver is not suffering from a disqualifying condition. If on insulin see under insulin treated diabetes.' Vocational drivers are individually assessed.

Patients who have islet transplants have often had recurrent severe hypoglycaemia with unawareness and may have periods of safety when on reduced or no insulin, followed by transplant failure and the need to restart insulin of which DVLA should be informed. DVLA states: '[a]s long as not on insulin and provided the driver is not suffering from a disqualifying condition medical review licence will be issued. If on insulin see under insulin treated diabetes.' Vocational drivers are individually assessed.

In both situations, the driver must notify DVLA. Generally these drivers would be known to DVLA as they would have been on insulin treatment and would have had short term medical review licences.

Travel at home and abroad

People with diabetes can travel wherever they wish. To reduce problems they should:
- ensure that their diabetes control is as good as possible.
- ensure that their general health is as good as possible.
- obtain relevant immunizations.
- ensure sufficient diabetes medication and equipment plus extra to cover loss or theft.
- ensure sufficient medication/dressings, etc. for other conditions.
- ensure that they have planned what to do if something goes wrong.
- ensure that they have travel insurance—the diabetes must be declared and the cover should include repatriation (e.g. by air).
- check the Diabetes UK website 🖰 <http://www.diabetes.org.uk> which has good travel advice, or phone Careline: 0345 123 2399.
- check with airline, airport, and local immigration about security/import rules.

Check the diabetes control and general health

Is the diabetes stable?

Review glucose balance and attempt to stabilize. Patients with erratic glucose balance may decompensate abroad and require admission or repatriation. Travelling with recurrent severe hypoglycaemia is ill advised. One study (*J Travel Med* 1999; **6**(1):12–15) found that two-thirds of patients on insulin had glucose instability on tropical holidays but only one-third of type 1 patients increased monitoring frequency. Several had a febrile illness.

Diabetic tissue damage?
- Diabetic foot problems
  - See podiatrist/chiropodist before travelling.
  - Take well-fitting comfortable shoes—lace-ups are best; sandals/flip-flops risk injury or gritty rubs.
  - Protect feet. Check noon and night for rubs, grit, blisters, sunburn, and treat urgently. Wash feet often and dry well.
- Untreated retinal new vessels. Treat before flying. Take ophthalmological advice.
- Cardiac disease—check if OK to fly.
- Renal disease—avoid dehydration.
- Peripheral arterial disease—protect feet and legs, keep warm in cold.
- Peripheral neuropathy—protect feet and legs, beware sunburn.

Other health problems

Diabetes may worsen other health problems. If other conditions worsen, this can destabilize the diabetes. Review these before departure.

Supplies (and extra)
- Give the GP practice and pharmacist enough time to provide prescriptions.
- Take double the diabetes and other medical supplies they expect to use.
- Medication for diabetes and other conditions in original packs/containers.

- Insulin (cartridges, vials, and spares). Insulated container for hot or very cold countries.
- Pens, syringes, needles, needle-clipper (and spares).
- Insulin pump (take spare pump), batteries, cannula, tubing, insertors, vials, etc. Pump patients should also carry syringes and needles or insulin pens with appropriate insulin and needles.
- Finger-prick glucose testing kit—finger-pricker, lancets, strips, meter (×2), spare batteries.
- Glucose—tablets, gel, boiled sweets, snacks, bottled water.
- Glucagon with syringe and needle.
- Diabetic card stating (preferably in the local language):
- 'I am a diabetic on insulin/tablets. If I am found ill please give me 2 teaspoons of sugar in a small amount of water or 3 of the glucose tablets which I am carrying. If I fail to recover in 10 minutes please call an ambulance.'
- Diabetes ID medallion or bracelet.
- Letter from doctor about diabetes.
- Copy of prescription.
- Medical summary from doctor if long trip or significant health problems.
- Travel insurance documents and/or EHIC.
- First aid pack (with instructions), relevant to destination including:
  - sticking plasters, bandages, wound dressing
  - wound-cleaning wipes
  - paracetamol or similar analgesic
  - anti-diarrhoeal (e.g. loperamide)
  - motion sickness pills
  - anti-emetic
  - antihistamine
  - course of antibiotics
  - antifungal cream
  - if relevant, sterile venesection, suture, and IV infusion pack
  - sunscreen
  - insect repellent
  - antibacterial hand-cleaning wipes or gel
  - copy of sick-day rules (⊃ p. 210; p. 211)

Immunization and prophylaxis

People with diabetes should have every appropriate immunization. It may temporarily upset glucose control, but not as much as the relevant infection would!

- Annual influenza immunization
- Pneumococcal immunization
- Anti-tetanus immunization
- Hepatitis B immunisation
- All standard childhood vaccines
- All immunizations for destination
- Antimalarials if relevant

The journey

Patients on diet alone or metformin only for diabetes have little diffi-culty travelling unless they have symptomatic tissue damage. Patients on glucose-lowering treatment must avoid hypoglycaemia while travelling. They may end up in the wrong place or be arrested while hypoglycaemic and confused.

Patients should get a clear travel itinerary with local and actual timings. Insulin-treated patients should test their blood glucose every 4–6 hrs while travelling (every 2 hrs if driving themselves).

Most questions arise about air travel. Travelling north/south does not usually need a change in insulin timing. Travelling west means that the 'day' will be longer so more insulin may be needed. Travelling east, the 'day' will be shorter and less insulin may be needed. Consider the day of travel as being from breakfast at home until breakfast in the destination. Patients should eat every 2–3 hrs. During the day they should reduce the insulins which are acting when travelling but be prepared to take a small extra dose (e.g. 2–6 units analogue fast-acting) immediately after any extra meal if the breakfast-to-breakfast time is > 24 hrs and the pre-food glucose is > 11 mmol/l. Before sleeping check that the SMBG is > 6 mmol/l and have a bed-time snack.

All diabetes medication and monitoring equipment should be carried personally in cabin hand-baggage that is always kept in sight. It is sensible to carry a copy of the prescription, diabetes card, and a doctor's letter, and keep medication and other diabetes kit in original packaging unless in use, e.g in pump/pen. Many airports have sharps boxes in toilets; ask cabin crew for a sharps box on the aircraft.

People with diabetes on insulin or GLP-1 agonists are carrying liquids. Security rules for different countries vary (do not forget transit airports). The Civil Aviation Authority UK states:

- 'Passengers may carry essential liquid medicines such as insulin for the period of their trip. These are permitted in larger quantities above the 100ml limit for liquids, but will be subject to authentication. Passengers must have obtained the prior agreement of the airline with which they are travelling and with their departure airport.
- For diabetic passengers who use insulin pumps and/or continuous glucose monitoring (CGM) devices, it is essential that they speak to the airline to obtain precise advice on the use of such devices on board the aircraft.
- Passengers must also take with them supporting documentation from a relevant qualified medical professional.
- It is essential that diabetic passengers carry adequate equipment (glucose meters, lancets, batteries) and medication in their hand baggage. It is also important that insulin not being used in the flight is not packed in the hold baggage as this may be exposed to temperatures which could degrade the insulin, in addition there is also the potential that luggage may be lost en-route.' <http://www.caa.co.uk/default.aspx/default.aspx?catid=923&pagetype=70&gid=924&faqid=1111>

Guidance for Air Travel and diabetes in the USA can be found at: ℘ <http://www.diabetes.org/living-with-diabetes/know-your-rights/discrimination/public-accommodations/air-travel-and-diabetes/what-special-concerns-may.html>

Most insulin pump and CGMS manufacturers advise that the devices and remotes/meters should be detached before going through an airport body scanner because X-rays may affect function. It is usually possible to request a different screening process (e.g. a pat-down search). Some airlines may not permit use of devices that use remote wireless technology on the aircraft.

INPUT (➲ p. 166) provides advice: ℘ <http://www.inputdiabetes.org.uk/airport-n-insurance/>

Make sure all electronic diabetes devices are fully charged.

Problems abroad

Food

Patients may worry about getting the 'right' food. A few weeks of a less than perfect diet is not a disaster. However, it is usually possible to find a local staple CHO—bread, potato, pasta, rice, maize, yams, beans, etc. Obvious fat and sugar can be avoided. Cooked vegetables and fruit are usually available. Uncooked fruit and vegetables should be avoided or peeled carefully or washed in newly opened bottled water to reduce the risk of gastroenteritis. Advise sparkling bottled water or diet drinks (open the bottle/can yourself; clean can tops first). Alcohol is self-sterilizing but advise moderation (➲ p. 77). Carry some food but beware local regulations (e.g. Australia, New Zealand, and Canada all ban import of some foods—declare all food if in doubt).

Infection

- Do SMBG four times daily if any infection. Increase glucose-lowering treatment if necessary.
- Minor wounds must be cleaned promptly and covered with a sterile dressing. Sepsis is common, especially on the feet.
- Fungal infections—athlete's foot and thrush are common. Use antifungal cream immediately. Women susceptible to thrush should take an imidazole pessary with them.
- Chest or urine infections should be treated promptly—hence the benefit of packing a course of antibiotics.
- Gastroenteritis is common and may precipitate DKA. Patients should:
  - take anti-diarrhoeal and anti-emetic promptly.
  - drink bottled water and non-diet canned drink.
  - check SMBG every 2 hrs.
  - increase insulin if necessary.
  - follow sick-day rules (➲ p. 210; p. 211).
  - get medical help promptly if the glucose rises and blood ketones > 3 mmol/l (➲ pp. 216–9).

Heat

- Britons are not always used to heat.
- It increases insulin absorption from injection sites risking hypoglycaemia.
- Increased sweating + hyperglycaemia may cause dehydration.
- Neuropathic areas can sunburn.
- Advise a cool-bag for insulin (➲ p. 161).

Cold

- Cold slows insulin absorption—it is released when the patient warms up, risking hypoglycaemia.
- Hypoglycaemia prevents shivering (➲ p. 198).
- Patients with PAD must keep extremities well-wrapped to avoid frostbite.
- Cold may precipitate angina.

Altitude (> 3000 m)

- Remote locations, mountain sickness, food availability, variable appetite, hyoxia, extreme exertion may all be harder to cope with for people with diabetes, but there is experience of successful high altitude activities among people with diabetes (*Diabetes Care* 2005; **28**:2563–72; doi:10.2337/diacare.28.10.2563).
- Glucose control may become erratic. Many glucose meters do not read accurately at altitude.

Medical aid abroad

Specialist diabetes care is available worldwide but access is variable. Some countries (e.g. the US) measure glucose in mg/dl (1 mmol/l = 18 mg/dl). The UK uses 100 units/ml insulin. Some countries may use 40 units/ml or 80 units/ml insulin which must be drawn up and given with a syringe that matches that insulin strength. The IDF can provide addresses of local diabetes associations. ✍ <http://www.idf.org>

Local medical resources vary. Patients must have adequate travel insurance and have declared their diabetes to the insurer. UK patients visiting Europe should carry a European Health Insurance Card (EHIC) card obtained free at: ✍ <http://www.ehic.org.uk>

It is wise to note local emergency and ambulance call numbers and arrangements on arriving in a foreign company, and program them into a mobile phone.

Summary

- Walking and cycling are good exercise. Ensure adequate food and reduce glucose-lowering medication if appropriate.
- Healthcare professionals should warn diabetic drivers of their need to check whether DVLA notification is required, and to tell their motor insurance company.
- Drivers with diabetes on long-term insulin must inform the DVLA of their condition, and those on other forms of treatment must check this website to find out if they need to notify. ✍ <http://www.gov.uk/driving-medical-conditions>
- Vocational drivers face more stringent requirements and must also check the DVLA regulations.
- Patients with frequent or unrecognized hypoglycaemia must not drive.
- Patients with some forms of tissue damage must not drive and may need to notify the DVLA.
- Diabetic travellers should plan for the unexpected.
- Planning includes a diabetes and general health check.
- Immunizations and prescriptions should be obtained in good time.
- Adequate diabetes and other health supplies should be taken, along with a first aid kit.
- Patients should carry a diabetic card, preferably in the language of their destination.
- Before travelling check with airline, airport, and immigration at departure, transit and arrival about security and import rules.
- Aim to avoid hypoglycaemia while travelling.
- Aim to avoid gastroenteritis while travelling.
- Protect feet while travelling.
- Having diabetes should not prevent happy travelling—pre-planning ensures continued enjoyment.

Chapter 23

Psychological and social aspects of diabetes

Introduction

Everyone with newly diagnosed diabetes is worried and some are very frightened, especially if they have relatives who have gone blind, had amputations, or died from diabetes. The experience at diagnosis influences the patient's attitude long term. All patients need a clear explanation in language they can understand, an opportunity to express concerns and ask questions, and support with further opportunities for discussion from an expert. Some anxiety increases adherence to treatment regimens but excessive anxiety may hinder this.

Adults with diabetes may also feel angry or guilty, miss favourite foods or relaxed eating, resent the effects diabetes self-care and healthcare have on their lives and livelihoods (e.g. taking medication, especially insulin, SMBG, medical appointments), resent the inefficiencies of healthcare or other systems, resent being told what to do, feel punished (e.g. by insurance companies), miss spontaneity, feel the diabetes pervades their whole lives 24 hrs a day, and the fear never goes away ('what if I go hypo?').

Optimal diabetes control requires self-motivation and knowledge for self-care. A feeling of autonomy and self-sufficiency can increase satisfaction with life for diabetic patients. Self-care without knowledge of diabetes and without taking beneficial action will not improve glucose balance. Weight gain (e.g. associated with hypoglycaemic therapy) can frustrate patients and reduce concordance with diabetes treatment (*Postgrad Med* 2009; **121**(5):94–107; doi: 10.3810/pgm.2009.09.2056). Apathy is also associated with worse HbA$_{1c}$, even in the absence of depression (*Diabetes Res Clin Pract* 2008; **79**:37–41; doi: 10.1016/j.diabres.2007.06.012).

Chronic stress and the issues discussed can contribute to anxiety or depression. Ultimately some people with diabetes will fulfil the criteria for formal mental health diagnoses.

Brain function

The prevailing glucose concentration affects brain function. This is acutely affected by hypoglycaemia, leading to changes in cognitive (and physical) function and emotion, and ultimately fits or coma (➲ pp. 184–6). Evidence for longer-term effects of hypoglycaemic episodes upon brain function varies. Overt permanent cerebral impairment is uncommon. A study in people with type 2 diabetes showed that those who had experienced severe hypoglycaemia had poorer late-life cognitive ability than those without this history (*Diabetic Med* 2012; **29**:328–36; doi: 10.1111/j.1464-5491.2011.03 505.x). Prolonged profound hypoglycaemic coma may cause permanent brain damage.

Hyperglycaemia also alters brain function. Anecdotally, patients or relatives report increased irritability (difficult to live with) and slower thinking with higher glucose. Different studies have measured this in variable ways with variable results. One study in type 2 diabetes showed that, short-term, a glucose of 16.5 mmol vs 4.5 mmol/l impaired information processing, working memory, and some aspects of attention. Mood also changed with reduced energetic arousal, and increased sadness and anxiety (*Diabetes Care* 2004; **27**:2335–40; doi:10.2337/diacare.27.10.2335). This suggests that teaching sessions may have greatest impact in patients with near-normal glucose levels at the time.

The ACCORD MIND study of baseline glucose control and cognitive function in type 2 diabetes found that higher HbA_{1c} was associated with lower cognitive function (Diabetes Care 2009; **32**:221–6; doi:10.2337/dc08-1153); however, intensive glucose lowering did not improve cognitive outcomes (*Lancet Neurology* 2011; **10**:969–77; doi:10.1016/S1474-4422(11)70188-0).

Dementia is discussed elsewhere (➲ p. 367).

Psychiatric disorders

Psychiatric disorders are common in people with diabetes. Diabetes in common in people with severe mental illness (➔ p. 415).

Psychiatric disorder is present in 37 % of adolescents with a 10-yr history of diabetes. Depression and anxiety are particularly common at all ages, Eating disorders and obsessive–compulsive disorder are also found. Patients with chronic poor glucose control were twice as likely to have a psychiatric disorder, and were more likely to have pre-diabetic behavioural problems than those with good glucose balance (*Diabetic Med* 2005; **22**:152–7; doi: 1 0.1111/j.1464-5491.2004.01370.x).

The presence of any psychiatric disorder makes diabetes care more difficult, and increases the risk of non-concordance with therapy, and subsequent problems with glucose control (hyper- or hypoglycaemia) and increased risk of diabetic tissue damage. Patients in psychiatric wards may have limited access to diabetes expertise and must be referred to the DST as fluctuations in their glucose control may worsen their emotional state. Patients may develop gross glucose instability and can die from ketoacidosis.

Psychotic diabetic patients with substance abuse are four times more likely to die than similar patients without diabetes (*Psychiatric Services* 2007; **58**:270; doi: 10.1176/appi.ps.58.2.270). Young people with diabetes have a similar frequency of substance abuse to the non-diabetic population (➔ p. 325).

Depression

Screen for depression (NICE CG 91, 2009):
- During the past month have you often been bothered by feeling down, depressed, or hopeless?
- During the past month have you often been bothered by little interest or pleasure in doing things?

⚠ Assess suicide risk. Diabetic patients, especially those on insulin, have ready access to fatal overdose. People with diabetes are at greater risk of death from self-harm than in non-diabetic people (➔ p. 248).

Patients with severe depression are more likely to develop type 2 diabetes (although more healthcare attention might detect this sooner). A review of 42 studies (*Diabetes Care* 2001; **24**:1069–78; doi:10.2337/diacare.24.6.1069) found that people with diabetes are twice as likely to be depressed as the general population, women (28 %) more than men (18 %). Depressive symptoms were reported by 31 % on questionnaires. Major depression was reported in 11 % of those formally assessed. Carers may attribute depression to a natural reaction to having diabetes, and some two-thirds of patients are not offered treatment. Depressed diabetic patients are less likely to adhere to their diet and treatment than those who are not depressed (*Diabetes Care* 2008; **31**:2398–403; doi: 10.2337/dc08-1341). Depression is associated with higher HbA_{1c}, and some studies have shown that anti-depressants improve this (*Diabetes Care* 2000; **23**:934–42; doi:10.2337/diacare.23.7.934). Having diabetes and depression has a greater impact on quality of life than having either alone. (*Diabetes Care* 2004; **27**:1066–70; doi:10.2337/diacare.27.5.1066). Depressed diabetic patients have higher healthcare costs than those who are not depressed. Depressed diabetic patients are more likely to die, especially from cardiovascular causes than those without depression (*Diabetes Care* 2005; **28**:1339–45; doi:10.2337/diacare.28.6.1339). Treatment for the depression reduces mortality (*Diabetes Care* 2007; **30**: 3005–10; doi:10.2337/dc07-0974). Depression is also linked with microvascular complications. Functional disability was reported in 58 % of non-depressed diabetic patients and 78 % of depressed diabetic patients (*Diabetes Care* 2004; **27**:421–8; doi:10.2337/diacare.27.2.421). This reduces ability to work.

Tricyclic antidepressants and selective serotonin-reuptake inhibitors (SSRIs) may affect the blood glucose in either direction, although it appears that tricyclics are most likely to raise it and SSRIs to lower it. Up to half of all diabetic patients with depression are unable to tolerate full-dose anti-depressant medication. Treatment of depression in type 2 diabetes improves HbA$_{1c}$ (*Ann Fam Med* 2012; **10**:15–22; doi: 10.1370/afm.1344).

Anxiety

Anxiety is common in diabetes. A review showed that 14 % diabetic patients had generalized anxiety disorder (a formal psychiatric disorder) and 40 % had elevated symptoms of anxiety (*J Psychosom Res 2002*; **53**:1053–60). Elevated anxiety symptoms were more common in women than in men (55 % vs 33 %). A large American study showed a 20 % higher prevalence of lifetime diagnosis of anxiety among people with diabetes vs those without (*Diabetic Med* 2008; **25**:878–81; doi: 10.1111/j.1464-5491.2008.02477.x). Anxiety is natural. It may be heightened in patients with hypoglycaemia who may run high glucose levels to avoid this. High glucose levels may also be associated with increased anxiety.

Phobias

Phobias are more common in diabetes than in the general population, but < 1 % of type 1 patients are needle-phobic (*Diabetes Med* 2001; **18**:671–4; doi: 10.1046/j.1464-5491.2001.00547.x). Refer patients to a psychologist experienced in treating diabetic patients.

Eating and body image disorders

Diabetic patients are advised to focus on what and how much they are eating as part of their care, and this may encourage abnormal fixation on aspects of eating, body image, and weight. All forms of abnormal eating behaviour, food restriction (anorexia), and binge eating (bulimia) occur in people with diabetes of all ages. Diabetes appears to be associated with an increased frequency of eating problems but measurement of frequency is difficult because focus on food is a required part of the management of diabetes and this may distort standard diagnostic tools. Using careful methodology, disordered eating behaviour and eating disorders were shown to be more common in young people with type 1 diabetes than in non-diabetics and are associated with poor glucose control (*Diabet Med* 2013; **30**:189–98; doi: 10.1111/j.1464-5491.2012.03771.x). Obese patients with type 2 diabetes may binge eat; 8 % of a diabetic bariatric surgery population showed this (*Eating Behaviours* 2011; **12**:175–81; doi: 10.1016/j.eatbeh.2011.04.007). Features of eating disorders should be sought, especially in patients who are underweight or overweight, or have poor glucose control, and in adolescent girls.

Refer all diabetic patients with any form of eating disorder or body image problem to the specialist diabetes team and to a mental health team specializing in eating disorders. These patients are at risk of severe illness or death from their behaviour. They tend to fail attendance, avoid help, and ignore advice. They may have other psychiatric problems and can self-harm. Try to stay in contact. Assign a key worker if possible. Non-mental-health staff should realize that such patients, who may be consciously or subconsciously manipulative, can cause distress and conflict between staff. Involve the experts early.

Up to a third of diabetic girls omit or under-dose insulin to remain slim, or lose weight via hyperglycaemia and glycosuria. This is sometimes known as 'diabulimia'. △ These patients are at risk of DKA, and may die.

Patients with a restrictive eating pattern may require very little insulin and are at risk of hypoglycaemia. They have little liver glycogen (so glucagon is unlikely to work in hypoglycaemia). Dietary ketosis is common. There is danger of fatal ketoacidosis if they also omit insulin. Those abusing laxatives can become severely hypokalaemic. Very thin patients may also have other hormone abnormalities.

Bulimic patients find that their glucose oscillates wildly. Those who vomit may have difficult knowing how much nutrition is retained. Those who binge and do not vomit will need extra short-acting insulin to cover this additional food.

Severe mental illness

Check HbA$_{1c}$ in every patient before starting any psychiatric drug, to reveal undiagnosed diabetes in those not known to have this, and to assess glycaemic control in those with diabetes.

People with severe mental illness are more likely to have diabetes than the general population. Diabetes is found in 10–15 % of patients with schizophrenia, and 8–17 % of patients with bipolar disorder.

🕮 <http://www.rcpsych.ac.uk/pdf/PCCJ_Holt_FINALONLINE_JAN[1].pdf> There appear to be several causes, e.g. obesity, lack of exercise, genetics, and medication.

A study of Medicaid patients with bipolar disorder found that the risk of new diabetes was greatest among patients taking risperidone, olanzapine, and quetiapine, hazard ratios 3.8, 3.7, and 2.5, respectively, vs conventional antipsychotic drugs (*Pharmacotherapy* 2007; **27**:27–35; doi: 10.1592/phco.27.1.27).

⚠ Glucose can rise rapidly after starting antipsychotic drugs and should be checked after 1–2 mths. Deaths from DKA or HHS have occurred. These patients should be screened at least once a year for diabetes. Weight gain and hypertension were also linked with greater risk of new diabetes.

Summary

- Everyone with diabetes experiences emotional distress to varying degrees. Staff should recognize this and provide appropriate support.
- Emotional factors influence diabetes self-care and outcomes.
- Primary and secondary care staff should liaise about individual diabetic patients with a psychological or psychiatric problem. Consider referral to the mental health service for expert help.
- Psychiatric disorders are more frequent in diabetic patients than in the non-diabetic population.
- Depression is twice as common in the diabetic population.
- Many diabetic patients have some form of anxiety.
- Phobias may occasionally limit insulin therapy and monitoring.
- Eating disorders may be more common in diabetes than in the general population and make glucose control difficult.
- Omission or under-dosing of insulin is common in diabetic girls who are trying to stay slim.
- Substance abuse increases mortality in diabetes.
- People with severe mental illness are at risk of developing diabetes.
- Atypical psychiatric drugs increase the risk of developing diabetes compared with typical antipsychotics.
- Management of diabetes in people with mental health problems (and vice versa) requires expertise. Such patients are at risk of self harm or death from diabetes emergencies.

Useful resources

- Diabetes UK & NHS Diabetes 2010. Emotional and psychological support and care in Diabetes ℘ <http://www.diabetes.org.uk/Documents/Reports/Emotional_and_Psychological_Support_and_Care_in_Diabetes_2010.pdf>

Chapter 24

Diabetes care in hospital

See also individual chapters

Introduction

This chapter is about the care of people with diabetes attending as emergencies or admitted as inpatients. Read the relevant chapters for more detailed management of these conditions.

In 2007/8, 6.2 % of patients discharged from English hospitals were coded as having diabetes using Hospital Episode Statistics. Mean length of stay (LoS) was 6.3 days (standard deviation, SD, 52 days) vs 3.5 days (SD 16 days) in patients without diabetes codes. 'Multivariate analysis showed an independent 15 % (0.8 days) overall increase in LoS for people with diabetes over people without diabetes. The diabetes-related LoS increase was 4 % greater for women compared with men, proportional to age > 20 years, and greater with greater socio-economic deprivation. 'By linking to the NDA, a further 3 % of patients were found to have uncoded diabetes; they did not have excess LoS. (*Diabetic Med* 2012; **29**:1199–205; doi: 10.1111/j.1464-5491.2011.03535.x).

By 2010/12, 11.2 % of hospital admissions in England had recorded diabetes. In 2012, the National Diabetes Inpatient Audit (NaDIA) found that in 2010/11 15 % (5–30 %) of hospital beds in England were occupied by people with diabetes. Median LoS in England was 8 nights for emergency admissions and 5 for elective admissions. Among admissions with diabetes 8.8 % were for foot ulcer or amputation (Kerr, (➲ p. 302).

Diabetes, whether known or newly discovered, has a major adverse impact on most inpatients. Compared with inpatients without diabetes, diabetic patients often have increased risks (Box 24.1) in addition to the condition with which they were admitted. Much of this risk is secondary to hyperglycaemia and pre-admission diabetic tissue damage. The adverse effects of their primary admission diagnosis exacerbate their complications. Dehydration worsens renal failure, hypoalbuminaemia worsens cardiac failure, and infection or steroid treatment increase glucose.

Patients with glucose > 11mmol/l are 3–4 times as likely to get infected wounds or UTIs as those with glucose in the non-diabetic range. Patients with newly diagnosed diabetes are particularly at risk. An American study showed that inpatients with newly diagnosed diabetes had a 16 % mortality, vs 3 % in known diabetic patients, and 1.7 % in those without diabetes. The newly hyperglycaemic patients also had a longer stay and were less likely to be discharged to their own home (*J Clin Endocr Metab* 2002; **87**:978–82).

People with recorded diabetes are more likely to die in hospital than those without diabetes recorded. All admissions to English hospitals for 2 yrs (2010/12) were analysed; 11.2 % had diabetes but 21.5 % of inpatient deaths occurred in this group (OR 2.207). When adjusted for age, sex, deprivation, method and reason for admission, and type of hospital, the OR was 1.137. Adjustment for comorbidities reduced the OR to 1.065 or an excess risk of inpatient death of 6.3 %. (However, many of the comorbidities would have been diabetes complications.) This excess risk translates to 2316 excess deaths in hospital in 2 yrs or 1.4 % of all deaths in all admissions. The excess risk is higher in smaller/medium hospitals, and in surgical patients with cardiac or urinary tract disease. There was considerable variation in excess mortality between hospitals and it seemed likely that local differences in patient care and systems contributed to this (*Diabetic Med* 2013; **30**:1393–402; doi: 10.1111/dme.12282).

Box 24.1 Risks for hospitalized diabetic patients

- ↑Infection risk (e.g. urinary tract, wound)
- ↑Risk of cannula/line/catheter-site infection
- ↑Severe infections which take longer to resolve
- ↑Antibiotic-resistant or hospital-acquired infections
- ↓Healing
- ↑Risk of fistula formation
- ↑Risk of thrombosis
- ↑Risk of ischaemic events-myocardial, peripheral vascular, cerebral
- ↑Risk of renal failure
- ↑Risk of cardiac failure
- ↑Risk of pressure sores, especially heel ulcers in vasculopaths
- ↑Metabolic complexity
- ↑Hospital inpatient stay
- ↓Likelihood of returning to their own home
- ↑Mortality
- ↑Cost of care

Every hospital managing inpatients with diabetes should have at least one diabetes inpatient specialist nurse (DISN). DISNs have been shown to reduce admissions, incidents and LoS, and improve patient experience (e.g. *Diabetic Med* 2008; **25**:147–51; doi: 10.1111/j.1464-5491.2007.02326.x). The DISN should be part of an inpatient diabetes team—diabetologist, dietitian, and podiatrist, with access to clinical psychology.

Education

Diabetes education for staff

Repeated education of all staff in safe management of diabetes is essential. All staff prescribing or administering insulin should do a Safe Use of Insulin training course, e.g. ✏ <http://www.healthcareea.co.uk/theinsulinsafetysuite>

The diabetes team should provide prompt support in managing patients and advice should be available 7 days a week. The diabetes team needs good liaison with all other departments. Link nurse programmes in which one nurse on each ward is responsible for passing on diabetes education to the others have helped in some hospitals.

Education for diabetic inpatients

A diabetic inpatient is a captive audience. Help him or her to understand how he or she came to be in hospital and how this might be avoided (if possible) in the future. Admission also provides an opportunity for revision and further diabetes education. A formal inpatient diabetes education programme may reduce readmission (Box 24.2) (*Diabetes Care* 2013; **36**: 2960–7; doi:10.2337/dc13-0108).

Box 24.2 Diabetes education for inpatients

- Assess current knowledge and understanding of their own diabetes.
- Review self-care. Review previous glucose balance.
- Involve family members (with patient permission).
- For new patients—provide full diabetes starter education (⊋ p. 59).
- Review knowledge of general lifestyle and preventive healthcare.
- What caused hospital admission? What actions might prevent another such admission?
- Teach about diabetes self-care and other treatment which will be needed after discharge.
- Involve the multidisciplinary team—ensure that all team members understand the current plan and have been trained in the same diabetes care protocols ('sing the same song').
- Refer all patients to the dietitian.
- Explain diabetes care and education arrangements in the community.
- Explain follow-up arrangements.
- Explain how to get help if problems arise.
- Communicate with ward staff about what has been taught.

Assessment of emergency attenders

This is relevant to management of patients seen in emergency assessment units or A&E departments (Box 24.3). One in three diabetic emergency attenders to an A&E department had actual or compensated DKA (*Diabetic Med* 2005; **22**: 221–4; doi: 10.1111/j.1464-5491.2004.01374.x).

Don't miss new diabetes. Check finger-prick glucose (venous later) (⊃ p. 98–105) in high-risk patients:
- everyone with an acute/emergency medical problem
- symptoms of diabetes
- White people > 40 yrs old, non-white ethnic groups > 25 yrs if overweight
- overweight people
- tissue damage or conditions known to be associated with diabetes
- on medication known to be associated with diabetes (e.g. steroids, thiazides, olanzapine, antiretrovirals)
- history of glucose intolerance
- past gestational diabetes or current pregnancy (⊃ p. 342–44)
- severe mental health disorders

See Box 1.3 (⊃ p. 6) for full list, and Table 1.3 (⊃ p. 10) for diagnostic criteria for diabetes.

All diabetic patients check as a minimum:
- presenting complaint
- duration of diabetes (long duration, more tissue damage)
- history of tissue damage, especially cardiovascular, eyes, kidneys, nerves
- current or recent infection (may be incompletely treated)
- treatment for diabetes and other conditions
- look at medications if available, including insulin, remembering that some insulins have very similar names but different actions
- recent SMBG and HbA_{1c}—verbal report or diary or lab if available
- check injection sites in insulin-/exenatide-treated patients
- current finger-prick glucose—too low (< 4 mmol/l)? Too high (> 11 mmol/l)? Send a laboratory sample to confirm and treat appropriately
- finger-prick glucose > 11 mmol/l—check finger-prick blood ketone level
- pulse, BP, respiratory rate, oxygen saturations, temperature
- assessment of presenting complaint as appropriate
- full assessment if unwell enough to require admission (⊃ p. 23–30)
- examine emergency and elective admission patients fully (⊃ p. 23–30) including checking for foot problems and pressure areas
- urine dipstick

Box 24.3 Investigations

- Finger-prick blood:
  - glucose
  - HbA_{1c} (if available)
  - ketones if glucose > 11 mmol/l (all emergency attenders).
- Urine:
  - dipstick glucose, ketones, protein, blood, leucocytes, nitrite
  - if no signs of a UTI—microalbumin:creatinine ratio.
- Laboratory venous blood:
  - glucose (repeat fasting if diagnosis unproven)
  - urea and electrolytes
  - creatinine
  - liver function
  - calcium and albumin
  - thyroid function
  - haemoglobin A_{1c}
  - full blood count
  - consider adding C-reactive protein (?infection), urate (?gout)
  - fasting cholesterol, HDL, LDL, triglyceride next day
  - (add tissue transglutaminase/anti-mysial/anti-gliadin antibodies if < 20 yrs old and not previously checked)
- Chest X-ray if chest signs or symptoms, smoker, recent immigrant, Asian (or local protocol)
- Foot X-ray if ulcer, possible infection or injury
- ECG if > 30 yrs old, or diabetes > 10 yrs duration, or chest pain any age
- MRSA screen
- Microbiology samples, e.g. urine, sputum, pus, blood, ulcer, other

Emergencies

For more detailed information read the relevant chapters.

Hypoglycaemia (Chapter 10, ➔ pp. 181–200)

- ⚠ Any diabetic patient on glucose-lowering treatment who behaves oddly in any way is hypoglycaemic until proved otherwise.
- Features of hypoglycaemia include confusion, sweating, shaking, blurred vision, aggression, coma, fits.
- Stop IV insulin infusion temporarily and restart once hypoglycaemia treated after reducing dose if necessary. For CSII see (➔ pp. 166–7).
- After treating the hypoglycaemia do not omit usual insulin if due, but review the dose. Omitting insulin in type 1 patients may cause DKA.

Patients capable of swallowing

Glucose is absorbed most rapidly in liquid form. Give 20 g glucose. Treat hypoglycaemia as soon as it is suspected. Check finger-prick glucose if possible; if not, give oral glucose immediately. The following contain about 10 g glucose:

- three glucose tablets (e.g. Dextrosol®)
- one tube 25 g GlucoGel® or Dextrogel® (glucose gel)
- one-third of an 80 g bottle of GlucoGel® (a whole bottle contains 32 g glucose)
- 50–60 ml or one-sixth of a 380 ml bottle of Original Lucozade® (a whole bottle contains 68 g glucose; other versions contain different quantities of glucose)
- 90 ml or one-third of a can of non-diet Coca Cola®
- *One-third of a carton of original Ribena® (dilute for children)
- *100 ml orange juice (without bits)
- two spoonfuls of sugar
- three sugar lumps
- three or four sweets (e.g. fruit pastilles or jelly babies)
  *avoid in renal disease if possible

Review oral hypoglycaemic or insulin dose.

Patients who cannot, or will not swallow safely
Conscious patients who refuse to swallow

- Firm encouragement to eat. GlucoGel® or Dextrogel® is best in this situation as it is difficult to spit out.
- Violent patients—keep back to avoid personal injury and try to contain the patient in a safe area. Inject glucagon into whatever muscle bulk can be accessed safely. The alternative is to muster sufficient help to achieve robust venous access and give IV glucose.

Unconscious patients, unsafe swallow, uncooperative

- ⚠ Risk of respiratory or cardiac arrest.
- Protect airway. Recovery position.
- If on IV insulin or CSII, stop it (➔ pp. 166–7) but leave cannulae in situ. (After management of the hypoglycaemia the insulin must be restarted in type 1 patients and inpatients unable to be managed on non-insulin therapies; review insulin dose).

- Give oxygen if convulsing or hypoxic.
- Safeguard patient and staff from injury.
- In non-clinical setting families/carers can inject glucagon (➲ p. 190).
- Gain IV access via a large vein, tape in cannula securely (take care—extravasated glucose can cause ulceration).
- Withdraw blood for laboratory glucose, urea, and electrolytes, liver function, and perhaps thyroid function or cortisol.
- Give IV glucose (repeat once if not recovered within 15 mins).
  Over 10–15 mins infuse 75–80 ml 20 % glucose IV or 150–160 mls 10 % glucose.
- 50 % glucose is not recommended nowadays—hard to use, hypertonic, and risk of ulceration from extravasation.
- Check finger-prick glucose at 10 mins. If not > 4 mmol/l recheck every 10 mins until it is.
- IV access impossible—inject glucagon IM.
- If patient fails to recover consider steroid lack. Take blood for subsequent cortisol level and inject 100 mg hydrocortisone IV or IM.
- Monitor Glasgow coma scale, heart rate, BP, respirations, oxygen saturations, and, of course, blood glucose.
- Feed patient if safe, or infuse 5 % or 10 % glucose slowly—rate depends on clinical situation.
- ⚠ Prolonged hypoglycaemia (e.g. after insulin overdose) requires continued infusion of both glucose and potassium with expert advice with ECG and potassium monitoring. Call diabetes registrar or consultant urgently. Risk of death (➲ p. 191).
- Monitor glucose and condition hourly until full consciousness regained and maintained. Keep under medical observation for at least 4 hrs.
- Do not remove IV cannula until patient ready for discharge.
- Hospitalize hypoglycaemic patients:
  - on sulfonylurea.
  - if elderly.
  - living alone and vulnerable.
  - who have ingested alcohol or drugs of abuse.
  - with renal disease, liver disease, or other significant concomitant disease.
  - with psychiatric problems.
  - with suspicion of overdose of insulin or glucose-lowering tablets.
  - if you have concerns about their safety.
- Patients on long-acting insulin should be considered for admission unless they are fully conscious and capable of monitoring themselves and their finger-prick glucose, and adjusting their food and insulin safely.
- Why were they hypoglycaemic? Educate patient (once glucose normal) and carers.
- Diabetes team follow-up.

Diabetic ketoacidosis (Chapter 12, → pp. 213–31) diagnosis Table 12.1.)

⚠ Any suspicion of DKA requires immediate 999 transfer to hospital.
- Always consider DKA in all diabetic patients.
- DKA is likely in vomiting insulin-treated patients and/or ill patients with glucose > 11 mmol/l (→ p. 216).

Initial management (→ pp. 217–18)
- Resuscitation: airway, breathing, circulation.
- Aim door to needle time < 15 mins.
- Good IV access.
- Take venous bloods.
- 1000 ml 0.9 % sodium chloride IV over 1 hr.
- After IV fluids flowing, start FRIII 0.1 units/kg/hr soluble insulin (e.g. Actrapid®, Humulin S®).
- Protect pressure areas, especially feet.
- Inform diabetes registrar or consultant diabetologist.

Tests
- Finger-prick capillary blood glucose + ketone (beware cold fingers, always send blood for laboratory venous glucose as meters have an upper limit to readings).
- Venous blood pH unless hypoxic on pulse oximetry.
- Urgent laboratory venous glucose, U&E, creatinine, FBC.
- Use point-of-care (POCT) biochemistry system (e.g. blood gas analyser) quality-controlled by laboratory to monitor progress.
- Later LFT, TFT, lipids, blood cultures, CRP.
- Dipstick urine.
- MSU, throat swab, microbiology swab any lesion.
- Pregnancy test in girls/women of childbearing age.
- 12-lead and monitor ECG thereafter.
- Chest X-ray.
- Consider abdominal X-ray.

Aims of treatment
Start initial resuscitation within 15 mins. Then:
- gradual return to normal.
- rehydrate over 24 hrs.
- use IV fluid and insulin to correct DKA (→ pp. 218–19).
- Aim for:
  - a glucose fall of 3 mmol/l/hr.
  - a blood ketone fall of ≥ 0.5 mmol/l/hr.
  - a venous bicarbonate rise of 3 mmol/l/hr (no help after 12 hrs sodium chloride infusion).
- Aim for the venous/arterial pH to rise gradually over 24 hrs.

Actions
- Consider ICU/HDU for each patient
- Good IV access
- Oxygen if hypoxic (unless respiratory disease risking CO_2 retention)
- Nasogastric tube if severe vomiting, gastric retention, coma

- Consider urinary catheter if incontinent or not passed urine within 1 hr, immobile, coma
- IV fluids and electrolytes
- Insulin
- Treat precipitating condition (e.g. antibiotics for infection)
- Prophylactic low molecular weight heparin
- Contact seniors and DST

Hyperosmolar hyperglycaemic state (Chapter 12, ➲ pp. 220–2 diagnosis Table 12.1)

Initial management
- Resuscitation: airway, breathing, circulation.
- Aim door to needle time <15 mins.
- Good IV access.
- Take venous bloods as for DKA.
- 1000 ml 0.9 % sodium chloride IV over 1 hr.
- Do not start insulin unless blood ketones > 1 mmol/l or ketonuria > 2+ and do not give stat dose of insulin (➲ pp. 220–1).
- Patients are often confused or aggressive—get help early if needed.
- Urinary catheter to measure fluid output accurately.
- Protect pressure areas, especially feet.
- Treat cause of HHS e.g. infection.
- Give prophylactic low molecular weight heparin if there are no contraindications (some diabetologists would fully anticoagulate).
- Review all treatment for comorbidities.
- Inform diabetes registrar or consultant diabetologist.

Infection

- ⚠ Consider infection in every diabetic patient—it may be much more severe and extensive than is apparent.
- UTIs, respiratory infection, deep soft tissue infection are commoner in people with diabetes than those without.
- Send samples of body fluids or pus for microscopy and culture.
- Do blood cultures before starting antibiotics.
- Examine the 'nooks and crannies', e.g. perineum, axillae, between toes.
- Intertrigo and oral and genital candidasis are common and can become secondarily infected.
- CRP and WBCC may not be raised, despite significant infection.
- There may be multiple organisms—a US study found that if these include Pseudomonas aeruginosa there was a higher mortality. Gram-negative monocultures also had higher mortality, as did patients transferred from another hospital and those with non-foot infections (*Diabetologia* 2010;**53**:914-23; doi: 10.1007/s00125-010-1672-5).
- There may be little evidence of infection (e.g. no fever, slight redness, vague malaise, little pain).
- Image suspicious or painful areas (e.g. X-ray feet).
- Infected areas may have poor blood supply (e.g. PAD) which may worsen because of the infection.
- Infection may recur after treatment.

- MRSA and *C.difficile* are a risk in diabetic patients because these individuals have multiple or prolonged infections and are in and out of hospital constantly.
- Diabetic patients, especially those on steroids, are at risk of necrotizing fasciitis, especially if the initial infection is between the navel and knees. This includes Fournier's gangrene (extensive necrotizing perineal infection mainly in men).
- Diabetic patients are immunocompromised so may have unusual infections, including fungal infections.
- Rarer internal infections may include gas-forming organisms (e.g. gall bladder, kidney, bladder).
- Check ear, nose, and throat for common infections and, rarely, malignant otitis externa and rhinocerebral mucormycosis.
- Hepatitis C is commoner in people with diabetes than those without.

Acute coronary syndromes (⟴ pp. 253–5)

- Common in people with diabetes, including premenopausal women
- May accompany other presenting problems
- May have past/recurrent/extensive ACS as diffuse coronary artery disease is likely
- Atypical symptoms are common in people with diabetes
- Any chest pain, discomfort, heaviness; breathlessness, syncope; acute malaise—consider ACS

ESC recommendations on revascularization for people with diabetes (2013) are:

- Coronary artery bypass grafting should be considered, rather than PCI, when the extent of the coronary artery disease justifies a surgical approach (especially multi-vessel disease), and the patient's risk profile is acceptable. (*Eur Heart J* 2010; **31**: 2501–55; doi:10.1093/eurheartj/ ehq277).The European Societies for Cardiology recommendations on revascularization for people with diabetes (2013) are:
- 'Optimal medical treatment should be considered as preferred treatment in patients with stable coronary artery disease (CAD) and diabetes mellitus (DM) unless there are large areas of ischaemia or significant left main or proximal left anterior descending lesions.
- Coronary artery bypass grafting (CABG) is recommended in patients with DM and multivessel or complex (SYNTAX Score >22) CAD to improve survival free from major cardiovascular events.
- Percutaneous coronary intervention (PCI) for symptom control may be considered as an alternative to CABG in patients with DM and less complex multivessel CAD (SYNTAX score ≤22) in need of revascularization.
- Primary PCI is recommended over fibrinolysis in DM patients presenting with STEMI if performed within recommended time limits.
- In DM patients subjected to PCI, drug-eluting stents rather than bare metal stents are recommended to reduce risk of target vessel revascularization.
- Renal function should be carefully monitored after coronary angiography/PCI in all patients on metformin.

- If renal function deteriorates in patients on metformin undergoing coronary angiography/PCI it is recommended to withhold treatment for 48 hrs or until renal function has returned to its initial level.'

(Eur Heart J 2013; **34**:3035–87. doi:10.1093/eurheartj/eht108)

- Give diabetic patients standard medical treatment for ACS. They may gain even greater benefit than those without diabetes.
- Do not give thrombolytic therapy to patients with unresolved proliferative retinopathy or current vitreous haemorrhage (rare).
- Patients with any glucose reading > 11 mmol/l should have careful glucose control using VRIII for at least 24 hrs with an appropriate concentration of IV glucose depending on fluid needs and eating ability. Monitor and replace potassium as necessary. Stop VRIII once glucose controlled and eating normally, and transfer safely to other glucose-lowering therapy (NICE CG 130) (➋ pp. 167–8).
- Avoid hypoglycaemia which can cause dysrhythmias or cardiac arrest. This means meticulous blood glucose monitoring, including at 2 a.m. and especially at weekends.
- Check for other tissue damage, especially PAD and cerebrovascular disease.
- Contact cardiology and diabetes team.

TIA or stroke (➋ pp. 266–7)

- Common in people with diabetes.
- May accompany other presenting problems.
- Check finger-prick and laboratory glucose to exclude hypoglycaemia which can mimic stroke.
- If glucose < 4 mmol/l give 150–160 mls 10 % glucose IV (➋ p. 189) and reassess patient.
- Manage as for non-diabetic patients with prompt referral to the specialist stroke team and transfer to the stroke unit.
- Assess for other CVD—does patient have ACS as well?
- Assess for other diabetic tissue damage—visual problems and neuropathy make rehabilitation more complex.
- May have past/recurrent/extensive strokes as diffuse cerebral artery disease is likely.
- Because of previous strokes and diabetic peripheral or mononeuropathy, neurology may be confusing in new TIA or stroke.
- Manage as for non-diabetic stroke/TIA patients (NICE CG 68 (2008).
- CT or MRI brain scan urgently.
- Use thrombolysis if indicated and appropriate expertise is available.
- Contact diabetes team promptly.
- Control blood glucose with usual medication if non-insulin agents, patient can swallow, glucose < 11 mmol/l, and medication dose can be adjusted to control glucose.
- If unable to swallow or glucose ≥ 11 mmol/l, set up careful VRIII (➋ pp. 167–8) with sodium/glucose/potassium solution in parallel (e.g. 0.45 % sodium chloride with 5 % glucose, and potassium chloride 0.15 %; or 0.45 % sodium chloride with 5 % glucose, and potassium chloride 0.3 %).
- If required, use enteral nutrition (➋ p. 267).

- Monitor finger-prick glucose hourly aiming to keep the glucose between 6 mmol/l and 10 mmol/l (seek local DST guidance) (➲ p. 105).
- ⚠ Do not allow patient to become hypoglycaemic. Monitor finger-prick glucose. Treat all glucose levels < 4 mmol/l.
- Contact stroke unit and DST.

Diabetic foot or lower limb (➲ pp. 301–14)

Read NICE CG 119.

Never underestimate the severity of a diabetic foot problem. Look for:
- ulcers or wounds (including between toes)
- infection—soft tissue, bone, systemic
- circulatory problems e.g. gangrene
- neuropathy
- bone—fracture, osteopenia, deformity, infection
- injury
- foreign body
- all of these

Refer all diabetic foot patients in hospital to the DSFT within 24 hrs. The DSFT should ideally see the patient within 24 hrs. Time is tissue. Admit if in doubt.

- Assess whole patient—there will be other diabetic tissue damage (➲ p. 249)
- Investigations as in Box 24.3 (➲ p. 423)
- X-ray foot. Show area of interest on request form. MRI? (➲ p. 311)
- Treatment must be prompt and vigorous, guided by the DSFT
- Review the patient often, at least daily if inpatient
- Pain relief
- Suspect infection in all patients. Treat if any evidence or strong clinical suspicion. Use your local antibiotic 'diabetic foot' protocol
- Take great care to prevent MRSA or *C.difficile* infection
- Debride dead tissue, send wound base swab for microbiology
- Remove any foreign body and re-image
- Avoid further pressure on the affected area(s)
- Protect other pressure areas
- Prevent deformity (e.g. Achilles tendon contracture)
- Elevation
- Prophylactic low molecular weight heparin; N.B. thrombo-embolism-prevention stockings may cause ulcers in patients with PAD or neuropathy
- Good nutrition—refer to dietitian
- Psychological support
- Optimize glucose control
- Optimize CVD risk prevention
- Treat other complications and comorbidities vigorously
- Vascular assessment and treatment
- Early surgery for major infection or ischaemia

Critical limb ischaemia or gangrene (⊃ pp. 264, 307–9)

⚠ These patients are at risk of death. They have extensive vascular disease (e.g. heart) and often microvascular complications.

Admit immediately all patients with:

- infection with purple/blue/black ischaemic areas
- gangrene toe/foot/anywhere else
- PAD and rest pain
- acute arterial obstruction—painful, pulseless, cold leg
- note that pain may be modified by neuropathy—the situation may be worse that it seems
- same day vascular assessment with DSFT

In hospital:

- very detailed clerking by diabetes team including careful assessment of cardiac status (most have IHD) and renal status (risk of renal arterial stenosis or renal failure due to nephropathy, infection, and dehydration)
- Investigations as in Box 24.3
- X-ray foot
- Treat infection vigorously
- Control glucose between 6 mmol/l and 10 mmol/l without hypoglycaemia
- Ensure optimal statin therapy (interact with some antibiotics, see BNF)
- Treat any intercurrent problem promptly. Consider cardiac opinion
- Ankle:brachial pressure index—may be misleading (⊃ p. 264)
- Refer to podiatry
- Refer to dietitian for full nutritional review
- Refer to physiotherapy for maintenance of movement and power
- Very careful protection of pressure areas—high risk of heel sores
- Urgent vascular imaging as agreed with vascular team and radiology
- Stop metformin before procedures using contrast (⊃ p. 121)
- ⚠ Risk of contrast-induced renal failure; hydrate carefully before any contrast procedure
- Revascularization or surgical procedures as indicated
- Excise slough, drain pus
- Amputate unsalvageable toes or limbs promptly
- Push for prompt effective care. There are often unacceptable delays in care of diabetic foot patients—timing of radiology lists, theatre lists, availability of different staff. Time really is tissue. Delays increase risk of worsening of original problem, nosocomial infection, depression, glycaemic instability.

Surgery

Read 'Management of adults with diabetes undergoing surgery and elective procedures'.

 <http://www.diabetologists-abcd.org.uk/JBDS/JBDS_IP_Surgery_Adults_Summary.pdf>

Trauma and surgery (open or laparoscopic) cause marked metabolic disturbance. Food intake and digestion change as patients fast or develop post-operative vomiting and altered bowel habit. GI surgery may cause longer-term gastric or digestive changes. Adrenaline and steroid hormones rise and sympathetic activity increases causing insulin resistance, liver glucose release, and body fat and protein breakdown (catabolism). This process may be worse in diabetic patients, e.g. protein catabolism after colorectal surgery is increased in patients with type 2 diabetes mellitus (*Anesthesiology* 2005; **102**:320–6). Blood glucose rises.

Surgical ward nurses and doctors may not be confident about diabetes care, and may be unaware of the potential consequences of erratic glucose control. Peri-operative hyperglycaemia increases the risk of surgical complications and impairs surgical outcomes. However, overtreatment of blood glucose ± inadequate monitoring may be disastrous. Diabetic patients also have tissue complications (e.g. CVD and renal impairment).

In a perfect world people with diabetes undergoing surgery would have non-diabetic blood glucose levels without hypoglycaemia before, during, and after the operation which would occur exactly when planned with care from staff trained in surgical, anaesthetic, and diabetic management. But we all work in the real world.

Good liaison between surgeon, anaesthetist, diabetes team, primary care, and clinical and administrative colleagues is essential for optimal results of surgery in diabetic patients. Doctors' schedules and different systems/locations for patient care may impede coordinated management, as may administrative issues (e.g. cancellations, waiting list initiatives). Pre-operative clerking is often done by inexperienced doctors, although some units have specially trained nurses. Many factors delay surgery and ill diabetic inpatients (e.g. with infected feet) may suffer fasting and VRIII for days. Diabetic clinic appointments may be scarce, and not all hospitals have DISNs who can see patients before admission and peri-operatively. GPs and practice nurses may not be kept closely informed. Patients may not realize that they need more than an annual diabetes review to get the best result from surgery—some staff may not realize this either.

Every hospital should have protocols for the perioperative care of people with diabetes undergoing surgery or procedures and should audit compliance.

Pre-operatively

Plan surgery in diabetic patients carefully with good liaison between surgeon, anaesthetist, DST, and GP.

For surgical emergencies contact the diabetes registrar urgently—if he/she is not available call the medical registrar. Resuscitate the patient before operating. If the patient has blood glucose ≥ 11 mmol/l ± vomiting ± abdominal pain, check finger-prick ketones. Do not operate on patients

Box 24.4 Primary or ambulatory care. Referring people with diabetes for surgery or procedures

- Do the benefits of surgery outweigh the risks in this person with diabetes?
- Have you done a recent full review of this patient's condition?
- Is the HbA_{1c} < 69 mmol/mol (8.5 %)? If not, refer to DST.
- Does the patient have frequent hypoglycaemia or lack awareness of this? If yes, refer to DST.
- Does the patient have diabetic tissue damage? If yes, will this increase the risks of surgery or require special care (e.g. renal or cardiac disease). Have you optimized management of complications? Consider referral to relevant specialist services.
- Have you included HbA_{1c}, BP, cholesterol, weight, complications of diabetes, other comorbidities, and all medications in the referral letter? N.B. patients with autonomic neuropathy can die under anaesthesia ($\bigcirc$ p. 282).
- If surgery or a procedure is agreed, have you and the patient had written guidance on medication adjustment for fasting, preparation, and other care? If not, get it.
- After surgery or a procedure, have you and the patient had post-operative discharge, diagnostic, and management information? If not, request it.

with DKA or HHS unless immediately life-threatening emergency—risk of death.

For elective surgery, notify the DST of the operation date as soon as possible to allow intensive improvement of glucose control if required. Agree a local pre-operative clerking and investigation plan and ensure that all concerned are aware of this. Agree referral and clear communications for patients requiring improvement in glucose or management of other problems found during pre-operative clerking. Tell the administrators. The 'system' may admit patients before they are ready, who are then sent home because of poor glucose control.

Do not delay urgent surgery unduly. Weigh up the risk of delay (e.g. of cancer spreading/obstruction, etc.) vs the potential risk of post-operative complications if sugary. Is the illness for which surgery is required impairing glucose control?

Call the DISN and/or diabetes registrar when the patient is admitted. Surgical outcomes are often worse in people with diabetes than in those without. Complications are more likely ($\bigcirc$ p. 419).

Use Box 24.3 ($\bigcirc$ p. 423) to decide pre-operative investigations—tailor these to the patient, the situation, and the procedure. For major surgery perform all the tests in Box 24.3. In general, perform the usual investigations for your patient's particular surgical situation and procedure, and add finger-prick glucose ± ketones), laboratory glucose, U&E, LFT, HbA_{1c}, ECG, and chest X-ray.

Day surgery

People with diabetes are less likely to have day surgery for problems usually managed in this way. Yet with good perioperative planning, most people with diabetes can be treated as elective day cases. Offer this if the patient will miss only one meal, has an HbA$_{1c}$ < 69 mmol/mol (8.5 %) in the past 3 mths, and fulfils usual local day surgery rules. Perioperative diabetes teams improve care and increase day surgery rates (*Diabetic Med* 2010; **27**:1289–94; doi: 10.1111/j.1464-5491.2010.03114.x).

Adjust glucose-lowering treatment

See Table 24.1.

Inform the patient, and medical and nursing staff of the perioperative treatment plan before admission. Ensure it is clearly prescribed.

Glucose, potassium and insulin

See Tables 24.1 and 24.2.

- Seek the DST's advice.
- Patients undergoing surgery need glucose as well as insulin to counteract catabolism. Infusion should be continuous not intermittent.
- Patients who will miss more than one meal or who cannot eat, need VRIII (➲ pp. 167–8).
- Adjust VRIII to achieve glucose levels of 6–10 mmol/l (acceptable range 4–12) (Table 24.2, and (➲ pp. 167–8).
- Monitor blood glucose by finger-prick hourly while on VRIII.
- Beware hypoglycaemia (➲ pp. 181–200). Treat it promptly.
- Run IV sodium/glucose/potassium solution in parallel (e.g. 0.45 % sodium chloride with 5 % glucose, and potassium chloride 0.15 %; or 0.45 % sodium chloride with 5 % glucose, and potassium chloride 0.3 %).
- Other fluids may be needed (e.g. blood) which may require adjustment of glucose/sodium/potassium infusion rate to optimize fluid balance.

Table 24.1 Adjustment of glucose-lowering treatment on day of surgery assuming no more than one missed meal (afternoon operation assumes breakfast has been eaten)

Medication	Morning operation	Afternoon operation
Long or intermediate-acting insulin once daily in **evening**	Consider reducing previous evening's dose by a third	Consider reducing previous evening's dose by a third
Long or intermediate-acting insulin once daily in **morning**	Two-thirds to full dose	Two-thirds to full dose
Twice daily fixed mixture insulin	Halve morning dose Usual evening dose	Halve morning dose Usual evening dose

(Continued)

Table 24.1 (Cont.)

Medication	Morning operation	Afternoon operation
Twice daily self-mixed short-acting insulin with intermediate-acting insulin	No short-acting insulin in morning Calculate total dose of both morning insulins and give half as intermediate-acting in the morning Usual evening doses	No short-acting insulin in morning Calculate total dose of both morning insulins and give half as intermediate-acting only in the morning Usual evening doses
Three or more insulin injections each day	Two-thirds to full dose of basal insulin Omit morning and lunchtime short-acting insulin	Usual morning insulin Omit lunchtime short-acting insulin Usual evening meal dose (adjusted to food)
Metformin (BNF/SPC but see*)	Stop 48 hrs before elective surgery. Restart ≥ 48 hrs following surgery or resumption of eating and only if normal renal function has been established If X-Ray contrast required, stop for 48 hrs. Restart if renal function back to baseline (➲ p. 121)	Stop 48 hrs before elective surgery. Restart ≥ 48 hrs following surgery or resumption of eating and only if normal renal function has been established If X-Ray contrast required, stop for 48 hrs. Restart if renal function back to baseline (➲ p. 121)
Sulfonylurea	Omit morning dose	Omit all doses that day
Meglitinides	Take with food when eaten (no meal, no tablet)	Take with food when eaten (no meal, no tablet)
Pioglitazone	Take as usual	Take as usual
DPP-4 inhibitors GLP-1 analogues	Omit on day of surgery	Omit on day of surgery
Acarbose	Take with food when eaten (no meal, no tablet)	Take with food when eaten (no meal, no tablet)

Book surgery first on the morning list for all patients if possible.

There is rarely any need for changes to medication on the day before surgery.

Check finger-prick glucose on admission, during and after surgery for all patients.

*For metformin NHS Diabetes consensus guidance states 'take as normal' but notes that lunchtime doses (if taken) should be omitted. 'If contrast medium is to be used and eGFR < 50 metformin should be omitted on the day of the procedure and for the following 48 hrs.'

Source data from 'Management of adults with diabetes undergoing surgery and elective procedures'. NHS Diabetes ⌨ <http://www.diabetologists-abcd.org.uk/JBDS/JBDS_IP_Surgery_Adults_Summary.pdf>

Table 24.2 Insulin infusion rates for VRIII

Finger-prick blood glucose (mmol/l)	Initial rate of insulin infusion (units per hour)
< 4.0	0.5
	(zero if long-acting background insulin has been continued)
	Treat for hypoglycaemia (⮫ pp. 188–93)
4.0–7.0	1
7.1–9.0	2
9.1–11.0	3
11.1–14.0	4
14.1–17.0*	5
17.1–20.0*	6
> 20.0*	7, pending advice if insulin infusion working
Check glucose meter (is it working properly?)	Check insulin infusion pump has not run out and is working; line is intact and connected to cannula; cannula is correctly inserted and patent
	Contact DST or medical team immediately

* If glucose does not fall despite increasing doses of insulin contact DST.

Adapted from NHS Diabetes. Management of adults with diabetes undergoing surgery and elective procedures.

🔗 <http://www.diabetologists-abcd.org.uk/JBDS/JBDS_IP_Surgery_Adults_Summary.pdf>.

- Monitor U+Es daily– some patients may need more sodium chloride or a different potassium concentration, others may have renal disease.
- Check all peripheral cannulae daily and change every 2–3 days—high infection risk in diabetic patients. Remove promptly if not needed.
  🔗 <http://www.nursingtimes.net/Journals/2012/08/22/b/k/e/210812Care-of-peripheral-venous-cannula-sites.pdf>
- Follow hospital protocol for meticulous central line care.

Post-operatively
- Control glucose well—6–10 mmol/l (acceptable range 4–12).
- Post-operative patients may be insulin resistant at first.
- Good nutrition—involve dietitian.
- Do not use glucose-free nutrition. Use the standard nutrition (parenteral or enteral—(⮫ p. 267) for your hospital appropriate to your patient with dietetic input and adjust the insulin to cope with the diabetes team's help.
- Meticulous pressure area care.
- Thromboprophylaxis as for non-diabetic patients but note that thrombo-embolism-deterrent stockings may cause pressure ulcers in vasculopaths or neuropaths.
- Meticulous cannula/line/catheter care.

- Meticulous wound care—increased risk of wound infection.
- Do not cross-contaminate a clean wound from a dirty one (e.g. a surgical excision and an ulcer on the other limb).
- Neuropathy and postural hypotension may complicate rehabilitation.
- Increased exertion (e.g. walking) with effort after bed-rest may cause hypoglycaemia. Reduce insulin as exertion increases.

Good post-operative glucose control from day 1 onwards reduces the risk of hospital-acquired infection (*J Parenter Enteral Nutr* 1998; **22**:77–81; doi: 10.1177/014860719802200277). Of 100 uninfected diabetic patients admitted for elective surgery, 31 % with glucose > 12 mmol/l on day 1 post-operatively (POD1) developed an infection vs 11 % with POD1 glucose ≤ 12 mmol/l). Excluding minor UTIs, patients with just one glucose > 12 mmol/l on POD1 were 5.7 times more likely to develop serious infection. Each millimole glucose rise > 6.1 mmol/l on POD1 increased risk of complications by 17 % after CABG (*Diabetes Care* 2003; **26**:1518–24; doi:10.2337/diacare.26.5.1518).

A larger study of 5259 patients (877 diabetic) found that post-operatively, renal, neurological, and gastrointestinal complications were more common in diabetic patients. Infection was not. Five-year event-free survival was lower in diabetic patients and mortality greater (*J Thorac Cardiovasc Surg* 2006; **132**:802–10). Another study showed that cognitive function was worse after cardiac surgery in diabetic vs non-diabetic patients (*Thorac Cardiovasc Surg* 2006; **54**:307–12).

Diabetic patients form a high proportion of those requiring vascular surgery. In diabetic patients, increasing area under the curve for the glucose above 6.1 mmol/l over the first 48 hrs post-operatively after infra-inguinal bypass was linked with increasing risk of poor outcome (death, major amputation, or graft occlusion at 90 days) (*Br J Surg* 2006; **93**:1360–7; doi: 10.1002/bjs.5466).

Intensive care

An ICU study showed that intensive glucose lowering reduced mortality. However, susbequent studies showed higher mortality. A meta-analysis stated '[i]n critically ill adult patients, tight glucose control is not associated with significantly reduced hospital mortality but is associated with an increased risk of hypoglycemia' (*JAMA* 2008; 300:933–44). NICE-SUGAR reported a large randomized study showing that that intensive glucose control increased mortality among adults in the ICU: a blood glucose target of 10 mmol/ resulted in lower mortality than did a target of 4.5–6 mmol/l (*N Engl J Med* 2009; **360**:1283–97; doi: 10.1056/NEJMoa0810625).

The greatest danger for glucose balance in these diabetic patients is likely to be when the patient is transferred to a general ward where one-to-one nursing is not available. Do not stop IVIII during transfer (➲ pp. 167–8).

Diabetes on the wards

Diabetic patients should be cared for in a diabetes specialist ward wherever possible. Hospitals should have an inpatient DST including DISNs who should agree a local referral protocol and shared care arrangements. Patients in whom diabetes plays a major role should be managed by the DST. In shared care arrangements it must be clear which consultant is ultimately responsible for the patient.

- Plan care with the patient—for the clinical problems and the diabetes.
- Patients who are well enough to control their diabetes treatment safely in hospital should do so (➔ pp. 439–40).
- Prescription charts should be clear (especially for insulin doses—use insulin charts). Check them regularly (pharmacists are best at this).
- Patients should be seen daily by a doctor (including at weekends).
- Test finger-prick blood glucose before each meal and before bed aiming for 6–10 mmol/l (acceptable 4–12). (Tailor this to each patient and avoid hypoglycaemia.)
- Reduce testing in stable patients (e.g. awaiting placement).
- Record blood glucose tests on a standard glucose chart used throughout the hospital and teach staff how to use it.
- Monitor pulse, BP, temperature, respiration. Diabetic patients can deteriorate rapidly (often after subtle signs of worsening have been missed).
- Prophylactic low molecular weight heparin for most patients. N.B. thrombo-embolism-prevention stockings may cause ulcers in patients with PAD or neuropathy.
- These are complex patients with many volumes of paper notes.
- Previous admissions may 'hide' behind new electronic record pages.
- Initial assessments should be clear.
- Record investigations cumulatively and visibly (e.g. last year's creatinine is relevant to this year's admission—has renal function worsened?)
- Produce a clear summary and management plan for each problem.
- Recognize interactions between types of tissue damage, and between different treatments.
- Write a full discharge summary; do not forget to include the diabetes
- All English hospitals caring for adults with diabetes should participate in NaDIA (➔ pp. 460–2).

Diabetes self-care

Experienced diabetic patients know much more about their diabetes and how to manage it than most healthcare professionals. They should self-manage their diabetes if well and able to do so. The Joint British Diabetes Societies have produced national guidance:

    🔗 <http://www.diabetes.org.uk/Documents/Reports/67190-Self-management-in-hospital0312.pdf>

1. 'Trusts should provide written information to explain the responsibilities of self-management to both patients and hospital staff.
2. The responsible nurse and the patient should agree, on admission, the circumstances in which the patient should self-manage. An agreement form should be signed by both the patient and registered nurse.

3. For elective surgical admissions, a care plan should be agreed at the pre-operative assessment clinic to establish whether the patient wishes to self-manage and the circumstances in which this may not be possible.
4. During the admission, the clinical circumstances should be assessed regularly to ensure that the patient's ability to self-manage has not been compromised by their clinical condition.
5. The DST should be involved if there is disagreement about the patient's ability to self-manage or if there are difficulties with diabetes control. Diabetes specialist nurse staffing levels should be sufficient to support this role.
6. Patients should be able to self-monitor their blood glucose but should make the results available to hospital staff.*
7. The insulin dose administered by the patient should be recorded on the prescription chart.
8. The hospital should ensure that the timing and content of meals are suitable for the patient with diabetes.
9. Facilities should be available for the safe storage of insulin in the ward environment.'

*Increasingly, hospitals are using centrally recorded glucose testing systems. If this is the case, another blood drop from the same finger prick can be used in duplicate.

Some problems on the wards
- Lack of experience of diabetes in medical and nursing staff
- Failure to realize how ill the patient is (e.g. neuropathy may blunt symptoms, cardiac pain may be atypical)
- Failure to realize that the patient knows more about his/her diabetes than staff do
- Failure to realize that the patient is not complying with treatment or dietary recommendations
- Unfamiliarity with different insulins
- Lack of awareness of the importance of timing of food and insulin or hypoglycaemic drugs in diabetic patients
- Delayed meals with too little CHO
- Evening meal too early
- Lack of snacks
- Lack of awareness of the variety of hypoglycaemic symptoms
- Delayed treatment of hypoglycaemia
- Overtreatment of hypoglycaemia (e.g. giving glucose when a diet-only-treated patient's blood glucose is 4 mmol/l)
- Errors in doing finger-prick glucose (e.g. wiping finger with alcohol)
- Ward glucose meter not checked or quality assured
- Failure to identify tissue damage (e.g. not noting the peripheral neuropathy which caused the fall which fractured the femur)
- Insufficiently prompt recognition and vigorous treatment of infection
- Failure to appreciate the severity of PAD or neuropathy
- Vulnerable feet bare on dirty floors—slippers/shoes essential
- Poor ulcer hygiene—especially with multiple large oozing ulcers

- Lack of awareness of visual loss from severe retinopathy or treatment
- Lack of awareness of hearing loss
- Failure to appreciate renal vulnerability
- Problems managing obese weak diabetic patients—insufficient bariatric equipment
- Inadequate bowel preparation for colonoscopy/radiology (dysmotility reduces effectiveness of laxatives)
- Failure to recognize gastroparesis (glycaemic instability, slow response to oral glucose for hypoglycaemia, slow absorption of oral medication, food in stomach despite fasting) (➲ p. 287)
- Inappropriate timing of fasting procedures or operations
- Cancellation of procedures requiring fasting, with consequent destabilization of glucose
- Many different clinical staff seeing the patient and incomplete (or absent) verbal and written communication. Good coordination is needed
- Communication problems with patient as many staff involved
- Failure to identify the diabetes at all!

Discharge planning

- Start on admission with complex and disabled patients.
- Assess family/community support available.
- Liaise with GP and community diabetes team (e.g. phone GP).
- Set up further appointments in podiatry or wound care.
- If a diabetic patient has been ill enough to require admission, at least one specialist diabetic clinic visit is usually a good idea.
- Many patients who have required admission have very complex medical problems and need continued specialist follow-up.
- Check patient's understanding of diabetes treatment and diet (admission may have been precipitated by misunderstandings or confusion).
- Go over the take-home medication very, very carefully—pharmacists are usually best at this.
- Provide a timely, detailed, and legible discharge summary. Give the patient a copy and make sure he/she understands what it says.
- Ensure that the community nurse really has agreed to come in and give the insulin (they rarely come more than twice a day and cannot always match their visit to meal times). Consider Tresiba®.
- Ensure that arrangements have been made for supplies of dressings and that the district nurse or other wound care staff know exactly how to continue the right dressing (changes in dressing type or application can lead to deterioration and re-admission).
- Ensure that arrangements for meals are in place.
- Check that equipment has been delivered.
- Check that home modifications have been made.
- Make sure that transport arrangements are in place.
- Ensure that all the staff and agencies involved know what is happening (this is much harder than it sounds).
- Ensure that everyone knows who to contact if problems arise.
- Ensure that the patient has all their appointments in writing.
- Phone the patient over next few days to see how they are getting on.
- Educate staff about managing diabetic patients.
- Use the opportunity to enhance patient education.

Summary

- People with diabetes occupy 15 % of hospital inpatient beds in England.
- Diabetic patients do not do well in hospital.
- Diabetic patients have increased risk of severe, prolonged, and complicated infection.
- There is increased risk of thrombosis.
- There is increased risk of cardiac and renal failure.
- There is increased risk of pressure sores.
- Diabetic patients have greater mortality, longer stay, and are less likely to return to their own home that other patients.
- Do not miss new diabetes in emergency attenders.
- Assess diabetic attenders or emergency patients carefully—do not forget blood glucose.
- Manage diabetic glucose emergencies promptly and vigorously.
- Manage sepsis promptly and vigorously.
- Manage diabetic aspects of acute coronary syndrome fully.
- Plan surgical admissions and use the relevant diabetes protocol.
- Control blood glucose well and safely post-operatively.
- Be aware of the problems of managing diabetic patients in a general hospital ward.
- Discharge planning must include consideration of food and administration of diabetes medication, especially insulin.
- Discharge planning requires particularly clear liaison with the community multidisciplinary team and primary care.
- All diabetic patients who have required emergency admission with a diabetes problem should have at least one follow-up appointment with the specialist diabetes team in secondary or primary care.
- Read JBDS and NHS Diabetes guidance.

Useful reading

Joint British Diabetes Societies for Inpatient Care guidance:
The management of Diabetic Ketoacidosis in adults (2010)
⚕ <http://www.diabetologists-abcd.org.uk/JBDS_DKA_Management.pdf>
The hospital management of hypoglycaemia in adults with diabetes mellitus (2010)
⚕ <http://www.diabetologists-abcd.org.uk/JBDS/JBDS_IP_Hypo_Adults.pdf>
The management of the hyperosmolar hyperglycaemic state (HHS) in adults with diabetes (2012)
⚕ <http://www.diabetologists-abcd.org.uk/JBDS/JBDS_IP_HHS_Adults.pdf>
Self management of diabetes in hospital (2012)
⚕ <http://www.diabetes.org.uk/Documents/Reports/67190-Self-management-in-hospital0312.pdf>
Glycaemic management during the inpatient enteral feeding of stroke patients with diabetes (2012)
⚕ <http://www.diabetologists-abcd.org.uk/JBDS/JBDS_IP_Enteral_Feeding_Stroke.pdf>
NHS Diabetes: Management of adults with diabetes undergoing surgery and elective procedures (2011):
⚕ <http://www.diabetologists-abcd.org.uk/JBDS/JBDS_IP_Surgery_Adults_Summary.pdf>
⚕ <http://www.diabetes.org.uk/Documents/Professionals/Reports%20and%20statistics/Management%20of%20adults%20with%20diabetes%20undergoing%20surgery%20and%20elective%20procedures%20-%20improving%20standards.pdf> (full report)

Local diabetes care

Introduction

People with diabetes want the right care at the right time from a kind, efficient, expert, and experienced team they know and trust. They want to gain access to their care easily at convenient times—one phone call and a prompt appointment; routine check-ups to fit in with their personal time-table; immediate emergency care from the specialist team. They do not want to have to tell their story repeatedly. They want good communication between the members of the district diabetes team. Best of all it should be one team 'singing the same song', friendly, and supportive.

Multiple reorganizations in healthcare and diabetes care in the UK have had varying impacts upon district-wide diabetes care. The Diabetes National Service Framework 2003–2013 provides a blueprint for diabetes district networks (➲ p. 45–6): ✒ <http://www.gov.uk/government/publications/national-service-framework-diabetes>

The Quality and Outcomes Framework (QOF) provides guidance about key indicators in primary care obtained at annual review (➲ p. 43). This has led to identification of diabetic patients within practices and improved outcomes. Clinicians should individualize care and not overtreat to target, whilst ensuring patients don't miss out. QOF is updated annually.

Planning diabetes care

Commissioning information is available at ℘ <http://www.diabetes.org.uk/Documents/nhs-diabetes/commissioning/commissioning-at-a-glance-guide-2nd-edition.pdf>

Commissioners will, of course, be guided by national commissioning regulations.

The Diabetes Commissioning Toolkit (2006) states that to plan district-wide care one needs to know:

- where are we now?
- where do we want to be?
- how do we get there?
- how will we know when we are there?

℘ <http://www.diabetes.org.uk/upload/Professionals/NHS_commissioning_toolkit_Diabetes_2d.pdf>

This is still relevant. The cycle advised is to review local service provision, taking into account national good practice and targets, decide priorities, design services, manage supply and demand, manage referral arrangements, review and manage performance, seek patient and public views, assess needs, review local service provision, and repeat.

Information needed

- Available local funding for diabetes care?
- Who is in charge of commissioning diabetes care?
- Who are the experts in diabetes able to advise commissioners? Check what resources and expertise with local knowledge are available. This includes consultant diabetologists and GPs with a special interest in diabetes. Others include people with diabetes or representative bodies, public health consultants, GPs with local overview roles, those responsible for specialist nurses, podiatry, dietetics, local hospital commissioning links, hospital biochemistry/pathology leads, information technology (IT) leads, data leads in CCG and hospital.
- Local people with diabetes
  - How many people are known to have diabetes?
  - Who they are? Age, male/female, ethnicity.
  - Where they are? Diabetes densities around the district. In what accommodation or circumstance—house, care or residential home, special needs, prison, detention centre, no fixed abode.
  - Any special needs or special issue groups locally?
  - Areas of social deprivation?
  - How many people are expected to have diabetes? In England use diabetes prevalence model for local authority or CCG: ℘ <http://www.yhpho.org.uk/resource/view.aspx?RID=154049>
- Elsewhere in UK, use:
  - ℘ <http://www.yhpho.org.uk/resource/view.aspx?RID=81090>
- Clinical issues—diabetes type, well or ill, use of emergency or specialist care?
  - Newly diagnosed annually, type 1 or 2, or other
  - Existing diabetes, type 1 or 2 or other

- Current prescribing patterns of diabetes drugs, e.g. insulin, and testing materials
- Complications—DKA or hypoglycaemia, eye, kidney, foot, heart, stroke, PAD, erectile dysfunction
- Hospital admission rates – emergency, elective, day case
- Pregnancy (including gestational diabetes)
- Residential and care home population (25 % have diabetes)
- Non-diabetes—illnesses requiring admission of diabetic patients
- HIV patients on antiretrovirals
- Psychiatric patients on diabetogenic drugs
- Multidisciplinary staff required for diabetes care (including new patients from case-finding programmes)
- Local staff currently available for diabetes care
  - Diabetologists
  - Diabetes specialist nurses (DSNs)
  - Diabetes educators (if separate from diabetes specialist nurses)
  - Diabetic specialist midwives
  - Diabetic specialist podiatrists
  - Diabetic specialist dietitians
  - Diabetic specialist wound care nurses
  - GPs with a special interest in diabetes (GPwSI)
  - Practice nurses with a special interest in diabetes
  - Pharmacists with a special interest in diabetes
  - GPs with some training in diabetes
  - Practice nurses with some training in diabetes
  - Dietitians
  - Podiatrists/chiropodists
  - Health psychologists
  - Pharmacists
  - Support staff for clinics
  - Staff who could help with diabetes care if trained
- Staff expertise in diabetes care
  - What training? Recognized professional training? Course(s)—recognized or not?
  - What revision/update? Attends national professional diabetes meetings? Belongs to national diabetes organization, e.g. Diabetes UK?
  - What experience?
- Time available to devote to diabetes care
  - Full time (e.g. DSN)
  - Dedicated diabetes sessions as part of role (e.g. GPwSI)
  - Mixed in with other work (e.g. dietitian with no separate diabetes clinic)
- About local facilities
  - GP surgeries
  - Intermediate outpatient facilities
  - Hospital outpatient facilities
  - Mobile facilities (e.g. caravan)
  - Roaming staff (e.g. visiting several clinics or practices, or homes). If roaming where is their base?

- Communications (patient confidentiality must be secure)
  - Laboratory and radiology results (paper, electronic)
  - Patient records, current and previous, diabetes and non-diabetes—within practice, across health care providers, shared with patient, etc. Paper? Electronic?
  - Communication with patients—verbal, written, electronic
  - Communication about patients—verbal, written, electronic
- About access
  - Mobile patients—pedestrian, cycle, bicycle/car parking, bus/tram/tube/train access
  - Immobile patients—care home/nursing home, hospital inpatients
  - Prison/remand homes
- If external provision of services is being considered, can all the information noted be provided?

Where are we now?
- Audit (pp. 460–2)
- Patient experience
- GP-based diabetes care—QOF
- Intermediate diabetes care
- Secondary care clinics
- Secondary care complication management—glucose emergencies and tissue damage
- Diabetic foot care
- Care of inpatients with diabetes
- Care of diabetic patients with non-diabetic illness
- Children
- Teenagers and adolescents
- Pregnant and pre-pregnant women
- Adults, including frail or elderly

What about the future?
- Local obesity
- Ethnicity
- Age range of population—especially elderly
- Changes in deprivation or not
- Organisational changes and impact—**before** they happen

Integrated care

People with diabetes require care throughout the health system. Fragmented care is bad for patients, for organizations, and for funding. Read 'Best practice for commissioning diabetes services an integrated framework', supported by major relevant organizations:
% <http://www.diabetes.org.uk/Documents/Position%20statements/best-practice-commissioning-diabetes-services-integrated-framework-0313.pdf>

'Integrated diabetes care is both integration of a health care system and co-ordination of services around a patient . . . In essence, diabetes integration is the whole health community joining in partnership to own the health outcomes of patients with diabetes in their local area . . .

Pillars of integration—
- Integrated IMT systems
- Aligned finances and responsibility
- Care planning
- Clinical engagement and partnership
- Robust shared clinical governance'

Best practice

See NSF and NICE standards of diabetes care (→ pp. 45–8).

Prevention of diabetes

All healthcare professionals should advise everyone to eat healthily, stay the right weight for their height, and exercise regularly and safely. High-risk people and those noted to have impaired fasting glucose or impaired glucose tolerance should received intensive personalized advice to prevent their condition worsening to diabetes (NICE PH 38) (→ p. 5).

Diagnosis of diabetes

All those in contact with patients in primary or secondary care should know who is at risk of diabetes and how to diagnose it (→ p. 7–15).

Comprehensive care

This means diabetes care from diagnosis to grave—from well-person diabetes checks to emergency admission to ICU. To achieve this, people with diabetes, those who care for them, and those who care about them need to get together. Patient care should not be impeded by artificial boundaries between care providers. People with diabetes, primary care, intermediate care, and secondary care should liaise to ensure continuity, and avoid duplication or omission of care.

Comprehensive care also means building clear pathways with other bodies such as social services, education authorities, local schools, care and residential homes, detention centres, and prisons. This includes education about diabetes and its consequences.

Initial assessment and management (→ pp. 23–30, 36)

Ensure local protocols for initial assessment and management, and guidelines for agreed education, diet, preventive care, medication, and monitoring. Base these on national guidelines and consensus, and adapt them for the local population.

Continuing care (→ p. 43)

In a district of 100 000 people (all ages) ~6000 will have diabetes, of whom ~ 600 will have type 1 diabetes. The numbers of people with diabetes will increase every year.

Continuing care is based on annual review with more frequent contacts if any of the risk factors are uncontrolled or problems arise. There is no evidence base for the one-year interval, but the consensus is that it is straightforward to organize and easy to remember. A year is a long time in the life of someone with diabetes. Poor risk-factor control causes tissue damage. Professionals should teach patients how to monitor their own health and ensure they know when to seek help.

Nowadays, many annual reviews are carried out by GP practice nurses. A great deal can be checked routinely, but it is very important that people with diabetes are given the opportunity to ask detailed questions and that they obtain informed replies. The patient may know more about diabetes than the professional, therefore all practice nurses performing diabetes checks should have training in diabetes and know when to seek further advice from a GP, DSN, or specialist care.

Diabetes education

People with diabetes and their families

All newly diagnosed diabetic patients should have a formal education programme tailored to their needs (➔ pp. 63–4). They should also have annual revision and update. The resources needed for diabetes education are a worthwhile and ultimately cost-effective investment.

Staff caring for people with diabetes

Those providing specific diabetes care must be trained, e.g. undertake a Warwick course:

    ✍ <http://www2.warwick.ac.uk/fac/med/study/cpd/subject_index/diabetes>

If staff cannot attend these kinds of courses, arrange local training (e.g. via local DSNs, diabetologists, or GPwSIs).

Specialist care

Identify local provision for the following specialist care (Box 25.1):

- diabetes
- endocrinology
- paediatric, teenage, and adolescent diabetes
- diabetic foot care
- diabetes in the elderly
- eyes
- kidney
- neurology
- cardiac
- PAD
- neurovascular
- stroke
- pre-pregnancy
- pregnancy
- erectile dysfunction
- genitourinary medicine
- gastroenterology/hepatology
- orthopaedic/musculoskeletal service
- elderly
- rehabilitation
- psychological
- psychiatric

Agree referral arrangements for emergencies and routine problems, and maintain links. Clinicians in primary, secondary, and community care should have prompt access to specialist advice without impedence by organizational or financial barriers. Patients should be able to choose to seek specialist advice or to remain under primary or community care. Similarly, patients in secondary diabetes care should be able to choose intermediate or primary diabetes care.

Box 25.1 Guidelines for referring diabetic patients for diabetes specialist care

- Children and teenagers up to age 18 yrs.
- All patients with type 1 diabetes unless specific trained expertise is available.
- Refer new type 1 diabetic patients same day.
- Patients with unusual type 2 diabetes, e.g. monogenic
- Brittle diabetes.
- Patients with insulin pumps or needing them.
- Patients who may benefit from CGMS.
- Patients requiring specialist education, e.g. CHO counting.
- Any patient attending hospital with hypoglycaemia.
- Any patient who has any accident/incident due to hypoglycaemia.
- Any patient admitted with high glucose, DKA, or HHS.
- Women planning pregnancy or pregnant (same day).
- Patient in whom primary/intermediate care cannot keep risk factors within target after intensive effort for 6 months (HbA$_{1c}$, lipids, BP).
- Glucose instability e.g. lows/highs even if HbA$_{1c}$ is within target.
- Patients with diabetic tissue damage such as sight-threatening or proliferative retinopathy, CKD ≥3, PAD, cardiac disease, painful or autonomic neuropathy. Many districts will have protocols for specific tissue damage to be managed in primary care.
- All diabetic foot disease
- Patients with learning disabilities (diabetes often coexists).
- Patients with psychological or psychiatric problems making diabetes care difficult. This includes significant non-concordance or suspected manipulation.
- Patients with drug-induced or exacerbated diabetes (e.g. steroids, psychiatric, antiretroviral drugs). It may be possible for the relevant specialist teams to work together to reduce the diabetogenic drug.
- Patients with significant other disease.
- Patients requiring intensive education.
- Patients who may be suitable for new or unfamiliar glucose-lowering treatment unless primary or intermediate expertise is available.
- Patients in whom bariatric surgery is being considered.
- Patients with eating disorders.

These guidelines should be adapted to local need and diabetes expertise.

Specialist and generalist care

In the UK there has been an initiative to deliver most diabetes care in primary care. Many patients will require specialist diabetes care intermittently or long-term, depending on local primary care expertise. In some other countries people with diabetes expect their care to be delivered by diabetes specialist services (but may have to pay for this). Diabetes UK and other relevant organizations produced guidance on the commissioning of specialist diabetes services. They estimated, for the UK, that a general population of 250,000 with a 5 % prevalence of diabetes requires at least:

- 3 consultants specializing in diabetes and endocrinology delivering 12×4-hr sessions dedicated to diabetes a week
- 5 DSNs
- 1 DISN per 300 inpatient beds
- 4 state-registered dietitians with a special interest in diabetes
- 2 state-registered podiatrists with a special interest in diabetes
- 1 consultant obstetrician with a special interest in the management of pregnant women with diabetes (2 obstetricians should share this to cover leave)
- I consultant in care of the elderly with a special interest in diabetes
- 1 professional with special expertise in psychological therapies
- ℘ <https://www.diabetes.org.uk/About_us/What-we-say/Improving-services--standards/Commissioning-Specialist-Diabetes-Services-for-Adults-with-Diabetes---Defining-A-Specialist-Diabetes-UK-Task-and-Finish-Group-Report/> (*Diabetic Med* 2011; **28**:1494–500; doi: 10.1111/j.1464-5491.2011.03410.x)

Each locality develops referral criteria to specialist care. DSTs provide specialist care in non-hospital settings or work entirely in community settings. Diabetes services across a locality (e.g. a CCG) must be integrated for optimal patient care and efficiency of service.

Admission avoidance

People with diabetes do not want to be admitted to hospital. Commissioners do not want this either. Admission avoidance includes preventing both the first admission, and readmissions. Much of this book is about optimizing patient care to prevent the complications of diabetes. This will reduce admissions. Some admissions occur because the local system does not act soon enough or with the appropriate expertise and perseverance to manage the patient out of hospital. These arrangements need to be organized and commissioned. Much of the process has been described.

JBDS has produced detailed guidance for CCGs on commissioning for admission avoidance. This includes reviewing benchmarking data, commissioning a whole-systems review of diabetes care across all health organizations (e.g. primary and secondary care, ambulance service, industry etc.) and commissioning a service model based on adequate diabetes specialist staffing and services (e.g. DISNs, DKA and hypoglycaemia prevention and care, children and adolescents, foot care, diabetes education). In particular healthcare professionals outside and inside hospitals need training in diabetes care, and there should be a diabetes specialist out-of-hours service.

🔊 <http://www.diabetologists-abcd.org.uk/JBDS/JBDS_IP_Admissions_Avoidance_Diabetes.pdf>

Potential gaps in diabetes care

Healthcare services and social care need to work closely together, particularly for people in the groups described in this section. For example, organizational and financial integration of health and social care in Torbay reduced admissions and improved other aspects of care. ℳ <http://www.kingsfund.org.uk/sites/files/kf/integrating-health-social-care-torbay-case-study-kings-fund-march-2011.pdf>

Diabetes UK has summarized some of the issues that disadvantage people with diabetes: ℳ <http://www.diabetes.org.uk/Documents/Reports/Diabetes_disadvantaged_Nov2006.pdf>

Social deprivation

Diabetes is a disease of social deprivation. Compared with the least deprived, people in the most deprived quintile are over twice as likely to develop diabetes (*Diabetic Med* 2008; **25**:1462–8; doi: 10.1111/j.1 464-5491.2008.02594.x; *Diabetic Med* 2013;**30**: e78–e86; doi: 10.1111/dme.12062). Diabetes prevalence calculations take this into account. ℳ <http://www.yhpho.org.uk/resource/view.aspx?RID=81090> Once diabetes is present, the most deprived are 1.7 times more likely to have a foot ulcer or amputation (*Diabetic Med* 2013; **30**:484–90; doi: 10.1111/dme.12108). Mortality increases in parallel with social deprivation. Commissioners for diabetes in areas with marked social deprivation should consider how to address diabetes in this vulnerable group.

Mobility problems (➲ p. 365)

Patients with mobility problems (e.g. amputees) may be unable to get to GP surgeries or specialist clinics. They are likely to have multiple health problems, especially if elderly, and if possible should be seen at least once in a specialist diabetic clinic (e.g. an elderly diabetes clinic) with appropriate ambulance or hospital car transport. Their care is time-consuming (e.g. 30–40 mins per appointment) and multiple resources are often required. These kinds of patients should be discussed with their GP so that the best arrangement can be made for each patient. Home visits by the GP and primary care team are very helpful.

Patients in care or residential homes (➲ p. 369)

Ideally, a local DSN, GPwSI, or diabetologist should visit patients in the homes for an annual review. About a quarter of residents will have diabetes. People will be in this accommodation because they cannot cope at home and they are likely to have multiple significant health problems. Their care should be audited. Diabetes UK guidelines (2010):
ℳ <http://www.diabetes.org.uk/About_us/What-we-say/Improving-diabetes-healthcare/Good-clinical-practice-guidelines-for-care-home-residents-with-diabetes/>

Patients whose first language is not English (➲ pp. 371–82)

Districts with high proportions of such patients should make appropriate provision for diabetes care. Diabetes is more common in people of South Asian or African–Caribbean descent than in White European populations. A few of these patients will be seeking asylum or on temporary visas. Frequent change of address and fear of authority can make continuity of diabetes care difficult. Diabetes health workers who speak the relevant language(s) are invaluable. Establish links with community leaders, and resources (e.g. Asian day centres).

Psychiatric patients (➲ pp. 409–16)

Whether at home or in hospital, psychiatric patients have a higher frequency of diabetes than people without psychiatric disease. Their psychiatric problem often prevents access to diabetes care. Ideally, each mental health trust should have a system for identifying diabetic in- or outpatients, and a planned arrangement to ensure that they are receiving annual diabetes reviews and interim care. Diabetic glucose problems or tissue damage can worsen psychiatric problems.

Diabetes is common in patients in secure hospitals (up to 20 %) who can benefit greatly from intensive diabetes support. Secure hospitals should ensure a formal link with a DST. Obviously, care is required with use of sharps and injectables to protect patients themselves, other patients, and staff.

Patients in prison or detention centres

Prisoners are entitled to proper diabetes care. In 1992 diabetologists provided diabetes care in Walton Prison, Liverpool, and demonstrated that the strict prison routine, diet, and supervision could provide good diabetes control (*BMJ* 1992; **304**:152–5; doi: http://dx.doi.org/10.1136/bmj.304.6820.152). There should also be a system to optimize diabetes care in immigration detention centres. Further information:

- Diabetes UK information pack: ℘ <http://www.diabetes.org.uk/How_we_help/Advocacy/Advocacy-packs/Having-diabetes-in-prison/>
- Nursing: *J Diabetes Nursing* 2009; **13**:390–5.
- Police custody: *Practical Diabetes* 2008; **25**:72–5; doi: 10.1002/pdi.1209.
- US guidance: *Diabetes Care* 2008; **31**: Supplement 1 S87-93; doi:10.2337/dc08-S087.
- IDF guidance: ℘ <http://www.idf.org/sites/default/files/attachments/DV_56-2_Bayle.pdf>

Itinerant or homeless patients

Such patients rarely have continuous diabetes care. Those who live on the streets may have erratic and inappropriate diet, infections, foot problems, and tissue damage. Use and storage of insulin may be difficult. One suggestion is to link with agencies already working with such groups to try to provide assistance in a clearly identified location and way, and to communicate this to the patients.

Non-attenders

Every clinic/surgery has non-attenders. Such patients often have high HbA$_{1c}$ and tissue damage. Some have psychological problems or communication difficulties. Contact them and re-book them. Nowadays, secondary care patients who have failed to notify inability to attend are often discharged back to their GPs. Check that there has not been an administrative error (e.g. wrong address, failure to note patient's phone message). Reminders (e.g. phone or text) before clinic increase attendance help.

Inform both patient and GP of the discharge. Ensure that the patient knows that he/she can come back (tell him/her the local system for this). Consider telephoning non-attenders before discharge in case an error has occurred.

⚠ Do not discharge pregnant women, those < 25 yrs old, or frail patients of any age. Telephone, text, or e-mail them.

Communications

Those responsible for commissioning, providing, and using diabetes care should have regular joint discussions to ensure that the care commissioned is appropriate to local needs and uses resources optimally. This means good communication across multiple organizations, often with changing structures and personnel, in response to governmental, regional, and local reforms, and financial issues. The importance of maintaining good communication, whatever the difficulties, cannot be overstated.

Give patients complete information about their condition and (with consent) copies of all letters. Agree the communication system preferred by the patient—telephone, text, e-mail, letter. Ideally there should be a district-wide approach. Some districts use patient-held records. Sophisticated electronic diabetes systems can provide this.

Agree communication systems between healthcare professionals. Ideally there should be one district-wide electronic information system. In a few districts these exist and work well. Changes in local organization of care, funding problems, or IT issues can hamper communication. Elsewhere in the world (e.g. Finland) such systems are commonplace.

Letters/electronic summaries should be sent promptly and contain accurate legible information. Check addresses frequently, as those of patients and professionals change. Remember that patients also change GP.

Laboratory services should be accessible by primary, intermediate, and secondary care at the point of care. Diabetes is a metabolic specialty and relies on timely laboratory results. Radiology results should also be accessible district-wide.

Audit and information

Audit processes and outcomes of care (Box 25.2). This requires a full register of all diabetic patients which must satisfy confidentiality and data protection requirements. In the UK, QOF requires all GP practices to have a register of diabetic patients. Clinical employers should ensure that systems are in place to facilitate audit. All such local or regional systems should suit local needs, have maintenance and update contracts, an identified skilled person responsible for them, and they should link readily to national systems.

Audit is embedded in diabetes care in most of the UK. This provides an essential source of information to target improvements in individual practices, localities and nationally. The National Diabetes Audit (NDA) includes England and Wales. In Scotland, this is the Scottish Care Information—Diabetes Collaboration (SCI-DC). NDA (adults) and National Paediatric Diabetes Audit (NPDA) are part of the National Clinical Audit and Patient Outcomes Programme that is mandated in the NHS Standard contract. ℜ <http://hqip.org.uk/ncapop-information-contact-and-publications-details-for-each-project/>

The NDA 'is the largest annual clinical audit in the world, integrating data from both primary and secondary care sources, making it the most comprehensive audit of its kind.' In 2011–12 it included 2.4 million people with diabetes. Data are reported at local and national level. ℜ <http://www.hscic.gov.uk/nda>

The NPDA aims to examine the quality of care in children and young people with diabetes and their outcomes. In 2011–12 it included 25,000 children and young people with diabetes. ℜ <http://www.rcpch.ac.uk/national-paediatric-diabetes-audit-npda>

National Pregnancy in Diabetes Audit (NPID) began data collection in 2013. It aims to support clinical teams to deliver better care to women with diabetes who become pregnant. ℜ <http://www.hscic.gov.uk/npid>

The National Diabetes Inpatient Audit (NaDIA) is a snapshot audit of inpatient diabetes care in England and Wales.
ℜ <http://www.hscic.gov.uk/diabetesinpatientaudit>

The NDA team are also rolling out audits of diabetes patient experience and foot care.

The first UK Service Level Audit of Insulin Pump Therapy in Adults *Diabetic Med* 2014; **31**:412–18; doi: 10.1111/dme.12325.

The National Diabetes Information Service (NDIS) provides a wide range of user-friendly information. The service is now included in the Cardiovascular Intelligence Network.
ℜ <http://www.yhpho.org.uk/resource/view.aspx?RID=102082>

Among NDIS tools are the APHO diabetes prevalence model, Diabetes Community Health Profiles (for local authorities and CCGs), and Diabetes Foot care Activity Profiles. The Variation in Inpatient Activity (VIA) tool summarizes LoS, readmissions, and day care by HRG, for people with and without recorded diabetes in hospitals in England ℜ <http://www.yhpho.org.uk/default.aspx?RID=102616>.

Box 25.2 Diabetes audit topics

- Define audit population, e.g. GP surgery, hospital clinic, whole district
- Number of patients with new and existing diabetes
- Demographics
- Type of diabetes
- Treatment
  - Diet alone
  - Non-insulin hypoglycaemic drugs
  - Insulin (injection, pump)
- Annual review done/not done
- Risk factors—checked. Within target? Treatment?
  - BP
  - Smoking
  - HbA_{1c}
  - Cholesterol
  - Creatinine/eGFR
  - BMI ± waist circumference
  - Eye check done and result
  - Foot check done, risk assessed, and result
  - Urinary albumin:creatinine ratio
- Complications
  - Cardiovascular—heart, brain (e.g. stroke), PAD
  - Retinopathy
  - Nephropathy
  - Neuropathy
  - Feet—infection, ulceration, deformity, amputation
- Emergency, A&E attendance, and/or hospital admissions
  - Diabetes-related, e.g. hypoglycaemia or DKA
  - Non-diabetes-related—diagnoses (e.g. HRG)
- Elective hospital admissions
  - Diabetes-related
  - Non-diabetes-related
- Diabetes care in hospital
- Offered diabetes education
- Attended diabetes education
- Patient and carer experience (this should be at the top of the list!)

Prescribing for diabetes in England is published annually. In 2013–14, 45 million items were prescribed for diabetes (BNF, section 6.1) at a net ingredient cost of £803.1 million. This accounted for 4.3 % of total items and 9.5 % of the total cost of prescribing in primary care in 2013–14. In 2005–06 there were 27.1 million items at a cost of £513.9 million. ℘ <http://www.hscic.gov.uk/catalogue/PUB14681>

The *Atlas of Variation in Healthcare for People with Diabetes* published by Rightcare summarizes some of the information from NDA, NDIS, and elsewhere: ℘ <http://www.rightcare.nhs.uk/index.php/atlas/diabetes/>

Detailed information about diabetes in Scotland, which has a comprehensive national data system and patient register (on which individual patients can see their own data) can be found at the Scottish Care Information Diabetes Collaboration SCI-DC ℘ <http://www.sci-diabetes.scot.nhs.uk/>

The Scottish Diabetes Survey produces annual summaries:

℘ <http://www.diabetesinscotland.org.uk/Publications/SDS2013.pdf>

International information is available in the IDF Atlas ℘ <http://www.idf.org/diabetesatlas>

Summary

- People with diabetes should have accessible expert diabetes care matched to their individual needs—the right care at the right time.
- Commission comprehensive integrated diabetes care across the local area.
- Involve people with diabetes, and clinicians who provide diabetes care in service planning.
- Follow the annual review process for risk-factor management and prevention and identification of diabetic tissue damage.
- Provide specialist care for those who need it.
- Ensure good communications within the diabetes network.
- Use the commissioning guidance available.
- Local care must fit local needs and circumstances but fulfill national requirements.
- Apply Diabetes National Service Framework standards.
- Apply best practice—but tailor care to the individual.
- Agree who should care for whom.
- Identify gaps in care and fill them.
- Use resources wisely—avoid omission or duplication.
- Use nationally available information about diabetes in your area.
- Audit the process and outcome of diabetes care.
- Ask patients how you are doing, and how they are doing.

Chapter 26

Links

AAGBI	Association of Anaesthetists of Great Britain and Ireland ℘ <http://www.aagbi.org/>
ABCD	Association of British Clinical Diabetologists ℘ <http://www.diabetologists-abcd.org.uk>
ACDC	Association of Children's Diabetes Clinicians ℘ <http://www.a-c-d-c.org/>
ADA (US)	American Diabetes Association ℘ <http://www.diabetes.org/>
APPG	Diabetes All Party Parliamentary Group for Diabetes ℘ <http://www.publications.parliament.uk/pa/cm/cmallparty/register/diabetes.htm>
BNF	British National Formulary ℘ <http://www.bnf.org/bnf/index.htm> BNF is now provided via Medicines Complete ℘ <https://www.medicinescomplete.com/about/subscribe.htm>
BCPA	British Chiropody and Podiatry Association ℘ <http://www.bcha-uk.org/>
BDA	British Dietetic Association ℘ <http://www.bda.uk.com/>
BOMSS	British Obesity and Metabolic Surgery Society including national bariatric surgery registry ℘ <http://www.bomss.org.uk/>
BSPED	British Society for Paediatric Endocrinology and Diabetes ℘ <https://www.bsped.org.uk/>
CDC (US)	Centers for Disease Control and Prevention USA ℘ <http://www.cdc.gov/diabetes/>
College of Optometrists	℘ <http://www.college-optometrists.org/>
CQC	Care Quality Commission ℘ <http://www.cqc.org.uk/>
DAFNE	Diabetes Adjustment for Normal Eating ℘ <http://www.dafne.uk.com/>
DESMOND	Diabetes Education and Self Management for On-going and Newly Diagnosed ℘ <http://www.desmond-project.org.uk/>
Diabetes.co.uk	A privately owned community website providing a patient forum ℘ <http://www.diabetes.co.uk/>
Diabetes UK	The largest diabetes charity in the UK. Includes both people with diabetes and healthcare professionals. ℘ <http://www.diabetes.org.uk>

Meds and kit	🔗 <http://www.diabetes.org.uk/upload/How%20we%20help/catalogue/Meds%20and%20kit.pdf>
Diabetes publications	A list of some key diabetes and endocrine publications 🔗 <http://www.diabetespublications.co.uk>
DMEG	Diabetes Management and Education. The professional group for diabetes specialist dietitians 🔗 <http://www.dmeg.org.uk/about.html.>
DISN UK Group Forum	Diabetes Inpatient Specialist Nurses group. 🔗 <https://www.yammer.com/disnukgroup/.>
DRN	Diabetes Research Network 🔗 <http://www.drn.nihr.ac.uk/>
DRWF	Diabetes Research and Wellness Foundation 🔗 <http://www.drwf.org.uk/>
EASD	European Association for the Study of Diabetes. 🔗 <http://www.easd.org>
EMA	European Medicines Agency 🔗 <http://www.ema.europa.eu/>
eMC	Electronic Medicines Compendium (includes the Summary of Product Characteristics (SPCs) and the Patient Information Leaflets (PILs)). 🔗 <http://www.emc.medicines.org.uk/>
Expert Patients Programme	🔗 <http://www.expertpatients.co.uk/>
FDA US	Food and Drug Administration 🔗 <http://www.fda.gov/>
FEND	Federation of European Nurses in Diabetes 🔗 <http://www.fend.org>
GMC	Specialty Curriculum Endocrinology and Diabetes Mellitus 🔗 <http://www.gmc-uk.org/education/endocrinology_and_diabetes_mellitus.asp> 🔗 <http://www.gmc-uk.org/>
HSE	Health Survey for England 🔗 <http://data.gov.uk/dataset/health_survey_for_england>
Healthtalkonline	Seeing and hearing the real life experiences of people with diabetes 🔗 <http://healthtalkonline.org/>
HSCIC	Health and Social Care Information Centre 🔗 <http://www.hscic.gov.uk/>
IDF	International Diabetes Federation "The International Diabetes Federation (IDF) is an umbrella organization of over 230 national diabetes associations in more than 160 countries." The main source of information about diabetes around the world. 🔗 <http://www.idf.org>

Information about diabetes in each member country, with contact details of diabetes organisations worldwide
🔗 <http://www.idf.org/membership/meet-our-members>

IDOP — Institute of Diabetes in Older People
🔗 <http://instituteofdiabetes.org>

INPUT diabetes — "A charity that supports patients by advocating for easier access to diabetes technology across the UK – from insulin pumps to smart glucose meters and continuous glucose monitoring."
🔗 <http://www.inputdiabetes.org.uk/>

Insulin Pumpers UK — UK limb of international charity
🔗 <http://www.insulin-pumpers.org.uk/>

JBDS — Joint British Diabetes Societies for Inpatient Care Group
🔗 <http://www.diabetologists-abcd.org.uk/JBDS/JBDS.htm>

JDRF — Juvenile Diabetes Research Foundation. An international funder of Type 1 diabetes research.
🔗 <http://www.jdrf.org.uk/>

JRCPTB — Joint Royal Colleges of Physicians' Training Board
🔗 <http://www.jrcptb.org.uk/specialties/endocrinology-and-diabetes-mellitus>

Labtests online — 🔗 <http://www.labtestsonline.org.uk/>

MDU Cautionary tales — 🔗 <http://www.themdu.com/>
Enter diabetes in search

MIMS — Monthly Index of Medical Specialties
🔗 <http://www.mims.co.uk/>

NaDIA — National Diabetes Inpatient Audit
🔗 <http://www.hscic.gov.uk/diabetesinpatientaudit>

National Obesity Forum — 🔗 <http://www.nationalobesityforum.org.uk/>

NCEPOD — National Confidential Enquiry into Patient Outcome and Death
🔗 <http://www.ncepod.org.uk/>

NDA — National Diabetes Audit
🔗 <http://www.hscic.gov.uk/nda>

NDIS — National Diabetes Information Service
🔗 <http://www.yhpho.org.uk/resource/view.aspx?RID=102082>

NHSBT — NHS Blood and Transplant (includes reports on pancreas transplant and SPK)

	℘ <http://www.organdonation.nhs.uk/statistics/transplant_activity_report/> ℘ <https://www.organdonation.nhs.uk/>
NHS Choices	℘ <http://www.nhs.uk/Conditions/Diabetes/Pages/Diabetes.aspx>
NHS Diabetes resources	℘ <http://www.diabetes.org.uk/About_us/What-we-say/NHS-Diabetes-resources/> ℘ <http://webarchive.nationalarchives.gov.uk/20130513172055/http:/www.diabetes.nhs.uk#>
NHS Diabetic Eye Screening Programme	℘ <http://diabeticeye.screening.nhs.uk/>
NHS England	℘ <http://www.england.nhs.uk/>
NIDDK (US)	National Institute of Diabetes and Digestive and Kidney Diseases, National Institutes of Health (NIH) USA ℘ <http://www.niddk.nih.gov/Pages/default.aspx>
NIHR	℘ <http://www.nihr.ac.uk/research/>
NPDA	National Paediatric Diabetes Audit ℘ <http://www.rcpch.ac.uk/national-paediatric-diabetes-audit-npda>
NPID	National Pregnancy in Diabetes Audit ℘ <http://www.hscic.gov.uk/npid>
NICE	National Institute for Health and Care Excellence ℘ <http://www.nice.org.uk/> NICE publications (which are being updated): ℘ <http://www.nice.org.uk/guidance/index.jsp?action=byTopic&o=7239>
PCDS	Primary Care Diabetes Society ℘ <http://www.pcdsociety.org>
RCGP	Royal College of General Practitioners ℘ <http://www.rcgp.org.uk/>
RCGP	diabetes resources ℘ <http://www.rcgp.org.uk/clinical-and-research/clinical-resources/diabetes.aspx>
RCM	Royal College of Midwives ℘ <http://www.rcm.org.uk/>
RCN	Royal College of Nursing ℘ <http://www.rcn.org.uk/>
RCN	Diabetes Nursing Forum ℘ <http://www.rcn.org.uk/development/communities/rcn_forum_communities/diabetes>
RCOA	Royal College of Anaesthetists ℘ <http://www.rcoa.ac.uk/>

RCOG — Royal College of Obstetricians and Gynaecologists
🖰 <http://www.rcog.org.uk/>

RCOphth — Royal College of Ophthalmologists
🖰 <http://www.rcophth.ac.uk/>

RCP — Royal College of Physicians
Joint Specialist Committee for Endocrinology and Diabetes
🖰 <http://www.rcplondon.ac.uk/>

RCPE — Royal College of Physician of Edinburgh
🖰 <http://www.rcpe.ac.uk/>

RCPSG — Royal College of Physicians and Surgeons of Glasgow
🖰 <http://www.rcpsg.ac.uk/>

RCS — Royal College of Surgeons
🖰 <http://www.rcseng.ac.uk/>

RPS — Royal Pharmaceutical Society
🖰 <http://www.rpharms.com/home/home.asp>

Safe use of insulin and non-insulin therapy — National Patient Safety Suite elearning
🖰 <http://www.healthcareea.co.uk/theinsulinsafetysuite>

SCI-DC — Scottish Care Information Diabetes Collaboration
🖰 <http://www.sci-diabetes.scot.nhs.uk/>

SIGN — Scottish Intercollegiate Guidelines
🖰 <http://www.sign.ac.uk/>

TREND-UK — Training, Research and Education for Nurses on Diabetes
Includes Diabetes Nurse Consultant Group
🖰 <http://www.trend-uk.org/>

UK Renal Registry — Annual reports include information about people with diabetes and renal disease
🖰 <http://www.renalreg.com/>

Vascular Society — 🖰 <http://www.vascularsociety.org.uk/>

X-Pert — Diabetes education programmes – X-Pert diabetes, and X-Pert insulin
🖰 <http://www.xperthealth.org.uk/people-with-diabetes/x-pert-diabetes>

YDEF — Young Diabelogists and Endocrinologists Forum
🖰 <http://www.youngdiabetologists.org.uk/>

Index

thiazolidinedione 131–3
when to use 114–15
young people 319
non-proliferative
retinopathy 271, 272
NovoMix® 30 154
NovoRapid (insulin
aspart)® 153
NSAIDs 368

O

obesity 42, 78–80
and cardiovascular
risk 251
assessment 78
young people 320
obstructive sleep
apnoea 292–3
oedema, at injection
site 156
oesophageal dysmotility 286
OGTT see oral glucose
tolerance test
older patients 357–70
access to care 360–1
carers and care
homes 369, 456
complications 365–6
concomitant drug
therapy 368
diabetes education 364
diet 361
exercise 361
falls 366
glucose targets 362
hyperglycaemia 206, 364
hypoglycaemia 364
insulin therapy 363
management 360–3
medication 360
medication review 361
mental function
changes 367
non-insulin
medications 362–3
patient information 360
presentation and
assessment 359
omega-3 fatty acids 263
see also lipid-lowering
agents
optic neuritis 270
oral glucose tolerance test
(OGTT) 13
oral hypoglycaemia
agents see non-insulin
medications
oral insulin 179
oral problems 285–6
orlistat 42, 81–2
osteoarthritis 297

osteopenia 296
osteoporosis 296
overeating 203

P

Pakistanis, type 2 diabetes
risk 373
palpitations 185
pancreas transplant 180
driving after 400
with kidney 279
panic 185
papilloedema 270
paraesthesiae 3, 185
patient anxieties 58
patient education 32, 55–66
agendas 57
best practice 452
consistency 62
coordination 62
factors influencing
learning 57–8
full education package 59
insulin 178
non-insulin
medications 115
structured
programmes 58,
59–62, 63–4
survival kit 59
patient folder 29
patient information 25–6
biguanides 122
driving 400
essential 56
metformin 122
older patients 360
sulfonylureas 128
patient support 65
pen injectors 162–3
pensions 392
perindopril 259–60
peripheral arterial disease
(PAD) 264–5
periungual telangiectasia 294
personalized goals 35–6
pharmaceutical company
helplines 65
phobias 413
phosphate, HHS 222
phosphodiesterase type-5
inhibitors 354–5
physical work 386
pioglitazone 131–3
surgery patients 435
young people 319
plant stanols/sterols 75
polycystic ovary
syndrome 334–5
polydipsia 2
polyuria 2

post-partum care 343, 346
post-prandial capillary blood
glucose testing 104
postural hypotension
282–3, 365
potassium
DKA 219, 225
HHS 222, 225
surgery patients 434–6
prasugrel 261
pravastatin 261–3
pre-pregnancy
counselling 338–41
pregnancy 15, 46, 342–4
fetal distress/death 228
fitness for 341
gestational diabetes 18,
345–6
hyperglycaemia 204, 206,
345–6
insulin therapy 150
medication 339–41
patient education 341
pre-pregnancy
counselling 338–41
risks 343–4
preproliferative
retinopathy 271
presentation 2–3
pressure sores 228, 366
pressure ulcers 294
prevention of diabetes 451
prisoners 457
proliferative
retinopathy 271
protamine zinc injection 155
proteins 75
pruritus 3, 295
psychiatric disorders
412–13, 457
anxiety 413
depression 412–13
phobias 413
severe mental illness 415
psychological/social
issues 409–16
brain function 411
eating and body image
disorders 414
psychiatric
disorders 412–13
severe mental illness 415
in young people 325
ptosis 270
puberty 324
pulmonary aspiration 227
pulmonary oedema 227

R

Ramadan 379–80
ramipril 259–60

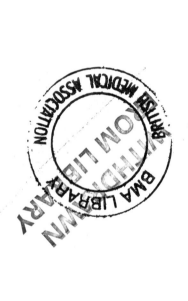